The Essential Guide to Practice Success for Acupuncturists

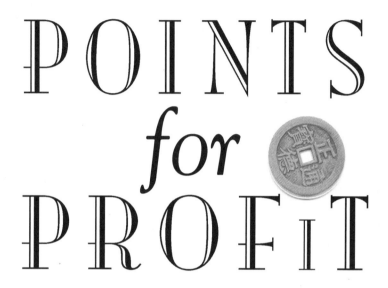

POINTS *for* PROFIT

Honora Wolfe
Eric Strand
Marilyn Allen

Fourth Updated Edition!

Published by:
BLUE POPPY PRESS
A Division of Blue Poppy Enterprises, Inc.
1990 N 57th Court, Unit A
BOULDER, CO 80301

First Edition, Februrary 2004
Second Edition, August 2005
Third Edition, June 2007
Fourth Edition, July 2009
Fifth Printing, July 2011

ISBN 1-891845-25-X
ISBN 978-1-891845-25-3
LCCN #2003117182

10 9 8 7 6 5

Printed at Edwards Brothers, Ann Arbor, MI
on acid free paper and soy inks

With Appreciation...

There were many people involved with the creation of this book. We'd like to thank everyone who helped us:

Bruce Staff for his gentle but steady pressure to get it written timely.

Bob Flaws for his research, creative suggestions, and editing of the final draft.

Cara Frank, Michael Gaeta, Ron Zaidman, Stuart Watts, and Misha Cohen for being our advance copy readers.

Joan Podgorski for a great book design.

Eric Brearton for design support and facilitation not to mention his unfailing good humor.

Christine Strand for her patience and support of Eric to get the writing done when he really should have been coaching soccer, seeing patients, or spending time with her.

The entire Blue Poppy staff for leaving Honora alone for a couple of months so that she could write.

Everyone who contributed their stories, information, and quotations:

Jonathan B. Ammen
Don Beans
Evelyn Kade Byram
Michael Buyze
Larry Caldwell
Judy Chaleff
Steven F. Otsuka Dardis
Valerie DeLaune
Dagmar Ehling
William Feather
Laura Freeman
John Frostad
Carol Green
Doug Grootveld
George Herbert
Valerie Hobbs
Geoffrey Hudson
Fred Jennes
Steve Kauffman
Gary Klepper

Peter Lichtenstein
Elizabeth Liddell
Andrew Lininger
Rande Lucas
Maria MacKnight
Eric Meyer-Reed
Neal Stuart Miller
Ogden Nash
Anna Nazos
Michael Nolan
Mary Ann Radmacher
Jean Jacques Rousseau
Ihara Sai Ka Ku
Susan Schiff
Michael Schroeder
Daniel Schulman
John Scott
Beverly Sills
Aman Tandias
Tierney Tully

Contents

SECTION ONE: GETTING UP AND RUNNING

SECTION TWO: WORKING ON YOUR OWN

SECTION THREE: GETTING PAID

SECTION FOUR: MARKETING YOUR PRACTICE

SECTION ONE

Getting Up and Running

Welcome & Introduction | 1

This book has been a long time in the making. While teaching classes on practice management and marketing all over the U.S. over the last several years, Marilyn Allen and I [HW] were asked scores of times, "Do you have a book on this subject?" We didn't. That was inevitably followed by, "Can you recommend anyone else's book?" We couldn't. Then, in the spring of 2003, Eric Strand, an ambitious, funny, and persistent young practitioner, showed up at one of our seminars and asked how he might be more closely involved with our company. After finding out how successful his practice was after only one year out of school, I asked him to help with the creation of what we truly believed our profession needed . . . a solid book on the business of acupuncture and Oriental medicine.

While there are many excellent books out there on every subject related to business that you can imagine, there hasn't really been a good one specifically for people practicing acupuncture and Oriental medicine. We hope this book will fill that niche. Furthermore, as we talk to practitioners all around the country, we hear a lot of chatter out there about business and money problems. People in our profession, as a group, seem to be struggling with these issues, and we feel that our combined experience as business people, clinicians, and marketers may help improve our chances, as a group, for long-term success. It is our belief that, by following even a part of the advice we give in this book, members of our profession will be able to create more successful practices and, hopefully, happier lives, whatever one's definitions of those things might be.

A book such as this one, which includes many legal and regulatory references, must be updated with each reprinting.

This fourth edition includes several changes. Sec. 4, Chapter 7, "Marketing Your Practice on the Internet," is totally expanded and revised; Sec. 1, Chapter 5, "Business Models" has been significantly revised; many other chapters have had substantive changes of various kinds. <u>Also, what was a CD is now a website.</u>

> **Tips on how to use this book and website**

1.**The ⊙ Icon.** As you go though this book, you will find a repeated icon that looks like this ⊙. Every time you see this, it means that there is something pertaining to the subject being discussed contained on the companion website. This website contains sample forms and letters (all down-loadable), a complete business plan outline, lots of web links, and a variety of other useful resources that we felt were not very useful on paper but would be valuable if made available to you in a form that you could personalize. To access the website, go to **http://pointsforprofit.bluepoppy.com**.

2. **Practitioner Pointers.** Another feature of this book is that we have included, wherever possible, quotes and stories from practitioners all around the country. These, we have to admit, were not easy to gather. People are busy, after all, and often don't have the time to think about what they want to say in a sound bite about practicing Chinese medicine. That being said, we have included these quotes throughout the book and hope you find them inspiring.

3. **Power Points.** These are specific bits of information that we want to draw special attention to. They are presented in boxed formats, separate from the main body of the text throughout the book.

4. **Points to Ponder.** At the end of each chapter, we have listed the most important points covered in that chapter. Not sure if you want or need to read the whole chapter? Read the

Points to Ponder at the end of the chapter to see what's there and why you might want to read the whole thing.

5. **Points for Teachers.** If you are using this book as a text for a practice management class, contact Blue Poppy for a teacher's guide to using this book. This companion information gives you ideas for student assignments and grading criteria. There is no charge for this guide when an order for the books is placed by your school.

6. **Related Products.** The publisher of this book has many other products to help you grow your practice including both live and distance learning seminars on specific subjects related to the business of Chinese medicine as well as brochures, intake forms, other practice building tools, and books about Chinese medicine written specifically for selling to the lay public.

7. **Business and Marketing Blog.** I [HW] try to blog on subjects related to business once a week or so. By going to http://www.bluepoppy.com and looking for the link on the home page for the Blue Poppy blog, you can read these at anytime. The blog is archived...so visit when you like.

Finally, we want to thank you for purchasing this book. We know there are a bazillion other books on business that you could have purchased instead of ours. We truly believe that something here will help you be a happier and more successful practitioner of your chosen profession. We wish you the best of luck with your practice, but we encourage you to remember that, most of the time, luck is at least 90% perspiration and only 10% inspiration.

First Things First: Setting Goals | 2

Buddha said, "Action follows thought as a cart follows an ox." Napoleon Hill said, "Think and Grow Rich." These statements are ways of saying that the mental activity of setting goals, when used effectively, helps us immeasurably to manage our behavior, prioritize our actions, motivate ourselves over the long haul, and set the bar high enough to help us excel. We begin our book with a chapter on goal-setting because this is where any business starts . . . as an idea, a thought, a dream. We believe it is important to get this part right, right from the start. So don't skip this chapter . . . it can make a huge difference in your life.

Goal-setting as a daily practice has always had a powerful place in the business world and is especially important for anyone starting a new small business, such as a private clinic. You may also find, after reading this chapter, that setting goals can have a substantial benefit to your personal life. Active goal-setting is really a combination of two things. First, it is a roadmap that you create as you travel it. Second, each small goal reached as you travel your map is a "prize" that you give yourself as you build a life in your chosen profession.

➤ Why do we need goals?

If suddenly tomorrow you woke up in the middle of the ocean in a boat, your only supplies being a compass, a box of playing cards, and a bag of Doritos, would you sit and wait, hoping to be rescued? Maybe you would zig-zag around the ocean turning east or west at the mercy of the winds. Or would you point your bow in one direction from your compass and sail (or row) until you found land?

Most likely, there is not a person among us who would see any sense in sailing around without direction with only a bag of chips to eat! And anyone who thinks that waiting for rescue is the best idea should probably not be a small-business owner. There is no one out there to pull you up, dry you off, and give you a hot meal when you are the boss . . . only yourself! No, the best bet as a castaway or as a business owner is to pick a direction and sail towards it as if your life depended on it. And, it is the positive action of setting goals that helps you give yourself direction and a map.

The power of a goal is tremendous. Setting a goal focuses your mind, your intention, your qi. Good goals give you a feeling of control over your world and

> **"If there is no wind, row."**
> —*Anonymous*

your destiny. They send the message out to the universe that you have a set of specific wants and needs and you are going after them. Goals help you focus your energy. Just like the acupuncture needle that you place in your patient, the focusing of your energy is doing work, only this work is for your life.

A goal successfully met increases your self-esteem. Few things make you feel as good as when you achieve a dream, and a goal is nothing other than a dream with a deadline. It is through goals that you stretch your potential, force yourself to reach just a little bit higher, take a bigger bite out of the universe of possibilities.

➤ Why we don't set goals

Setting a goal in and of itself is not a difficult task. Indeed, figuring out what you want and setting your sights upon achieving your dreams can be a simple activity. So why don't more people set goals?

First of all, most people are unaware of the power of setting goals. Another reason many of us do not set goals is because it is, consciously or unconsciously, scary. It requires some courage to honestly review your life, acknowledge what we want, and commit *out loud,* at least to ourselves never mind to others, to the journey to achieve our dreams.

Finally, and possibly the most common, if least acknowledged, reason that people do not set goals is that you may fail. It is possible that you will set a goal and not meet it. You may fall short in patient visits, income level, or personal achievement within the profession, and that is something many people cannot contend with. However, it is by pitting our current self against the possibilities of our future that we continue to grow, learn, and enrich our own lives and the lives of those around us.

> "Persistence and determination alone are omnipotent. The slogan 'press on' has solved and always will solve the problems of the human race."
> —*Calvin Coolidge*

➤ Dream into your Goal

What is a goal, really? It is an idea about what is worthwhile in life, a concept, a dream. So when you sit down to write a list of goals, start with the basics first. What do you value in this life? What do you believe is important: free time; family; money; philanthropy; travel? Once you have clearly defined what your values are, it is easier to extrapolate what goals might help you live those values. Whether you want to be a great parent, a trusted friend or spouse, or a well educated healer, or, if you have more tangible dreams like a nice house, a new car, prep-school for the kids, or an early retirement, these are the values and dreams that help you define your goals and put a plan in motion.

➤ **Wise goals are S*M*A*R*T**

Knowing why we should set goals is a good start. Knowing how to set a good goal is the next piece. Making goals, good ones that push us to our best without defeating or discouraging us, is something that takes a little work. However, by following the advice of renowned salesman and author David Sandler (see the Resources for Going Further section at the back of this book), the task of setting good goals can be made easier. Sandler says that goals need to be S*M*A*R*T—**S**pecific, **M**easurable, **A**ttainable, **R**ealistic, and **T**ime-bound.

Make your goals *specific*. State exactly what it is that you want to accomplish. For example, "I will make $100,000 net before taxes in the year 200X," or, "I will see 30 patients per week by the end of June this year." The more specific your goal, the more you will be able to focus your energy and resources towards its fruition.

Make your goals *measurable*. Can you go back at the end of the time period and check your progress? Be it dollars, patients, classes you want to take, or places you wish to visit, you have to be able to ascertain the difference between what you stated you would do and what you have actually done.

Make your goals *attainable*. They need to be possible. "I will see 100 new patients next week" is probably not attainable if you are only seeing 10 this week. Even if you had people lined up outside the door of your clinic and around the corner, it is probably physically impossible to treat that many patients in a week and do it well. So don't set *pie in the sky* goals. Set goals that are attainable. Otherwise you will defeat yourself and become discouraged before you even start.

Make your goals *realistic*. Attainable and realistic go hand in hand, although there is a difference. While you may be able to see 100 new patients in a month, it is doubtful you could see them without sleep or food for the duration. In other words, don't set a goal to be the first acupuncturist in space if you aren't a colonel in the NASA space program. Your goal must be within the realm of possibility.

Make your goals *time bound.* Set a deadline: this week, the end of this month, the 2nd of February, every Wednesday, by December 31st of this year, etc. If your goal has no deadline, then there is no way you will be able to *measure* your progress. You want to be able to ascertain if you did what you set out to do.

➤ More than just an idea

Goals can be like puffs of smoke or clouds on a blustery day unless you write them down. Putting your goals on paper does two things. First, it sets your intention in motion. By writing down your goals, you are making them real for yourself. Second, they are less likely to be forgotten. If your goals are written down, you are less likely to sweep them aside when another idea pops into your head. But, of course, it's okay to add more goals on to the ones you have written. In fact, Mark Victor Hansen, author of *The One Minute Millionaire* and *Chicken Soup for the Soul,* says that you should write down up to 100 goals every day, so that they stay clearly present in your consciousness.

There is more power in written goals than in spoken ones. Write them all down, both personal and professional. We suggest that you pick your most ambitious business goal, write it on a business card and laminate it. Then wrap the card in a hundred dollar bill and place it in your wallet. Keep it in your wallet until you meet your goal. You may spend the bill in an emergency, but it has to be replaced within 24 hours. Carrying that Ben Franklin around can give you a different feeling about yourself, about what's possible for you, and can affect the way you carry yourself and operate in the world.

Personalize your goals. Use words such as "I" or "we." By making your goal a personal endeavor, you increase your natural inclination to do something towards its fruition. If the goal is just some fuzzy hope for the future, it is likely that neither your mind nor the universal mind will be able to grab it by the horns and make it happen.

Do not use words like "try" or "should," "would" or "maybe." Goals should be positive and firm, not flimsy or wishy-washy. "I will," "we are going to," or "I will have" are all statements of intention. Do not be afraid to state what you will accomplish and by when it will be so.

> "You may be disappointed if you fail, but you are doomed if you don't try."
> —*Beverly Sills*

Keep it simple. Goals can run the gambit of complexity. In the beginning, keep them simple. Small steps in targeted areas will help to achieve the bigger goals. Instead of setting a goal to reach an overall clinic income of $75,000 within X months, set smaller short-term goals which will be stepping stones to that ultimate desire. Patient visits per week, new patients per month, outbound calls per week, marketing activities per week, etc. are all small stepping-stone goals on the path to the larger ones. When you achieve the small ones, it gives your conscious and unconscious mind the support and belief that you can achieve the greater ones as well.

Have fun with it! Goal-setting is all about improving your life and realizing your dreams. Having a goal should not make your life miserable. This is about challenging yourself to do better. By setting that carrot a little further out of reach and then growing to grasp it, you will continue to improve the quality of your clinic and your life. Also remember that it's okay and probably good to change your goals as you go. What you think is important will very likely change from year to year. Only you can decide what your goals will be and what the path to realizing them should look like.

➤ Time Lines

The length of time for reaching a goal that you set can vary from this week to next month to next year. In fact, it's useful to have short-term, long-term, and lifetime goals.

Short-term goals

Short-term goals are no longer than six months and better if kept to no more than three months. Goals in this time frame are usually smaller, stepping-stone goals. They are the action-steps which, when pieced together, will help you achieve a long-term goal. You should write down these goals every day and add to them with flexibility as you go.

Long-term goals

Goals with a deadline anywhere from six to 12 months are considered long-term. These goals should be larger in scope or level of achievement and usually will be the result of completing your smaller, short-term goals. These are the goals we set for serious financial change or personal improvement in our lives.

Lifetime goals

Obviously these are goals that you wish to accomplish at some point in your life, the sum total of what you create or achieve. Establishing lifetime goals can be fuzzy, and achieving them will be difficult if you don't have short- and long-term goals established in order to get there. Each consecutive set of goals that you accomplish will help you on your path to achieving your lifetime goals.

▶ The Seven Areas

Just as the benefits of acupuncture and herbal medicine are not just for the sick, goals are not just for your business. Although setting goals will help you make your clinic all that you desire, there are more things to life than work. In fact, there are (at least) seven areas in which we can and probably should set goals.

Family goals can be as simple as "spend one hour every evening just being with my kids this week" or as complex as "reestablish a friendly relationship with my estranged brother." A family goal is one that relates to your relations and activities with people who are part of your family.

Financial goals are about money or your financial stability within the mysterious world of flat, green qi. These goals include things like saving for a new car, establishing and regularly funding a retirement account or a college fund for your children, or creating enough patients to buy your own clinic space.

Spiritual goals reflect your life on the inside. This can include religious observance, qigong or meditation practice, creating time for reading or reflection, or just being in nature. It can be anything that nourishes your spirit, gives you strength, and supports you in your quest as a healer and human being such as, "I will spend 30 minutes of quiet sitting in my garden each week through the month of May."

Work goals include a wide variety of things. The area of clinical success may be the easiest part of your life in which to begin setting goals. "I am going to see five new patients per week, every week, by the second week in September," for example, is a specific, measurable, realistic, and time-bound short-term goal. But other work-related goals may include improving your clinical or diagnostic skills through continuing education, perfecting a new clinical technique, reviewing one herbal formula per week, or reading a new clinical text each month.

Certainly, business goals are an easy set of goals to start with. How many patients are you seeing per day, per week, per month? By focusing on your new patient load, you will be surprised at how easy it is to grow the size of your practice. Start with what you are seeing in the way of new patients now. Double that number and come up with a time-line—the end of next week, for example!

Social goals are those areas that have to do with outside relationships or activities. "I will have 100% member turnout for the Chamber of Commerce luncheon next month," "I will sponsor a child for the Big Brother organization," or "I will join the local XYZ volunteer fund-raising group." These are the type of goals that enrich and create the colors in the fabric of your life. While such activities can also be seen as part of your marketing, work alone is rarely enough for a satisfying life.

Health goals such as "I will do one trade for massage each Friday through the year 2004." Part of being a healer is making sure that you are taking care of yourself as well. Too often, we forget how much stress and strain we undergo in the routine business of just being a human, much less operating a small business where your focus is always on the health and care of others. Make sure to set goals in this area. Only by keeping yourself in optimum health will you be able to provide the best service and care to those that enter your clinic door.

And finally, *Education*. This is an area of life that is all too easily forgotten, even if you are required to fulfill a certain number of CEUs each year. The goal here is to improve upon your current knowledge base and is one of our favorites. While no one can ever know everything, you can take lifelong learning as a worthy goal. How about, "I will enroll in, study, and conquer one Blue Poppy distance learning course in the first quarter of next year," or, "I will continue study in the field of Oriental medicine, attaining my doctoral degree by the summer of 2007."

A Final Note

Mark Victor Hansen says you should be able to write 101 goals in 20 minutes. This may not happen at first, but, the more you write, the better you will get at it. What's more, you will find yourself meeting those goals more and more often. Remember, as you write goals, that there is no shortage of patients out there and no shortage of money. Think about what you want, put your mind to it, and you can make it happen.

Take some time and look at the seven areas for goal-setting listed above. Write at least one goal for each area. Maybe get a small, attractive notebook to write down your dreams and goals every day. Then see if you can write five specific, measurable, attainable, realistic, and time-bound goals for your clinic or your professional life. Don't worry if you think they might sound crazy to anyone else. This work is to help you. It's also okay to write down the same goals day after day until you reach them. Trust your crazy dreams and remember, whether you think you can or think you can't, you're right.

POINTS TO PONDER FROM CHAPTER 2

- Goal-setting is a powerful tool you can use to help you plan for and then create your own success.

- People often don't set goals due to fear of failure.

- Good goals are S*M*A*R*T: specific, measurable, attainable, realistic, and time-bound.

- It is effective to have short-term goals (1 week to 6 months) and long-term goals (more than 6 months).

- There are at least seven areas for which it is useful to have goals. These are family, financial, spiritual, educational, health, social, and work.

- It is useful to keep a small notebook or scrapbook for writing your goals. Write as many goals as you can every morning. Read them to yourself every day. After a few months, go back and read the goals you were writing then and see how they have changed and which ones you have achieved.

What Could You Be Doing While You're Still in School? | 3

While you are in school, there are many things you can and should do to ensure a smooth transition from student to full-time practitioner. In this chapter, we offer a wide variety of projects to improve your quality of life during the first weeks and months out of acupuncture school. The more groundwork for success you have laid in advance, the closer you will be to the practice you desire the day after graduation. You will also experience far less stress.

First and foremost, get the most out of your education! Do the work, be curious, be serious, and get a firm grasp on the theory behind the medicine. Don't just go through the motions. Consider that if you think school is hard, being in private practice is *much, much harder.* Each new patient is a challenge, and you have to take care of everything for yourself, every day, including chart notes, research, marketing, bill paying, your patients' needs, and yourself! Also, as we will discuss in later chapters, *you* will be your best marketing tool, and the better you know this medicine, the better and more self-assured your treatments and your marketing efforts will be.

Second, start thinking about and visualizing your life after school. Make these visualizations as real, detailed, and concrete as you can. Write them down. Keep a planning/brainstorming notebook of all your ideas and dreams, networking contacts, phone numbers, and leads. Then think about the first concrete steps you will need to take in order to manifest your "dream" clinical practice. Some of these will very likely include the following.

> ## Your roadmap

One of our favorite American icons, Yogi Berra, said, "You've got to be careful if you don't know where you are going, because you might not get there." So, even if you are not entirely sure of where or how you want to practice, some basic plans now will help ease the transition from student to practitioner. Narrowing down the areas in which you would like to practice is a good first step. Start with the region of the country that most appeals to you. This leads to some chores.

1. Look up the statutes and regulations regarding acupuncture and the use of herbal medicine in the states in that region. While most states now allow acupuncture, there are still a few which require that the treatment be performed by a medical doctor or under a doctor's supervision. Once you know the regulatory climate in the state in which you want to practice, you can start to look at other factors.

2. Check out the demographics of various cities and towns. There are many websites that will give you a wide variety of demographic information for areas all over the country. Call Chambers of Commerce or visit their websites. This is always a good first step to setting up any kind of business in a new town. Chambers of Commerce are designed to give you all kinds of statistics regarding population and expected growth, median income, the primary industries, major medical facilities, educational and cultural climate and opportunities, and, also importantly, the average age. All this information will help you determine the size and nature of your potential market and also possible practice specialties that would be fruitful.

3. What is the feel of the community? Any area you decide to move to should first and foremost be one where you can be a comfortable and active participant. What's the political climate and does it fit with your personal beliefs? (Donkeys and elephants may not be happy working and playing together.) What religious affiliations are possible and does your preference have a presence there? Is it a supportive environment for raising a family if you so desire?

4. Begin taking a serious look at the amount of capital you will need to start up your practice and consider possible sources of funding. What pieces of equipment and furniture do you already have? What more will you need? How much will you need for signing a lease, business insurance, licensure fees, installing a phone, computer hardware and software, printing forms, signage, and initial marketing? What will you need in reserve to pay personal bills for the first six months? How much do you have and what sort of family or personal financial support structure will you have in place when you graduate? Be as realistic as possible.

➤ Competition

You also need to know who's there already. If it is a large city, you can go to the library reference department and look through the actual yellow pages. Go online to the NCCAOM site and do a practitioner search there. Write down any names and phone numbers you can get. If you can also get addresses, that's even better. You may wish to contact them, possibly get some part-time work from them, rent space from them, ask for referrals for a specific specialty you plan to pursue, and otherwise try to set up a nice working relationship before you move into the area. There may be some sort of support or study group already in place. Some practitioners won't be happy about your move into "their" area, but don't let that disturb you too much. Others will be supportive and more helpful than you may think. They might even offer you a job!

Also do some web searching at sites other than the NCCAOM, especially if you live in a state that does not require NCCAOM certification. Try as many web searches for acupuncture in that area as you can. I like using www.dogpile.com since it uses all other search engines at the same time. Try going to www.yellowpages.com and looking up acupuncture for the zip code(s) of your chosen area. Anyone that has a Yellow Pages ad should come up.

Other resources may be www.acupuncture.com, www.acupuncturetoday.com, and the website for the licensing organization for the state in which you want to practice. ●

This exercise is designed to do three things. First of all, it lets you see where everyone is located. If 70% of all acupuncture clinics are on the west side of town, perhaps you should look at the east side. Or you may find that the little town of 13,000 people that looked so attractive already has 100 acupuncturists. That's not likely, but you may not like the numbers you see. And last, with this contact information, you will be able to get in touch with at least some of the already established practitioners in the area (if there are any) and check the current rates for acupuncture in that area. This helps you determine your own rates and whether or not you can make the living you need and desire.

➤ Should I be one — or one of a hundred?

No matter where you decide to hang your professional hat, you will undoubtedly have to spend some of your time educating the community as to the benefits of our medicine. However, if you settle in an area where there are other acupuncturists (or even if you don't), you can help yourself greatly by finding and serving a niche market. This means specializing. Specializing may *feel* like a limiting factor for you in the beginning, but it can produce patient interest in the community and lots of referrals from other acupuncturists or Western medical practitioners who are not as proficient in that specialty. Remember that there is no lack of human suffering with almost any condition, specialty, or body part. And it is easier to know a lot about one area than a little about a lot of areas. If you get really, really good at one thing, people will find out about it and refer to you when appropriate. We will discuss specializing in much more detail in Chapter nine of this section. I [HW] once had an arm surgery from an orthopedist who *only* did surgery on arms, and he had more than plenty of patients! So give specialization some serious thought.

While specialization is a wonderful way to carve out your niche in an area, make sure to get extra training in your area of interest. The reason we mention specialization in this chapter is that it may be easier to get that kind of training while you are still in school. Do some special research and talk with your instructors.

➤ Pick a name

It is never too early to begin searching for your name. The name of your business is a very important decision. It will represent you to the community and your patients, appearing on your signage, letterhead, business cards, website, everywhere. While a good name can help build a positive patient flow and bottom line, a poor one can contribute to you being alone in your office.

Why does your business name matter? Because it is your brand identity. It announces who you are and what you do. And it can lump you in with or raise you above your competition. When selecting the name of your business, you will want to keep a few important questions in mind:

- Does it make my business easy to market? The more information your business name conveys, clearly and concisely, the fewer explanatory words you need in ads, on signs, etc. In other words, if the name of your clinic is *Skin Care Acupuncture Clinic,* your Yellow Pages ad does not need any extra lines of type to tell people what you do. It's already in the name. Just pay to have it listed in red and call it good!

- Is it easy to remember, spell, and pronounce? *Whole Family Health Center, Boulder Herbal Medicine Clinic,* and *Orange Park Acupuncture Clinic* . . . these are all pretty easy to remember, right? They are short, concise, and can be pronounced by anyone who drives by your clinic. Why is this important? Hundreds, even thousands of people may drive past your clinic sign every day, but, if the name is weird, hard to pronounce, or hard to remember, you may lose that future patient to the guy down the street. We do not suggest that you use Chinese words like *An Shen* (calm spirit) or *Jin Shan* (golden mountain). These may sound pretty and may have meaning for those of us "in the club," but they mean nothing to and may even put off the average American patient.

- Does it convey a clear understanding of what you do? *Womencare Acupuncture Clinic* and *Athletic Edge Acupuncture Center* are good names that communicate to your patient population both that you do acupuncture and that a selected group of people would benefit from your services. Look for ways to add the words "acupuncture," "Oriental medicine," "herbal medicine," etc. to convey your purpose.

- Does it market you to the specific niche you want to serve? Again, this is a great way to separate you from the average. Niche marketing can fill your clinic quickly. Every athlete who sees *Athletic Edge Acupuncture Center* will have a pretty good idea what you do!

Once you select your clinic name, try it out on friends and family and see what their reactions are. Ask them to spell it without seeing it. Try it on the cute waiter at the coffee shop. You may just score your first patient before you even leave school!

➤ Check name availability

Now that your mind is brimming with ideas, go to the web site for your Secretary of State and search for name availability. Whether you are planning to be a sole proprietor, an LLC, or you are going to be huge and want to incorporate, you need to choose a business name that no one else already has. Most of the Secretary of State web sites are either www.sos.XX.us, with XX replaced by the initials of your state, but a few are www.ss.XX.us.

If your chosen name is available, call the number on the website or try to apply for the name online. Find out what the reporting/renewal requirements are for maintaining your business name. (Typically, you have to renew your name once per year or once every other year.) I [ES] registered my business name almost one year before leaving school and then printed business cards with my cell phone number and gave them to everyone! To this day I still get calls on my cell from those first business cards.

➤ Get a job

Another good idea for the beginning acupuncturist is to find someone looking to hire you. These days, more and more physicians are looking to augment the services they can provide in-house to their patients. Multidiscipline treatment facilities are the wave of the future in health care. The more of these that are out there, the more patients will realize how convenient it is to be able to go to a single clinic for their standard medical care, chiropractic, acupuncture, and other alternative medicine treatments.

A friend of mine [ES] is an acupuncturist in Denver, Colorado. He moved there straight from school, took a job at a multi-discipline clinic, and, within a week, was seeing a full load of 30-40 patients. It was a nice setup for him since the company also pays for all of his herbs, needles, and other supplies and they are paying for his malpractice insurance. Best of all, he is part of a staff of healing professionals in a nice, clean office with a receptionist who calls him on the intercom and says, "Mr. Hillman, your next patient is here."

This *can* be done. However, your timing must be right. Draft a letter describing yourself and your skills/specialties, desired position, and date of availability. ● Add referral letters from your academic dean or a few professors. You do not want to send the letter too early. Your letter might spark someone's desire to add acupuncture to their office now, not six or eight months from now. If you are still eight months from graduation, that may be too long of a wait. I recommend sending out feelers no earlier than four months from your expected licensing date. Offer to come and meet the practitioner(s) personally. Make sure to include some research reports on the increased effectiveness of Western medicine when combined with acupuncture and Chinese herbal medicine. ●

If you want a more Western medical setting to work in, that is also possible and happening more and more all the time, especially if you have had any experience in the Western medical world (RN, PT, Med. Tech., etc.) Go and talk to some hospital administrators and employment offices or directly to as many MDs as you can. This may take some persistence and repeated phone calls, but, if you don't give up, positions like these are being created all the time. See Section 1, Chapter 7 for more information on this subject.

In addition to Western medical or multidisciplinary clinics, you may find jobs with other acupuncturists. Ask your school administration to give you names and contact info for all alumni in the area where you wish to work. (Personally, I [HW] think there is something not quite right if they won't give you that information, but that is only my opinion.) You may also want to place a small ad in your school alumni newsletter if one exists. Contact the graduates in or near your chosen area and ask for a job. Be flexible about hours and duties. You may have to work odd hours, put herbal formulas together, or answer phones some of the time, but that could get you some free rent, observational experience seeing how another person runs their practice, and other benefits that help you get a toehold in your new community.

See the Resources section at the back of this book for websites and other books to get more guidance on negotiating skills. You may want to sharpen that saw a bit before you enter into negotiations with any kind of clinic that wants to hire you. One pointer with regard to negotiating anything: remember that the party most willing to walk away from the table has the edge in any negotiation. So don't act desperate. We have included an entire chapter about getting a job in Section 1 of this book.

➤ Paperwork is easy

Something that is very easy to get out of the way while you're still in school is creating the various forms you will need to use as a practitioner. There are some form examples on the companion website for this book, but don't let that limit you in designing your own forms. ● Look at the forms used in your school clinic as well. Maybe you can get some examples from recent graduates who may have become friends during school. Just remember that they need to be easy to read and understand for you, your future front desk staff, and anyone else who may be reading them, such as insurance companies or lawyers.

There are many forms that you will need to run a clinic, communicate with patients and insurance companies legally and effectively, and perform and properly record patient care. From patient intake and follow-up, to patient information and clinic policies, to HIPAA and financial policy forms, you can begin filling a computer or paper file with these immediately. It will actually give you some peace of mind to know that you can start practicing effectively and legally on the day after graduation. If you are a computer user, once you have your clinic name and address, you can place that information at the top of the forms. Below is a list of forms you will need, examples of which are on the companion website and which are discussed in more length in other chapters.

Patient management forms ⬤ http://pointsforprofit.bluepoppy.com
- intake forms
- patient health history
- liability waiver
- insurance form
- notice of privacy policy (HIPAA)
- acknowledgement of receipt of privacy policy (HIPAA)
- individual rights for authorization (HIPAA)
- disclosure form (HIPAA)
- informed consent (HIPAA)
- fax log (HIPAA)
- sign-in sheet
- patient information
- clinic policy (financial, cancellation, etc.)
- follow-up care (report of findings)
- herb instructions (bulk, patent)
- referral information sheet

Business/legal examples and forms
- hardship waiver form
- INS form 9
- IRS forms W2/W4/SE/S4

➤ Write some text for brochures

Brochures function as your clinic's voice when you are not available for comment. They are one way to extend your reach into your community. People love to take brochures. They take them home for more information, they take them to work to put up on the company bulletin board, and they give them to their friends and family. To be most effective, your brochure should contain just enough information to get people interested about acupuncture and Chinese medicine and its ability to treat a certain disorder but not so much technical jargon that they feel lost, bored, or stupid.

When designing your brochures, you want to include certain information. You may want one that just tells people what your clinic can do for them in a general way. This can have at least one picture of you. Get a classmate to take pictures of you working in the school clinic since people don't know what your clinic looks like in any case.

First of all with a brochure, make certain that prominent parts of it are based on *benefits* to the patient, not the *features* of your clinic that you think are important. For example, instead of a bullet point that says:
- Four spacious treatment rooms with modern equipment (feature)

We think it's more effective to have two or three bullet points that say:
- Clean and quiet treatment rooms insure *your privacy* (benefit #1)
- Modern equipment to guarantee the most *effective therapy for you* (benefit #2)
- Plenty of space to allow you the most *convenient scheduling* (benefit #3)

Second, you may want to make one or several brochures tailored to a specific disorder or set of disorders that you would like to treat, for example, gynecology, back pain, headaches and migraines, allergic rhinitis, etc. You might include a brief description of acupuncture and its uses worldwide and/or its history. It may also be useful to add a small piece of research proving acupuncture's effectiveness with your specified disorder. Last, include your clinic name and contact information and maybe a small section on the back panel about you if there is space.

Remember, the key is to make the brochure easy to read for the layperson yet informative enough to grab the attention of a potential patient. The other alternative to drafting your own is to look around and find someone to make brochures for you or to purchase premade brochures. There are several companies selling a variety of brochures these days.

Business cards

Sometime during your last year in school it is time to create a business card. Once you have decided on a clinic name and a general location, you can start work on a business card. You may not be able to accept patients yet, but you can start generating interest by letting people know the business name, the general area, and when you are expecting to begin your practice. Use your cell phone number to start this off. Remember, business cards are cheap and you can always print another 1000 cards when you have an actual clinic address and phone number.

As you can see by the example to the right, this beginning business card, while not perfectly complete, told people what we were, when we were going to be opening, a website for more information, and a phone number for questions. That phone number still gets calls

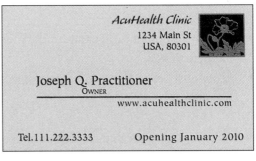

to this day. This simple $60 purchase netted almost 30 patients. Maybe not as many as one would like, but it helped us to hit the ground running. We actually had patients the first week we were open! Looking back, those first cards, the cell phone time, and the cost of our simple website, altogether $350–400, produced about $4500 in business in the first three months of our practice. That's not a bad return on investment and is certainly better than you can do on Wall Street in three months time.

Once you are really in practice, you will need new cards with other pieces of information. However, this is not the time to worry about that. When you are ready to get your "real" business cards, see Section 4, Chapter 5.

➤ Logo or no logo?

A company logo is another item that you can begin working on months before you graduate. You may decide to start without one and that is also fine. It may take you awhile to decide how you want to describe yourself pictorially. Whenever you decide to create this image, a good logo can require some time and effort to produce and you may want to enlist the help of a professional. One good recommendation is to call the art department at the local college and sponsor some sort of competition. Graphic arts students need to assemble a portfolio for potential employers. Getting their designs used by a real business is good for them and can be inexpensive for you. Talk to the graphic arts instructor and see if they have any ideas for a contest or if there is a talented student that would like a side job.

A logo is a visual symbol that should tell a story to your potential patients. It is useful to try and think like a layperson who may know nothing about Chinese medicine, culture, language, or art when you create this design. If a picture is worth 1000 words, you need to make sure the picture that represents you is worth the words you want it to convey. If you decide to use a Chinese character, for example, it may be wise to put the English translation in small italic type right below the picture or on the back of your business card.

P O W E R   P O I N T S

What other things could you do while still in school?

- Choose advisors such as accountant, attorney, banker, insurance broker, computer consultant, if you don't already have them.

- Look into answering services, call forwarding services, and other ways for you to stay in touch with patients and potential patients quickly and conveniently.

- Shop for business liability, health, disability, and malpractice insurance.

- Find out Worker's Compensation regulations, levels of reimbursement, and paperwork requirements in your state.

- Check out computer sign painting companies (Signs may be on a door, window, car, or on wood, plastic, or metal.) These prices may vary widely so shop around before you buy.

- If you like computer software systems for running your practice, take a look at the three or four that are out there for acupuncturists' offices, perhaps order a "test drive" copy or visit their websites. ⊙ This needs to be part of your equipment budget.

- Buy some CMS 1500 (insurance billing) forms. ⊙

- Will you need janitorial services, snow removal services, laundry services, grounds maintenance, medical waste disposal? You could get them all lined up with pricing budgeted before you graduate.

- Will you need appointment cards, telephone message pads, preprinted super bills, prescription pads, or other printing services? Again, prices vary widely, so shop around.

➤ Equipment

A major financial outlay when setting up a clinic is physical equipment. As a practitioner of acupuncture and herbal medicine, you are going to need two types of equipment: 1) items required to perform the duties of acupuncture (tables, needles, herbs, moxa, etc.), and 2) those required for running and managing a medical practice of any kind (computer, printer, fax, phone, etc.). When you are a student, money is not often the most readily available resource. However, a little money can go a long way on eBay and other online auctions, and there is another tool that you may be able to use—family.

Ah, family. We love them, and then we do something weird like run off to become acupuncturists. On top of that, then we ask for stuff to get our practice going! "Hey Mom, you know what I really want for Christmas? Acupuncture software for my new business . . . Here's all the info," says Johnny with a sly smile. Or how about a new business phone (with answering machine and caller ID) for your birthday?

- **Computer:** You will need a computer. Computers, although impersonal and filled with electromagnetic gamma rays (or something like that), are going to make patient management, financial recordkeeping, and in-house publishing of brochures and the like much easier. Keeping all your records on paper is very 19th century and a lot more work.

- **Printer:** If you follow our advice regarding the computer, then you will most assuredly need a printer. We recommend getting a color, all-in-one printer-fax-copier-scanner. For the extra money you will spend, the extra use you can get out of it is incalculable.

- **Phone:** You are hoping people will call to make appointments, right? Smoke signals and carrier pigeons are great, but have gone out of favor with most folks. Modern, Western patients want to call the clinic to set up their appointment. They want to be greeted by a friendly person, scheduled patiently, and to leave a message should the need arise. We strongly suggest a phone with caller ID and as many other bells and whistles as you can afford. We cannot count the number of times a new patient has called after business hours and requested a call back but then left no phone number.

- **A good sturdy table** for each treatment room is important. Really nice ones may have shelves underneath or attachments for table paper, or even hydraulic mechanisms to raise and lower them.

- **Desks, chairs,** waiting room furniture, carpets, decor, and shelving for herbal products. Wow, this is getting to be a long list, but it's better to know the reality in advance. A lot of this you may be able to get used or discounted online. Also cruise local garage and yard sales regularly and stay in touch with Office Depot and similar retailers for seasonal sales.

POWER POINT

Make a few photocopies of both your state and national license and diploma before you have them matted and framed for the wall. Keep a clean copy of each in a file. Then, when you apply to an HMO to be certified or when you need to show an herb company that you are who you say you are, you don't have to take them down off the wall and struggle to get another copy made.

These are just a few recommendations. For a more complete listing of suggested business equipment and acupuncture supplies, see the Resources section at the back of this book and the supplier section on the companion website. One caveat: While eBay is great for discounted-but-new products, we don't recommend buying old computer equipment. A used acupuncture table, desk, chair, work table, or shelving could be fine to recycle into your practice, but a three year-old computer is two months away from the scrap heap. Printers, if they are good ones, have a longer life than a computer, but take care when buying used computing equipment.

➤ Think about your herbal pharmacy

A bulk herb pharmacy is a great asset in any Chinese medicine clinic, especially if you become one of the few places in town with this feature. The downside of a bulk herb pharmacy includes the initial cash outlay, storage space and related costs, inventory management, and the fact that you will always come up against needing a medicinal you don't have that would be great for this patient right now. So, what to do and how to do it?

First of all, we do not recommend purchasing any herbs (bulk or otherwise) until you are ready to begin dispensing them to actual patients. Although properly packaged dried herbs have a decent shelf life, you will spend more in the long run buying a few herbs here and a few there. Storing boxes in your home or apartment can be a hassle. They may get damaged or you may find yourself opening the packages and using them before you are ready to open your clinic, which shortens their shelf life. We recommend, instead, doing some leg-work during your last year in school, checking out several sources, their prices and shipping policies, and then making a one-time large purchase as close to your opening day as you can. You can often get a nice discount as a first-time buyer. There are now distributors all over the U.S. so you can usually find sources that will get products to you very quickly and often with free shipping with a large enough order.

Next, preselect your list of the most important herbal medicinals. A bulk pharmacy, if you are trained, comfortable with, and legally allowed to dispense herbs, can vary drastically in size. Many school dispensaries have a bulk selection numbering in the range of 300–400 ingredients. While that is a very nice setup, it is not entirely necessary to carry that many herbs when you first open your doors. One hundred fifty medicinals can get you off to a very nice start. Just because you have graduated does not mean that you suddenly need *wu gong* (centipede). Sure, it looks cool in the glass jar, but if you haven't used it yet, you may not need it for some time.

A good idea, therefore, is to begin making a list of herbs that you use on a fairly consistent basis. While doing your clinical internship, keep notes on all of the formulas you write and dispense to your patients. See if you can whittle your selection of herbs down to 100 or 150. The list you create will establish your initial order just before you open your clinic doors.

Another option is to order the ingredients of 10-15 base formulas and a few others to then modify those formulas. These base formulas might include *Xiao Yao San, Xiao Chai Hu Tang, Si Jun Zi Tang, Si Wu Tang, Ba Zhen Tang, Liu Wei Di Huang Wan, Jin Gui Shen Qi Wan, Zuo Gui Wan, Er Chen Tang, Ping Wei San, Si Ni San,* and *Xue Fu Zhu Yu Tang.*

A step up from this would be to purchase a book on Chinese herbal formulas and choose from among the recommendations contained within. Blue Poppy has a few books on this subject, as do other publishers. The one I [ES] found helpful was *Seventy Essential TCM Formulas* and *260 Essential Chinese Medicinals.*

> **Wait until the last minute for . . .**

The last few things you want to do only a few weeks before you are ready to open your practice are:

- Call to have all your utilities and phone turned on by a specific date.

- Start accepting appointments from those friends that have been waiting.

- Place an announcement about your opening in the local papers.

- Take your brochure and other forms to the printer.

- Order some needles! And maybe some herbs, too. (For more information on setting up a dispensary, see Section 2, Chapter 1 and Section 3, Chapter 6.)

- Mail out announcements to local physicians, chiropractors, health food stores, hospitals, HMO groups, Human Resource departments for all local companies larger than 50 employees, friends, stores or services for any special niche market you plan to serve.

- Start planning your first open house celebration.

Finally, you can make all this work fun. Think of all this research, writing, and equipment prowling as the foundation of your success and stepping stones toward fulfilling your dreams. This is your own personal journey toward your chosen goal. So enjoy each day and each task as much as you can.

POINTS TO PONDER FROM CHAPTER 3

- Don't wait until you graduate to figure out your next move. You can complete lots of stuff now to help you hit the ground running, such as:

- Find a home for your practice, research the demographics online, at the library, and on the phone.

- Determine a niche market that will keep you interested for years to come and figure out how to find and best communicate with patients.

- Find out if there are other practitioners (acupuncturists, MDs, DCs, others, that you could work for part-time).

- Decide on a name, logo, and write promotional brochure text for your practice.

- Forms, letters, HIPAA compliance paperwork, and other patient records paperwork can be created while you're still in school.

- Start searching for and collecting equipment for your practice.

- Take notes on what things you want to carry in your herbal dispensary.

- Create a list of friends, media contacts, MDs, DCs, PTs, L.Acs, Human Relations Dept. directors, insurance company executives, stores, and other service providers that you will want to contact when you open your clinic.

Legal Stuff You Need to Know and Do | 4

> ## What you start with

Operating a business takes ambition and drive, yes. It also takes some amount of start-up capital, an office in which to work, and some little pieces of paper, the number and variety of which will depend on the state in which you practice. What do you need to put on your wall? What can stay in your closet collecting dust as a fond memory?

Diploma

After 3–4 years of putting the rest of your life on hold in order to focus on learning your new trade, the only thing you come away with for your business is a diploma. Almost all states that offer a license to practice acupuncture now require you to graduate from an accredited school of Oriental medicine. Graduation equals diploma. Depending on your state, your diploma will be needed for a variety of uses: state licensure, malpractice insurance, and certification. Therefore, it is highly recommended that the day you receive your diploma, take it to the local print shop and make 10 copies *at least.* Then, drop it off at the frame store to get it mounted and framed properly for display in your office. Take the copies and put them in a file. When you get to the last one in a couple of years, you can use that one to make more.

Certification

Some states, but not all, require you to be certified by the NCCAOM—the National Certification Commission for Acupuncture and Oriental Medicine. If this is true for you, you can visit them at www.nccaom.org or call them at (904) 598-1005. We recommend contacting this organization as early on as possible. There is an application process as well as both written and practical exams for acupuncture, as well as written exams for herbal medicine and Oriental bodywork. All of this will cost you some extra green qi. So call early and be prepared mentally and financially.

Business License

If required at all in your state, this license is maintained through your local government. Contact your city hall to get this process started. There may or may not be a fee, renewal requirements, etc. It usually is straight-forward and does not cost much since most cities and towns want new businesses both large and small.

Re-sale License

If you live in a state with sales tax and either your services or herbal products are *not* tax-exempt, then you need a re-sale permit. This allows you to act as a middleman for the state, collecting sales tax and sending it to them on a regular basis. For information on your specific state and how to apply for such a license, go to http://www.sos.XX.us and follow the links. For $35 you can get legalzoom.com to do all the paperwork for you!

➤ What pieces of paper should go up on your wall?

Once you are up and running, you will no doubt have a number of pieces of framed "artwork" that has your name plastered across the bottom as a certified, licensed, or registered such-and-such. Of all of these, some of them have to go on your wall and the rest are for decoration and personal glory. So, how do you know which ones have to hang in your lobby and which ones hang only in your personal shrine? Easy. Anything that has to be visible to those walking into your office will have a line printed across it saying "must be posted." Alternatively, it may say "must be visible" or "placed in a conspicuous place." It all means the same. Usually your state license to practice, your business license, and your re-sale license, if you have a state sales tax, need to be out where people can see them. Now, aside from those things that *have* to be on your office wall, you may want to consider putting your diploma in a very nice mat and frame and hanging that where your patients can see it. If you have a certification such as that from the NCCAOM, put that up as well. Remember that, no matter how far away from Western medicine *you* may want to be, the people that walk into your practice have been raised within that system. They want to see certain things that make them feel safe and confident in your abilities. And, when it comes to hanging things on the wall, get it done right. A nice matting and frame job will last forever and really shows a professional touch.

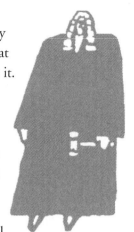

Where can you practice?

As of this edition of our book, there are only 4 states that do not have some type of acupuncture statute. However, not having an acupuncture statute does not *necessarily* mean that you cannot practice there. The Kansas law will allow you to practice only under the supervision and referral of an MD, DO, or DC. The laissez-faire state of Wyoming has no statute and does not regulate acupuncture at all. Of particular note is Louisiana, which does have an acupuncture statute, but allows practitioners only to work *directly* for a physician.

States that say no:

These are the states with a definite *no* where it comes to acupuncture: Alabama, North Dakota, Oklahoma, and South Dakota. Please note that laws are changing all the time may be changing as we write this. NCCAOM.org, Acupuncture.com, and Acufinder.com keep a *reasonably* up to date list.

States that say maybe:

Kansas: No statute. Acupuncturists must work under referral and supervision of an MD, DO, or DC.
Wyoming: Not regulated; do your thing and stay out of trouble.
Ohio: No herbal medicine in the scope of practice, but they are working on getting the legislation changed.

➤ **What can you call yourself in your state?**

For most states the standard is some version of "Acupuncturist."
That may be Licensed Acupuncturist (L.Ac.), Registered
Acupuncturist (Reg.Ac.), Acupuncture Physician (A.P.) or
Certified Acupuncturist (C.A.). Regardless of the prefix or suffix,
you are still an acupuncturist by any other name. The following
is a list of states that fall outside the lines of this conformity:

Florida: There is some amount of confusion and acupuncture-
title-mayhem in Florida. Evidently you can be an L.Ac., R.Ac.,
A.P., or a DOM. Hmmm—did someone punch the wrong
ballot? After reviewing the Florida Department of Health's
acupuncture site for over an hour, I have no more clarity to the
difference in title, meaning, or educational background.

Louisiana: Acupuncture Assistant. You have to actually work *for*
a physician.

Nevada: Here you are either a DOM (Doctor of Oriental
Medicine) or an Acupuncture Assistant. You become a DOM by
practicing for six years either someplace else or in Nevada under
another DOM. You become an Acupuncture Assistant by
working under a DOM in Nevada. If you are interested in
practicing in Nevada and have been working someplace else for
six years or more, please contact the Nevada Department of
Regulatory Agencies before moving to make sure you've got any
other requirements met. (775) 684-0222.

New Mexico: Doctor of Oriental Medicine

Rhode Island: Doctor of Acupuncture

➤ **How to get licensed in your state**

In order to get licensed in your state, you have to contact the
licensing authority. They will have a list of items that they want
from you, possibly including a copy of your diploma and your

Clean Needle Techniques certification as well as an application and, most assuredly, a check. It costs something in every state to get your license. That's just how it goes.

For an up-to-date listing of states' licensing requirements and who to contact, check out:
http://www.acupuncture.com/statelaws/statelaw.htm#1

➤ Malpractice Insurance

With the rapidly changing views of acupuncture across the nation, more and more people are flooding to our doors, curious about the benefits of our services. While this is very good for us in terms of building a patient base and doing what we love, it also means that insurance companies want to panel us or at least set reimbursement standards for our services. It opens us up wider to the possibility of getting sued. Malpractice insurance, therefore, is your way in, your way out, and the way to protect yourself and any clinic partners that you may have.

The way in: More and more insurance companies are looking to add the services of alternative medicine and specifically acupuncture, both to benefit their patients and their bottom line. While many companies are dealing directly with individual acupuncturists, still more are contracting with middleman MCOs (managed care organizations). This provides them with an instant, pre-credentialed list of providers for their payers as well as keeping their own costs down.

PRACTITIONER POINTER

"Ten years or so ago, I was accused by my state's Board of Medical Examiners of practicing medicine without a license. The charges were dropped but what a nightmare! I can't recommend too highly hiring a top-notch lawyer to protect you from frivolous lawsuits and having a good malpractice policy to protect you from your own mistakes."

—*Bob Flaws, Boulder, CO*

39

What this means is that those of us who are willing to jump through a few hoops (and take a small cut in pay) need to become paneled by the MCO. To do this, you need to have, among other things, malpractice insurance. The coverage amounts vary from one to another MCO, but the fact remains that they will require you to have and *maintain* your coverage while treating the patients they send your way.

The way out: Here in the good old U.S. of A., we belong to the most litigious society in the history of mankind (so far as we know). We sue our neighbor for the emotional trauma of watching him crush a bird's nest (and win). We sue the owner of the house whose skylight we fell through while we were trying to break in (and win). We sue the restaurant for making their hot beverages hot when we spill them on our lap (and win *big*). Is this a great country, or what?

The point is this—nobody out there reading this book thinks that you could ever do anything harmful to another person while practicing within your scope. However, that does not mean that you may not make a mistake or that someone will not make something up. When that happens, malpractice insurance will kick in and give you a way out. As long as you were acting within the guidelines of your abilities, training, and profession, your malpractice insurance will be there to cover your losses and to prevent you from losing everything you have built.

The way: Malpractice insurance, whether required in your particular state, is really a cost of doing business that all of us should carry. Every other medical provider out there carries it. Not because they are negligent or sloppy and not because they are fearful of false claims being brought against them. They maintain the coverage because it is the professional thing to do, and it protects their practice and their families as well as their patients.

As acupuncture licensing and insurance coverage grows across this country, you can rest assured that we are going to be scrutinized from top to bottom, from our individual abilities to our profession as a whole. While it is more than okay to have your style of medicine well-rooted in past history and tradition, we live and practice in modern times. As such, we need to wear the shoes of responsibility and professionalism that conform to the expected standards of our culture. That includes carrying adequate malpractice insurance coverage.

➤ Where to get malpractice insurance

The number of companies offering malpractice insurance for acupuncturists has fluctuated over the course of the past decade. At the time of this writing, there are four companies out there that are easily found with a quick web search, although there may be more. There are important coverage questions to ask, the answers to which vary widely between companies. You need to know whether these companies cover (either in the policy itself or as a policy rider): injection therapy, direct moxibustion, obstetrics-related acupuncture and whether it must be directly supervised by an obstetrician. Also, some companies offer less expensive policies for part-time or first-year practitioners. The companies (in alphabetical order) are:

American Acu. Council – www.acupuncturecouncil.com

Eastern Special Risk – www.easternspecialrisk.com

Scott Danahy Naylon Co. – http://scottdanahynaylon.com

Wood Insurance Group – www.woodinsurancegroup.com/

➤ General liability insurance

As a business owner with people walking in and around your clinic, it is ethically and economically prudent that you carry general liability insurance. This is just as standard as your homeowner's policy or the insurance you purchase as a renter. General liability insurance will cover trips and falls, scrapes and breaks that may occur on your property or the property that you are leasing. Almost every insurance company out there can give you a quote for this type of coverage. It is usually not expensive. Go with who you know or who you trust.

> ## HIPAA (Health Insurance Portability and Accountability Act)

Ah, yes—the ethereal HIPAA. Its wispy rules floating like pink, puffy clouds in the sky just out or reach of understanding. Well, I'm here to tell you that I caught one [ES]. I brought it down, put it under my TDP lamp, and asked it question after question until it dried up. Afterwards, I sat back with a grin thinking, "This stuff's not that hard at all."

When trying to understand HIPAA, forget trying to remember why it all started. None of that matters anymore, unless you've got a governmental regulation history fetish. What matters is knowing which practitioners it applies to and what it means for them. Some sources say that HIPAA applies only to health care practitioners who transmit a patient's protected health information (PHI) electronically for billing or checking eligibility for coverage. Straight up, that's it. However, even if you don't bill insurance electronically yet or transmit patients' PHI over the Internet, all of us collect a certain amount of protected health information from our patients in the normal course of our practice. For that reason, we all fall under at least the privacy and accountability part of the HIPAA laws. But it is not that onerous or difficult to comply.

Basically, you now must tell the patient *in advance of* their first treatment how you will both protect and use their PHI. You have to protect the computer files and records you may have (*i.e.,* password protected database and computer, fire wall if connected to Internet), and you must try to prevent unauthorized access to medical records (*i.e.,* behind front desk with staff or locking medical file cabinet). You have to make a note in the patient's chart each time you disclose any information (*i.e.,* faxing records to their doctor or insurance company).

On your clinic form for collecting patient information you must ask:

- if a certain phone number and address is okay for you to use to contact them.

- for their permission to send out newsletters and postcards, and give them a way to opt out of the mailings.

- permission in advance to send birthday or appointment reminders.

POWER POINT

What is the definition of PHI?
A patient's PHI is anything that "relates to the past, present, or future physical or mental health or condition of an individual, the provision of health care to an individual, or the past, present, or future payment for the provision of health care to an individual." [Public Law 104-191, August 21, 1996 – Health Insurance Portability and Accountability Act of 1996. http://aspe.hhs.gov/admnsimp/pl104191.htm.

Patients need to be given a *privacy practices notice* to read and sign, and they need to be able to read your clinic's privacy policy whenever they want or take one with them if they so desire. Also, if your clinic has a website, your privacy policy must be on that as well.

Now, all of this is done to protect the patient and their right to privacy. However, the gloves come off when it comes to trying to secure payment for services, in running your clinic, and anything done for the care of the patient. This means that if your patient owes you money, you do not have to ask to send the bill to their house or try to contact them on their phone numbers. You can share their name, address, social security number, and amount owed with any collection agency that you use.

There are a few other parts and pieces to HIPAA compliance. For a more detailed description of HIPAA regulations and how to comply, see Section 2, Chapter 9.

▶ Maintaining patient records

Taxes, financial receipts and patient management information— these must all be maintained for a certain number of years. The IRS says that financial receipts, such as credit card sales receipts, and deposit slips need to be maintained for three years, or for two years after the taxes they support have been filed, whichever is longer. The best bet is to keep all supporting documentation for at least three years after the taxes have been filed. Tax records, however, *should* be maintained for 10 years. Federal audits can go back seven years. The best course of action is to save everything. These records shouldn't take up yards of space. Keep them all together in a neat, organized fashion and just keep every year's records. There's no reason not to keep this stuff.

Where patient medical records and evidence of their visit (*i.e.,* sign-in sheets) are concerned, this varies from state to state. There is no federal law or guideline set for patient medical records maintenance. However, each state's statute of limitation is a good guideline to follow. Your state's medical association may have a suggested length of time for maintaining medical records as well. Your malpractice insurance company will tell you to keep the records forever, since patients have two years from the discovery of a problem in which to file a suit. While it might be difficult for a complainant to prove malpractice five, six, or even seven years after seeing you, you never know what a crazy person will do or what case a lawyer will be willing to take!

Therefore, medical records should be maintained indefinitely or, where this is impossible, then for at least as long as the statute of limitations (7–10 years for medical claims issues). This does not mean that a practitioner needs to maintain all medical records in the same location. Instead, clean house at the beginning or end of each year by going through your charts and pulling any of those of patients who have not come in for two years. Place those in a box, label the contents as Inactive Patients and store them in a safe, dry location. You can consolidate each year, keeping all records in alphabetical order or keep each year's pulled charts together alphabetically. Type a list of the charts contained in each box. Keep one copy of this list inside the box and one at your front desk or otherwise easily accessible location. When that patient returns in two years, you know right where their old charts are and can easily retrieve them.

If you use a patient sign-in sheet (not required but good to have if you bill Workers' Compensation), keep them for at least seven years. A good idea is to maintain all of one year's sign-in sheets in a binder, labeled with the year on the side. These don't take up much room and can be easily stored on a shelf or in a box in the back of a closet.

In the case of the death of a patient, it is a good idea to maintain those charts either indefinitely or for the term of the statute of limitations as set by your state (typically 7-10 years). In the case of the death of the practitioner (you), the medical charts need to be dealt with by whoever is in charge of settling your estate. While the medical records contain information on the patient, they remain the property of the practitioner and, as such, part of your estate. A good idea, therefore, is to designate in your will how such medical records should be dealt with. Typically, the surviving patients should be notified of the practitioner's passing by public notice in the local paper or through a mass mailing to each patient on the practitioner's patient roster. The medical records should be kept long enough for people to come and claim them if they so desire, say 60-90 days. Otherwise, the charts can be destroyed.

➤ Patient charting requirements

Remember the golden rule of medical charting; *if you don't write it down, it didn't happen.* Write down everything that occurs with patients, including phone conversations as well as any specific referrals that you suggest. Each chart note page should contain the patient's name, their age, sex, the date of service, and a signature of the practitioner. Your notes have to be legible and in blue or black ink. If you need to add something to a chart-note after the fact, write it on a separate piece of paper with the date the information was added and sign that page.

While taking notes, if you have to make a change or if you write something in error, line it out with one straight line and write your initials indicating you are noting a change or error. The information must still be legible. Don't scribble or erase and don't use white-out.

POINTS TO PONDER FROM CHAPTER 4

- Put your school diploma, any state or national certifications, and your tax licenses on the wall in your clinic. It is a legal requirement and gives your patients confidence.

- Check the website we refer to and find out your state laws and what, if anything, you are required to send to your state regulatory agency to practice there.

- You cannot practice acupuncture legally in Alabama, North Dakota, or South Dakota, and only directly under an MD in Oklahoma.

- Consider malpractice insurance. There are many good reasons to get it.

- For HIPAA, basically you must make a sincere effort to keep your patient records confidential and you must tell your patients how you are going to do that. See Section 2, Chapter 9 for more detail.

- Maintain patient records for the period of time that is your state's statute of limitations.

- Keep your patient records neat. No scribbling, no white out, date and patient name on every page.

Methods of Practice and Business Models | 5

▶ The Basics

Organizing a new business can be tough enough without worrying about what type of legal protection and taxability is best for you. While you read through this chapter, understand that the information below is to help you begin the process of this decision or to help give you a nudge if you are on the line. Furthermore, while most new business owners begin their journey as sole proprietors, you may decide at any point to change that status when another form of doing business becomes more appropriate. The information in this chapter is designed to help you understand the pros and cons of each business model and the tax and legal implications.

▶ Taxes

The structure you chose for your business will ultimately determine the way you and your business are taxed. We all have to pay taxes—most of us pay some kind of tax to the city, the county, the state, and to the feds. On top of taxes, we pay social security, unemployment insurance, workers compensation, and Medicare. It's best to do it with a smile because, at least to some extent, it is unavoidable. While there are many things as a business person that you can write off your taxable income quite legally (more on that in the Section 2, Chapter 1), you should actually hope that you make a lot of money and that you will be able to pay your taxes happily. We all grumble about taxes, but, if you want to be in business, at the end of the day (actually the end of each quarter), you will be sending something to Uncle Sam and possibly a few other government entities as well.

Robert Kiyosaki, author of the ***Rich Dad, Poor Dad*** series, says to think of yourself as being "in partnership with the government." We need good roads, schools for the kids, and we most certainly need police and fire crews. This is all supported by your tax dollars. (No, this is not a book to teach you how to fight the system, nor is it a book on radical politics.) Living within the system with as much intelligence as you can will relieve you of much stress and anxiety. That being said, the way you pay your taxes will vary depending upon the type of company structure you chose for your clinic.

➤ A word on being sued

In the descriptions below, you will find that the corporate structure provides you with some level of personal protection, while the others leave you dangling in the breeze. While a corporation may protect your personal assets from being considered when damages are assessed against you, it does nothing for keeping you from being personally named in a suit.

If someone wants to sue you, they can. If I walk into a supermarket tomorrow morning and slip on the wet floor, I can sue not only the store, but, in the suit, I can name the clerk who mopped the floor, the manager of the fruits and vegetable aisle, the store manager, and the lady standing next to me who did not lend a hand for good measure. Being named in a lawsuit does not mean that there will be a decision against you. But anyone *can* be named.

When operating your business, the protection that you are granted as a corporation or one of the corporate variations is for your personal assets and holdings only. In other words, if you are sued and there is a judgment against you, then your malpractice insurance and your company holdings can be gone after but not your home, your savings account, or your retirement house at the beach. If you are going into business with a partner or two, you may want to consider some type of corporate structure since this will provide your personal assets protection if and when someone in the group makes a mistake.

Also, it is important to realize that having this protection only protects you when you are acting on behalf of or within the confines of your business and you are doing so without malice or negligence.

Let's take a look at the pros and cons of each business model.

➤ Sole Proprietor

A sole proprietor is just that: someone working for and by themselves. A married couple can be considered a sole proprietorship but, otherwise, if two people combine to run a business, then they must form a partnership or some other business entity. In a sole proprietor model, the business and the person operating it are one entity from a legal and tax point of view. You get all of the profits and assets that come from your business, but you also *personally* assume all debts and liabilities. If someone sues you and you lose, your personal assets are on the table as well as the business. There is no veil of protection or legal separation between you and your business.

The biggest advantage to being a sole proprietor, and why so many people organize one, is that it is the simplest and least expensive form of ownership. Within the limits of the law, you are in complete control of your business and can do whatever you want with it and with the profits that you generate. If the business needs to be dissolved—poof, it is gone.

As far as the taxes go, all of the profits are reported on the owner's personal income tax form 1040. You will need to file a Schedule C: Profit or Loss from Business, and, since you will be making money, you have to file quarterly self-employment taxes

(Schedule SE). Doing this prevents you from having to make one huge tax payment each April 15th. Also, the general rule of thumb is that, if you are going to owe more than $500 in taxes, you are required to make quarterly self-employment tax payments. Otherwise you may have to pay a penalty.

Some disadvantages to being a sole proprietor include:
- Not all of your expenses will be deductible, especially those pertaining to employee benefits such as health insurance.
- Above a fairly low amount of income, you are likely to pay more taxes to the federal government.
- There is nothing to limit your personal liability in a lawsuit.

Partnership

Wherever there are two or more gathered in the name of doing business together, then shall they be called a partnership. A partnership is merely two or more people combining their business efforts, with the same benefits and disadvantages as a sole proprietorship. There is no protection of personal assets, nor is there a legal distinction between the owners and the business.

When entering into this type of business arrangement, the partners should have a legal agreement that sets forth how decisions will be made, profits will be shared, disputes will be resolved, how future partners will be admitted to the partnership, how partners can be bought out, or what steps will be taken to dissolve the partnership when needed. Yes, it's hard to think about a "break-up" when the business is just getting started, but many partnerships split up in moments of crisis, and, unless there is a defined process, there will usually be even greater problems than just those arising due to the crisis itself. Partners also must decide up front how much time and capital each will contribute as well as how the profits will be divided.

Depending on the level of initial contribution into the partnership, it is possible to pay one partner a greater percentage than the other. Be careful with this at the beginning or leave a clause in your contract that requires this issue to be reconsidered in X number of months. If it is stipulated that each partner gets 50% of the profits, you will each be responsible for that amount on your taxes. This means that, even if one of you is producing more income for the business than the other, you each get the same level of "draw" each month. A draw is the amount of money you choose to withdraw from the company account to pay yourself each month. In a partnership, you are a partner, not an employee. Therefore, you cannot pay yourself based on performance.

There are three types of partnerships that can be considered: 1) joint venture limited partnership, 2) partnership with limited liability, and 3) a general partnership.

- The general partnership is the most common setup in which partners divide management and liability responsibilities and profit and loss shares as set by the partnership agreement.

- A limited partnership means that some (or even most) of the partners have a limited liability, usually not more than the extent of their investment. However, this also means that the same partners have limited input into managerial and day-to-day business operation decisions. This is not a very good choice for your medical practice.

- Finally, a joint venture refers to a temporary partnership, usually for the duration of a single project or a limited length of time. Other than this, the joint venture partnership is operated the same as a general partnership.

As with sole proprietorships, the profits of a partnership flow directly to the partners' personal income tax returns, and self-employment tax payments should be made on a quarterly basis.

At the end of the year, each of the partners will receive a Partnership Return of Income (Form 1065) and a Partner's Share of Income, Credit and Deductions (Schedule K-1). Again, not all employee benefits are available as deductions to the partnership.

Despite having explained the ins and outs of partnerships, none of us suggest that you should form this type of business! While working with a partner can be very beneficial and satisfying, especially if you have complimenting traits, if one of your partners borrows money in the name of the company and then skips town or does anything that is illegal, all of the partners are on the hook! There are other forms of buisness that allow you the joys of working with others without these shortcomings.

➤ Corporations

A corporation, chartered by the state in which it is head-quartered, is considered by law to be a unique entity, separate and apart from those who own it. A corporation can be taxed, it can be sued, and it can enter into contractual agreements. The owners of a corporation are its shareholders. The shareholders elect a board of directors to oversee the major policies and decisions. The corporation has a life of its own and does not dissolve when ownership changes.

Forming a corporation may give you the best legal protection against lawsuits. However, this does not mean you have *carte blanche* to run a sloppy clinic, and anyone can be held liable for personal actions, whether they happened at work or not. That being said, at some point, you may wish to operate your business under a different structure than a sole proprietorship.

When you are ready to set up your corporation, it can be helpful to look either for books on forming one or online for companies that help you to do so inexpensively in your state. Ultimately, your corporation or company will have to be recorded in the state in which you intend to practice. Most states perform this function through the corporation division of the Secretary of State's office. Below is a breakdown of the types of corporations and their implications.

1. C-Corporation

This is the original "big-boy" corporation. All other corporate entities are either based on or scaled down versions of the C-Corp. Usually for very large companies, this structure provides personal protection to the owners and the benefit of being able to easily gather capital. A C-Corp, however, has the drawback of double taxation, which means that profits of the corporation are taxed first and then any dividends paid to the shareholders (that would be you in this case). In other words, the corporation pays taxes on profits and then you must pay personal income tax after being paid those profits by the corporation. You can look up the requirements in your state, but we won't spend further time on this since it is rarely a good choice for small medical clinics.

2. S-Corporation

For all intents and purposes, the S-Corporation is legally the same as a C-Corporation. The difference is that the S-Corp is allowed "pass through taxation," thus avoiding the double taxation mentioned above. Instead, dividends (called distributions in the case of an S-Corp) are recorded and taxed only on the members' personal tax return. The best thing about this is, while you have to pay yourself some salary, *you can pay yourself partially in distributions in addition to salary, on which you do not pay any Social Security or Medicare (FICA)*, which is a 15.3% savings on those distributions! (LLCs, discussed below, have the same benefit if they choose to file as an S-Corp.)

An S-Corp has the same requirements for organizing as a C-Corp. There are required annual meetings and reports and an elected board of directors/officers. The corporation must have at least one shareholder. Forming this type of corporation also requires some legal assistance for those who have never done it before or who are organizing a health-related company but is usually less expensive than a C-Corp.

3. Professional Corporation (PC)
The Professional Corporation was invented for private practitioners in the health industry. At one point, it offered the same types of benefits that an LLC now offers. However, since its inception, the cost and effectiveness of a PC has been surpassed by the LLC (discussed below). The PC offers its members personal protection from the liabilities of other members of a group office as well as allowing for the flexibility of operating as a C- or S-Corporation.

This type of corporation is restricted to those in the professional world: doctors, accountants, architects, acupuncturists, etc. In California, it is your only option besides an S-Corp (LLCs are not allowed). All persons operating under the PC must be licensed in the field in which they are practicing. A PC must have a board of directors/officers, is required to hold recorded annual meetings, and must establish bylaws for operation.

4. The enigma of an LLC
Ah yes, Grasshopper, when you can put an LLC into one category or another, you may leave the temple. A Limited Liability Company offers those who chose it the flexibility to operate as a partnership but affords the protection of a

> ## PRACTITIONER POINTER
>
> "My business has been set up as an S-corp from day one. Is it the best way? I really don't know. I have spoken with quite a few accountants and they have all advised me to do this for the greatest tax benefit. They leave the medicine to me and I leave the business/taxes/legal stuff to them.
>
> —*Susan Schiff*
> *Delray Beach, FL*

corporation. The tax structure of an LLC can be that of a corporation or a partnership, although this must be delineated at the time of organization. Like a corporation, an LLC can own property or enter into contracts. However, since the company may or may not dissolve when ownership changes, most contracts will include the name of your LLC as well as the individual names of the members.

While the LLC is the newest business model out there, it is now permissible in most states (but not for acupuncturists in California!). Less expensive and requiring less paperwork than a corporation, LLC owners are called "members" and, like a partnership, they share the profits as well as any losses. The shares are divided among members based on percentage of ownership. (Members must put actual assets into their LLC to be a member.) An LLC can be taxed like a partnership (each member reporting their share on personal income taxes) or like a corporation (partners receive salaries and distributions from company profits). This decision is made when filing for an EIN (Employer Identification Number – use IRS Form SS-4).

If an LLC chooses to be taxed as a partnership, the same tax forms as for a partnership are used and members are paid their share of the profits in lieu of salaries, reporting quarterly to the IRS on a Schedule SE with an estimated tax payment. The main difference here is that most employee benefits are deductible from the profits of the company, while, in a partnership or sole proprietorship, they are not. At tax time, members receive a copy of the form 1065 and a K-1, dividing the profits or losses from the company at the end of the year.

An LLC protects its members from double taxation but, unless members file as an S-Corp, they will pay more taxes (Social Security/Medicare) as discussed above under S-Corp. There is less paper work required for an LLC than the other corporate choices; no meetings or annual reports. It is a good choice to consider if you are opening a clinic with one or more partners.

➤ What's best for you?

As we said at the beginning of this chapter, it can be challenging to think about business model options when you are first starting a practice and are more concerned with getting patients, buying equipment, keeping dinner on the table, and getting the kids to soccer practice. Because of this, we know that most practitioners start out as sole proprietors. Many of you may never change your business model over the life of your practice, which is fine. The questions to ask yourself include, "Do I have many personal assets that I want to protect more than my malpractice insurance will? Do I wish to have partners in my business? Am I making enough that the impact of Social Security and Medicare (FICA) tax would be less with an S-Corp or an LLC filing as an S-Corp?" Depending upon your answers to these questions, another model may be a better choice and we think it is important to have knowledge about what your options are. We also advise that you discuss these options and any questions you might have about them with an attorney or tax accountant or both as your practice grows and develops.

POINTS TO PONDER FROM CHAPTER 5

- Because there is much to think about when you first start up as a business, most practitioners start as sole proprietors without thinking about other business models.

- Each type of business has a different way that taxes are assessed and a different level of legal separation between the owner's assets and the business's assets.

- As a sole proprietor, there is no separation between your personal assets and your business if you are sued.

"Points to Ponder" continue on the next page

You are also personally responsible for all debts and liabilities of your business. However, closing your business is as easy as locking the door, unplugging the phone, and tearing up your business cards.

- Partnerships require a great degree of trust in that you are legally responsible for each other's business conduct. In a partnership you create a contract about how to share the profits or losses experienced by your business. Otherwise . . .

- Partners should make sure that their business charter or contract clearly delineates the financial terms when the business is dissolved.

- There are three types of corporations, an S-Corp, a C-Corp, and a PC or Professional Corp. Most private professionals who wish to incorporate for legal protection or tax advantages, should consider either an S-Corp or a PC.

- An LLC provides almost the same level of legal protection as a corporation while avoiding the problem of double taxation. It also has some of the same features as a partnership. For people wanting to open a group clinic with a clearly defined financial and legal relationship between and among themselves, the LLC is an option to consider seriously.

- There are lots of books and websites on the pros and cons of each business model. Beyond the basics, it's a good idea to consult either an accountant or attorney when setting up and filing papers for anything other than a sole proprietorship.

Clinic Partners | 6

Owning your own business is a *tough business.* Being the sole manager, owner/operator is, at least for many people, even tougher. While working alone does have its advantages, it is also accompanied by challenges that may be detrimental to your small-business health.

Working alone gives you ultimate power. When faced with a predicament or risky decision, you have only to sit, think, and decide, with no one else's opinion or suggestion to get in the way. There is also the benefit of not having to share, split, or otherwise divide the income that your business generates. However, working alone means just that—you are alone in all your efforts, time availability, potential for income generation, and creative juice and ideas.

Having a partner that you know, trust, and respect can make your clinic a more rounded experience for patients and an easier life for yourself. For instance, say you have a young family and are soon expecting a new member. Wouldn't it be nice to be able to take a few weeks off to be with your new family? On the more traumatic side, what if there is a death in your family and you need to fly to the Midwest for a week? Do you think that you can just up and close your doors for a week or 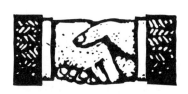 more without losing current or potential patients? A clinic partner who can cover those patients who need continuing care and keep your doors open for new seekers of your services is invaluable.

More than covering for each other, a clinic partner will push you to be more creative or give you a reality check if you are too far out there. Bouncing ideas off of someone who has just as much at stake in the business as yourself can take the smallest idea and blossom it into a profitable event. Two minds are better than one. Especially when you are not afraid to speak your mind and tell someone their idea is too crazy to succeed, or so crazy that it will.

Sharing educational costs is another benefit of having a partner in your clinic. Every year there are literally hundreds of educational events across the country, many of which overlap or coincide with each other. Some classes one of you may find interesting, but the other will not. Having that partner who is willing to divide and conquer the information available out there is a huge benefit to both practitioners as well as the patients. As each continuing education event is completed, the information is brought back to the waiting partner who kept the clinic up and running while you were away, and you both learn something new. The next time, the other partner goes, learns, and returns to disseminate. By the way, you can also share a clinic library, but label whose books are whose!

More practitioners mean more income. As strange as that sounds, it is true. Thinking that having a partner will mean you make less money is an inaccurate assumption. In fact, having two practitioners out in the community building present and future patients will grow your clinic by leaps and bounds. More patients equals more clinic traffic, more referrals from satisfied patients, and, in the end, more income for you and your partner.

Finally, another huge reason to have a partner is the benefit to the patient population. In your career as a healer, there will undoubtedly be times when you will be faced with a patient that does not "gel" with you or your treatment style. Instead of referring that person to the clinic down the street, there is another practitioner in your office. The patient is satisfied, and you don't lose that potential income to your clinic. Another side of this issue is the patient whose progress plateaus – they just stop getting better. When this happens, you have the option to refer your patient to your partner. This keeps the patient interested in both the medicine and your clinic. "Mr. Jones, I'm going to have you see Charles next week. I think that a fresh look at your condition will get the results we are hoping for." A great way to partner in such cases is to discuss the patient's situation before the next visit. Let your partner read your notes to get an idea of what's been going on, ask questions, and discuss further treatment options. In this way, the patient wins and so do you.

Take a look inside

Before starting your search for a partner to work with, you have to take a very deep, very serious look at yourself. Being introspective about who you are, the nature and direction of the clinic you want, and your style of business management and patient interaction will allow you to find a perfect match for your clinic partner. Be honest with yourself in determining your strengths and weaknesses. If you don't, you may find yourself in a working and financial relationship with someone you cannot stand.

Start with your person-ability. Are you a people person, or would you rather stay in the background? Part of establishing and building a successful practice is the ability to meet, greet, and talk with others about your clinic. Finding a partner who is good with crowds, can socialize easily with folks in all walks of life, and is not afraid of selling themselves (and your clinic) is a huge asset to you if you are less like this. The gift of gab is extremely important for at least one of you to possess!

One of you needs to be good with numbers. Many early practitioners begin by keeping their own books and records. Keeping track of expenses in a check register is but a small portion of the financial exercises required for every small business. Being able to work with numbers, be it the accuracy of your math skills, the vigilant recording of accounts receivable and payable, or the ability to understand basic accounting terms and programs, is essential. Even once you have grown your business enough to require an accountant or bookkeeper, you will still need to keep track of daily transactions and balancing the till at the end of the day.

The important idea here is to find the person who makes up for areas where you have deficiencies or where you aren't as strong as you would like to be. Working with someone else can round out your practice with stronger management skills, good patient contact and control, and give you an excellent sense of financial stability.

➤ Management

Whether you think you need one or not, someone has to be the ultimate brains behind the organization. Working with another person, day in and day out for 10 or more years is going to be difficult without some business structure. If that is something you feel comfortable with, great. Find someone who is a little less organized and needs that input. Otherwise, if you are deficient in this arena, try to partner with someone who has had some type of managerial experience or possibly someone who has owned their own business in the past. Even if they went out of business on a bad note, sometimes those are the best lessons we ever learn.

Since this is a business deal between you and one or more other practitioners, the initial business structure should be set down on paper in advance of opening your doors. If you are already in practice and are looking to add the strengths of another to your clinic, then it is a good idea to take a week or so to go over the business structure and set some operational procedures that everyone can agree on. Especially if you are already running your own clinic, you need to be open and accepting of the input your new business partner will ultimately bring to the table. While your way may be working for you, there is always room for improvement.

POWER POINTS

Areas where you may need operational procedure guidelines:

- Herbal medicinal and supplement pricing and distribution
- Inventory management
- Profit-sharing agreement
- Hiring and firing procedures
- Confidentiality of all patient information
- Record-keeping and patient management
- Marketing activities
- Holidays and holiday pay
- Conflict resolution procedure
- What happens when one party wants to leave the business
- What happens if one partner dies or is incapacitated

➤ Operating agreements

Once you find that special someone who can not only tolerate your idiosyncrasies but enjoys your companionship to boot, it's time to sit down together, perhaps with an attorney, and draft a contract or operating agreement. This agreement, although seemingly trivial or unnecessary in the honeymoon stage of your new relationship, will be an invaluable asset when and if it becomes time to part ways. No matter how famously you get along now, things can and do happen which invariably cause a rift. It is then that you will be very happy that you have a contractual guideline for dealing with the issue at hand.

There are a variety of standard agreements on most legal software that you can purchase at an office supply store, or you can use the services of an attorney. Regardless of the format of your contract, it is highly recommended that you have an attorney look over the document before both parties sign it. By using an online service or a legal forms CD, you may be able to write your own agreement, but you don't want it to have "holes" in it that can cause problems later. So getting it checked is a good idea.

Of important note here is that there is no requirement to have a partnership agreement unless you are operating your business formally as a Partnership. What we are recommending here is to have some sort of contractual relationship with anyone with whom you work. If you establish a corporation of some type, then you will have corporate by laws that govern behavior where the company is concerned, but it is still recommended that you establish some sort of working agreement to hammer out the details.

➤ What should be in my operating agreement?

Basically the information contained in an operating agreement is all of those things that you would set forth in an employee handbook. It's just that this one is for the owners. The key is to include as much information about the way "things" are going to work, how profits and loses are to be divided, an outlined procedure for selling one's interest in the partnership, and most importantly, conflict resolution. How will disagreements be resolved between the partners? If you do not stipulate it now, it can be very expensive for you later.

Capital, profits and losses

Include sections on capital acquisition and the distribution of profits and loses. Whether the capital to start up your company comes from one or both of you equally or from an outside source, be sure to indicate how capital is brought into the company. Also, if you both have an equal share/stake in the company, you should assign profits and loses equally. I [ES] once had someone tell me that you cannot assign losses. This is incorrect. With the addition of a simple statement, losses as well as profits can be assigned—especially if those losses are incurred from the normal operation of the business. An example of such a statement is:

> The profits of the business shall belong to the (partners/owners/whatever you are called) equally. All expenses incurred in the course of operating the business and any losses arising therefrom shall be paid out of the earnings of the business, or in the case of a loss, the losses shall be paid by the (again partners/owners, etcetera) in equal shares.

This statement is extremely important when you are setting up a new business with a co-owner. If you go out of business in a year because of bad management, poor marketing, or some other reason, without this section you alone could be responsible for covering any losses you may have incurred. A special note: be wary of anyone who is more than willing to share the day-to-day operating tasks and the profits equally but who balks at sharing the losses. Profits and losses are a part of business. If you want to be one of the bosses, you have to take all of the risks as well as the benefits.

Accounting

An accounting section of the operating agreement instructs that proper accounting methods must be adhered to and that, at the end of the year (this is only true in case of a partnership or an LLC operating as a partnership), you and the other partner will receive a schedule K-1 telling you what your share of the profits are. And that is what you pay taxes on. If, on the other hand, you are a corporation, then you receive paychecks throughout the year and that is what you pay taxes on.

➤ What not to do

This section of the operating agreement is probably the most important. It sets up the list of what you cannot do. For example, no partner may borrow money, endorse notes, or become security for another person in the name of the business without the agreement of the other partner.

This section can be as large or as small as you need it to be. Again, if you are a corporation, then much of this will be covered in your bylaws. However, there are still a few areas that may not be covered. You may wish to restrict each other to this one business, stating that no partner may be engaged in any other trade or business other than "the Business." This may seem silly, but when you are in your 9th month of business and the other partner decides to work as a bartender five days a week, leaving you to run it all but still expecting half of the profits, you will have some recourse.

You may also wish to establish a section stating that the one partner cannot assign or sell their interest in the company without the other partner's agreement. And, in case one partner does wish to sell, that the remaining partner has a "first right of refusal" to buy said interest. This will prevent one of the owners from selling off their shares of interest in the company to just anyone with the capital to buy it. This section will also delineate the procedure for evaluating the worth of the business so that the shares can be sold. Again, if this is a corporation, then there are shares of stock involved and much of this will be addressed in the corporate by-laws.

➤ What's in a name?

If one partner decides to bail on the company but both of you started it, who keeps the name? Typically, the remaining owner keeps the name, but this needs to be stated clearly in your operating agreement.

➤ First right of refusal

A first right of refusal means that when one partner wants to sell their interest in the company, they must first offer it to the remaining partner. Usually it assigns some preset number of days that the remaining partner has to decide to buy or not. Then, the leaving partner is able to sell to whomever they wish (unless you have certain "cannots" established above—like the new partner must be a licensed whatever, with so many years' experience, and no outstanding or unsettled lawsuits or malpractice claims against them) at the same or higher price than agreed upon in this document. If the departing partner wants to lower the price, they have to offer that price to the remaining partner before it can be offered to someone outside the business.

➤ Option to purchase on death or incapacity

This section will ensure the perpetual viability of the company should one of the owners/partners perish or become incompetent to work (coma, brain-damage, etc.). Without this section, you may run into some difficulty when dealing with your partner's mourning family. You may also find that your partner's family wants to run half of your business. Protect yourself and your business from this eventuality.

Make sure that this section includes certain guidelines such as:
1. The surviving partner can purchase the interests from the deceased or incapacitated partner.
2. If a price cannot be agreed upon, then the matter shall be arbitrated.

3. The surviving partner keeps the business name if they keep the business.

4. If the surviving partner has no further desire to maintain the business, its assets are divided equally amongst the partner and the family.

➤ Arbitration

The means by which two or more people settle a dispute outside of litigation in the courtroom is called arbitration. This provision is extremely important for any business to have amongst the owning members. Should you and your newly befriended partner come to be at odds regarding the operation of the business, you need to have a predetermined method of resolving the issue. Doing so will keep the business operating smoothly, will ensure an agreeable end to the conflict, and will keep the cost of the disagreement to a minimum.

Ideas to include in your arbitration section are that you both have to agree on an arbitrator. If you cannot agree, then you go with three arbitrators: one that each partner selects and a third selected by the two arbitrators. The decisions of the arbitrator or two of the three arbitrators must be final and binding upon each partner, their respective heirs, executors, or assigns.

➤ Amendments

Finally, the closing paragraph of your operating agreement should contain a section on changing the operating agreement as the two of you see fit in the future. If you decide to add, remove, or edit the pre-existing contract, this section will give you the authority to do so. Without this, you will have to rewrite and sign a new contract should even one word be edited.

POINTS TO PONDER FROM CHAPTER 6

Partnerships can be very satisfying and advantageous for a variety of reasons. Companionship, stability, group intelligence, shared responsibilities, expanded services to your clients, coverage of your practice when you go on vacation or if you have a personal emergency... Those are just a few.

- Before entering a partnership or group clinic arrangement, however, consider what you bring to the table as a partner and what you want from the other party or parties to balance your strengths and weaknesses.

- Once you decide to open a clinic with one or more partners, make sure you have a clearcut agreement about everything you can think of, and do it in writing. You may prepare an agreement using legal software, but getting it checked out by an attorney is not a bad idea.

- For more information on business models including Partnerships in the legal sense of that word, see Chapter 5 in this section.

Working for Other Practitioners, Clinics, or Hospitals | 7

While we discussed this idea briefly in Chapter 3 above, we feel this subject deserves more thorough treatment. Statistics from the world of chiropractic medicine indicate that new chiropractic graduates who take employment for a year or two with an experienced doctor before going out on their own grow their practices faster and easier when they do eventually go solo. This is logical. Getting experience with how an office is managed, how patient records are kept, how to maintain successful financial arrangements with insurance companies, how problem patients are dealt with, how to manage a front office staff, hiring and firing practices, HIPAA record-keeping, and all the many details of running an office can only make any practitioner's transition into private practice that much easier.

This type of situation, while less common in the world of acupuncture and Oriental medicine, has advantages for the established practitioner as well as the new graduate, which we discuss below. We encourage more practitioners with experience to provide these "mentoring" opportunities if their offices have the space to do so.

PRACTITIONER POINTER

"When I got out of school, my most powerful experience was working directly in the clinics of two practitioners who very generously took the time to teach me many things. This included information about how they ran their clinics as well as how to handle difficult patients and avoid legal or interpersonal problems. I believe that if every experienced practitioner shared their knowledge in this way, many more young practitioners would succeed and prosper."

—Laura Freeman
San Rafael, CA

If this sounds attractive to you as a student or a new graduate, there are a few strategies you can use to find a practitioner that will allow you to get your feet wet in their clinic.

➤ How to find a practitioner to hire you

You should begin your search during your final year of school. You don't want to find that someone-to-hire-you too many months before graduation, but you need to put together all the possible ways to find them early enough not to miss deadlines on any publications in which it might be useful to advertise.

1. Can you obtain a list of alumni from your school? Explain to your school administration what you want to do with the list and why. If they won't give you the list, perhaps they will send your letter or postcard for you if you pay the postage. Some schools guard this information very carefully and may not be willing to help you, but some will be more forthcoming or may even have an employment placement office.

2. If you cannot get an alumni list, is there an alumni newsletter sent out from your school? If so, find out the upcoming publication deadlines and if you can place a classified ad in the newsletter. You want to place your ad in the issue of the newsletter which will go out 3-5 months prior to your graduation.

3. Is there a state association newsletter and/or email list or chat group in your state? Most states where there are schools do have a state association. Similarly to #2 above, find out their advertising deadlines and place an ad in that newsletter as well. We'll talk about what your ad might say below.

4. If you have no other possible way of getting to practitioners, go to the NCCAOM website and look up every practitioner in the state or city or area where you wish to practice. Those

practitioners may not have graduated from your school, but you never know where opportunities will arise.

5. If you are open to moving anywhere in the U.S. for a short period of time, you can place a classified ad in a national publication as well. With *Acupuncture Today*, for example, you can advertise in their paper publication as well as on their website.

6. There are several online Chinese medicine bulletin boards out there. Consider posting your request on as many of those bulletin boards as you can find as well as Facebook, Twitter, LinkedIn, MySpace, and Craig's List.

We suggest you create a file for this project. In that file keep info about publications, websites, deadlines, (e)mailing lists, copies of the letters you sent or ads you placed, notes on phone conversations, and any "nibbles" you have received from your efforts—everything pertaining to this project. If you keep a calendar, put notations to yourself about follow-up phone calls, newsletter deadlines, or any other work that you need to do to make this job that you seek a reality. Be as organized as you can.

So, what should your ads, postcards, letters, or emails say to spark the interest of one or more practitioners to hire you? Below are some possible scripts you might use.

➤ Classified ad or web bulletin board posting

"Hey, practitioner! Too busy to file paperwork, manage forms, do outbound calls to patients, or market your practice as much as you'd like? I can help with all this and more. July '09 graduate seeks full or part-time position in established practice. Will work in reception, pharmacy, or clean bathrooms. Will trade work for use of clinic during evening or weekend hours. I am motivated, flexible, and creative. If you are interested in discussing this with me, call 111-222-3333 or email me at newgrad@acuweb.edu."

➤ Postcard Copy

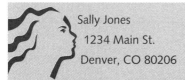

Sally Jones
1234 Main St.
Denver, CO 80206

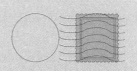

Sarah McLaughlin, Dipl.Ac
White Mountain Clinic
2345 Broadway
Colorado Springs, CO 80902

Too Busy to do your Paperwork? Help is a phone call away.

Dear Practitioner,

If you are too busy to file paperwork, manage HIPAA compliance forms, do outbound calls to patients, or market your practice as much as you'd like, I can help with all this and more. I am graduating from XYZ Acupuncture College in July 2009 and looking for a full or part-time position in an established practice. I am happy to work as a receptionist, in your pharmacy, or clean bathrooms if that is your need. I will work for money or a partial trade for use of your clinic during evening or weekend hours. I am motivated, flexible, creative, and open to your ideas. If you are interested in discussing this with me, call 111-222-3333 or email me at newgrad@acuweb.edu. Help is just a phone call away!

Thanks for your consideration, and I look forward to hearing from you.

Sincerely, Sally Jones

➤ Email or letter copy

Email tends to be informal and you could use either the same or similar text to the postcard or classified ad above. For a letter, however, you might want to be more formal or more thorough. You could include a photo of yourself (a photo can also go in emails or on postcards), a copy of a research paper you did in school, or even a Curriculum Vitae if you have an impressive before-acupuncture-college resume. If you have already created a business card, include that as well. If you have a Presentation Folder, you could offer to follow up with one if they want to see it. A letter you can download and rewrite to your own specs is included on the companion website in the marketing section. ⊙

➤ How to negotiate your situation

This can be tricky, especially if you have never negotiated for pay or perks or trades in the past. The first thing to figure out is exactly what you want from the situation in terms of money, space, business and patient management experience, and clinical experience. Make a list of your goals and desires for this position and tape the list to the inside front of the file where you keep all your other notes. Next, make a list of all the work that you would be willing to do and feel capable of doing in order to secure such a position. That's where you start. Then:

1. Remember that one of the secrets of negotiation is that whoever is the most willing to walk away with no deal usually gets the most from any negotiation. While this does not put you in a great position if you really need the work, try your best not to feel desperate for a job or behave or speak as if you are desperate. If you are talking on the phone or by email, keep your list of goals and your list of job capabilities in front of you. Be as flexible as you can, but don't give your services away for nothing in return.

2. Decide what you need to make per hour in cash or trade for this to work for you. While a great deal less than what you can earn as a practitioner, it might be worth your while to accept $12 per hour for work as a receptionist/pharmacy operator/janitor/office person position 20 hours per week if you also have use of the clinic rooms during evenings,

weekends, and/or the practitioner's day off. If you are starting from scratch, you don't have any patients yet anyway and a rent-free clinic or at least one room with all the equipment you need (tables, phone system, TDP lamp, etc.) could be a great leg up. It'll give you time to get your feet wet while having a little safety net for awhile.

3. Any practitioner with brains is going to want a minimum 1-2 year commitment from you. It is very disruptive to have practitioners or office staff coming and going from your clinic every few months. Don't even think about trying to find a job like this if you are not in a position to work for someone that long.

4. If the deal is to be for an off-peak hours rent trade only but you really like the clinic and want to work there, decide if it would be preferable to simply rent space for a year or if there are very specific jobs you could do for a minimum number of hours that would be worth it to the practitioner and to you. This gives you more time to be out there building your practice.

5. You will need to have a clear-cut arrangement concerning product sales and profits, use of computers, file cabinets, and other office equipment, access to supplies such as table paper, cotton swabs, etc., who is allowed to turn the heat up or down, and as many details of the clinic operation as possible. All agreements that you make with the practitioner, partnership, or corporation should be in writing.

6. If you are selling medicinals that belong to the practitioner from whom you rent or the clinic in general, try to negotiate at least 10% of the profits for yourself for any sales to your patients. This gives you the incentive to sell them and creates more profit for the clinic as well. Offer to create a system that allows everyone to easily keep track of office sales. This will help with inventory control in any case, no matter who gets the profits.

7. You may want to consider having a clause in your contract stipulating that you want to use your own line of herbal products after a certain number of months and that you will create the space or carry the products around in your car if space is not available. Cumbersome, yes, but this may be your only real option if the clinic space is very limited, the clinic doesn't sell herbs at all, or the practitioner(s) use lines of herbs that don't meet your needs. This could be the case, for example, if you are doing a completely different specialty than anyone else who works in this clinic.

8. Most practitioners will want to meet you in person. This is important for both of you. We don't advise taking a job in a clinic you've never seen or with a clinician you've never met.

9. Consider a three-month trial period at the end of which the final contract will be negotiated between you or you go your separate ways.

10. If this is happening in the town where you plan to locate permanently, consider specializing. Practitioners will be more open to your offer if you are planning to specialize in a specific niche different from their own. For example, if you want to do dermatology and skin care, it might be a nice addition for a practitioner who specializes in gynecology, and it will not be in direct competition with them.

For practitioners reading this chapter and feeling skeptical, we offer the following thoughts. If you are in practice but do not have an office staff or receptionist or anyone to put together formulas for your patients, consider making an offer to create a job like this for someone from the next graduating class at the closest acupuncture college. The advantages are more than they might appear to be on the surface of things:

1. Instead of just part-time office support, you get that support from someone who understands Chinese medicine and can knowledgeably answer your patients' questions.

2. You get someone to manage your herb inventory and put together powder or bulk orders who understands Chinese herbal medicine and who is less likely to make mistakes or require extensive training.

3. You get someone to see your patients, answer the phone, fill patient prescriptions, and generally hold down the fort while you are on vacation without sending patients to another clinic.

4. You are freed up to see patients and not have to run the front desk, request payments, answer the phone, or manage herb inventory at least for a certain number of hours per week.

5. If your new assistant sees patients during hours you are not there, your clinic is open more hours of the week with more phone traffic and more foot traffic to buy products and spread the good word about your services. More traffic makes more business for everyone.

6. If you collect all or most of the profit from increased sales of herbal or other products, after a few months this could cover most if not all of what you pay your assistant. Then all the rest of the advantages they bring to your clinic are gravy.

7. If you hire someone whose specialty is different from yours, you can broaden the services you offer to your patients without competition between you. This can increase your clinic's word of mouth buzz.

8. You are offering an invaluable service to the profession by helping train a new practitioner how to run a successful clinic. The more successful practitioners there are, the more political clout we have, the more public support we have, and the stronger all of us are as a group.

So as you can see, such an arrangement can be profitable and satisfying for all involved. We encourage both students and practitioners to create such mentoring partnerships. Depending upon your situation, and if both sides have integrity and work together, everybody can win with this one.

➤ Working in an MD, Multi-Practice Clinic, or Hospital

Working in a Western medical environment is becoming more common in our industry. These situations do exist and there are more MDs interested in hiring an acupuncturist to work in their clinic than you might believe. Although we have no specific evidence of it, this may be especially true for MDs who have some training in acupuncture but not in Chinese herbal medicine or, having done training in acupuncture, realize they don't really have the time to make it work financially if they do it themselves. There are also some specialties that may be more amenable to combining your services with theirs than are some others, notably orthopedic surgeons, rehabilitation specialists, neurologists, "holistic" general practitioners, and infertility specialists. (Do a search for members of the American Holistic Medical Association in your area as a place to start!)

While there may be some complexity when negotiating to work in such an environment, if we want to really be accepted in the mainstream of medical care in this country, such arrangements need to become more the norm than the exception. It may take some persistent networking to find a sympathetic MD to hire you or take you on as a clinic partner. However, from what we have found with practitioners who are working in hospitals or multidisciplinary clinics, it is always a question of making yourself known as a credible resource, offering to do hospital in-service talks, or otherwise putting yourself continually in the path of MDs in as many ways as you can. If you persevere in your search and show people that you can communicate in a way that makes sense to them and that your services are valuable to their patients, you can and will succeed.

There are at least two factors in our favor. First, MDs outnumber us more than 20 to one, DCs by more than three to one. Second, MDs are being asked almost every day by more and more of their patients the same question, "What do you think, Doc, should I try acupuncture for this problem?" That being the case, if a reasonably open-minded MD has any extra space in his or her clinic, they might be quite open to the idea of having an on-staff acupuncturist at least renting space in their clinic and having the office staff schedule their appointments.

In calling several practitioners who are working with MDs or in hospitals, we hear variations on the similar theme. One practitioner found her position because she joined a Women's Health Discussion Group that included two gynecologists interested in complementary alternative medicine (CAM). When one of these gynecologists joined a multidisciplinary clinic, they asked the group to hire her as the staff acupuncturist. As such, she paid a pro rata share of her patient visits for overhead costs for which she had full-time receptionist/ front desk services and lots of referrals from her clinic partners. She kept the proceeds from all herbal product sales.

PRACTITIONER POINTER

"I work out of a chiropractor's office that is 650 square feet. The office has a good location. His receptionist makes all my appointments and the bathrooms are always clean! I work when he doesn't which is Fridays, Saturdays and evenings as needed. I have the option of using the space during other times if a patient really needs to be seen immediately. I pay him $400 a month, which is more than paid by doing *tuina* for his patients every Thursday from 4-8 (he pays me for this). Doing the *tuina* has worked out well and continues to bring me acupuncture patients."

—Elizabeth Liddell
Philadelphia, PA

Another practitioner made a conscious decision that he wanted to work in a Western health care environment even if it took him a few years to create that reality. His strategy involved several steps, including hiring a resident at a nearby hospital to work in his clinic doing basic Western diagnostic intakes in conjunction with his acupuncture. Patients were charged extra for this service. The resident made a little income "on the side" besides his hospital salary and the acupuncturist had something more than most to offer his patients. This acupuncturist had two such residents work for him over a three-year period. In the meantime, he arranged to do talks and in-service trainings for the hospital at which these interns were employed. Due to his friendship with one of these docs, he was later offered a salaried position at a hospital special services satellite clinic.

A third practitioner in California became an active player in his city's Chamber of Commerce. By attending events, working on fundraising committees, and networking with all types of people, he has developed a practice almost completely based on orthopedic surgeon referrals.

A fourth practitioner in Minnesota works full-time in a satellite clinic for a large city hospital doing mostly postoperative pain cases. He has to see three patients per hour, but he has as many clinic rooms as he needs, has all his supplies purchased, sharps disposed of, appointments made, and billings done for him. He takes home about $65K a year, has learned to work comfortably in this environment, and likes the regular paycheck.

> "If opportunity doesn't knock, build a door."
>
> —Anonymous

If you are negotiating for work in such a clinic, there are several ways that you might make it work. You could simply pay rent, collect your own fees, and charge whatever you want for services. Or you can pay a flat fee to the clinic for each patient seen if they are scheduling your appointments and collecting your fees for you. However, for the most credibility, it is best to actually be a salaried employee. Recently, a practitioner who had been approached to work at a hospital called me [HW] to ask what salary package I thought he should try to negotiate. I suggested he consider what he would want per hour if he did not have any overhead other than malpractice insurance, annual CEUs, and professional association dues, which would actually be the case in his situation. We agreed that if all his supplies and insurance billing were to be included in the package, he would be quite happy with $50 per hour for the 25 hour-week contracted for. Although unable to use herbal medicine in this hospital, that came to over $60,000 before taxes for working four days a week, six hours a day. Not too shabby for someone only two years out of school. However, why not see if you can get the hospital to subsidize your malpractice insurance as part of your pay package?

> For more details on creating a good contract with a hospital, see Appendix B in the back of this book.

Another practitioner on the East Coast is an RN. She considered going back to a local hospital to get a part-time job while she grew her practice. During her interview process, she discovered that some of the people at the hospital were more interested in having her services as an acupuncturist than as an RN. At first, however, they were afraid that they would not be able to afford the "equipment" necessary for acupuncture care, but she was persistent with her phone calls, gave them needle and other product cost information, and, at the time we go to press with this book, she is negotiating her salary to work as many hours as she wants at this hospital.

We hope these stories inspire you to go out and put yourself in as many situations as you can where you get to show and tell about Asian medicine, acupuncture, and your services in particular to the Western medical community. The opportunities are there. But it is up to you to go and find them.

A word about non-compete clauses

Commonly seen in contracts is a non-compete clause stating that for so-many-years-and/or-so-many-miles from the clinic where you worked you will not set up practice after you leave. The legality of these varies widely by state (and even from one judge to the next!). However, a one year term is frequently enforceable if the agreement is enforceable for other reasons. Reasons for allowing enforcement vary but often are tied to the protection of trade secrets. Thus, if an employee does not know company secrets (which may include customer data), the agreement is not going to be enforced if it comes to a court battle. Some states don't allow non-competes at all in the medical area; others do. If presented with such a clause in a contract that seems excessive, it's best to seek legal advice.

POINTS TO PONDER FROM CHAPTER 7

- Statistics show that practitioners who are able to work under the wing of another practitioner are more likely to survive and prosper than those who do not.

- Contact your school alumni and others practicing in the area where you want to work. Get a list from school or place an ad in the alumni newsletter, state newsletters, national publications, and web resources.

- Create a nice letter or postcard to send to every practitioner in the area where you'd like to practice.

- Before you negotiate, make a list of what is and is not negotiable. Beyond that, be as flexible as you can.

- For practitioners already in practice, there are some advantages to creating an "internship" job in your clinic. Check out our list.

- If you want to work in the world of Western medicine, it is being done more and more. The key is networking, networking, and persistent networking. Read some practitioners' stories and take notes.

Going Where Your Skills are Needed | 8

This topic could be a paragraph or two in another chapter. However, we feel strongly enough about this to give it its own chapter heading, even if it is only two pages. Consistently and repeatedly, we have heard the same things from practitioners who have had the largest, most successful practices the most quickly. There seem to be two major categories of practitioners who do the best. First are those who specialize in a very specific area of practice. If they are clever enough to decide on a specialty prior to graduation, they can often have several job offers, clinic partner offers or referral networks put in place weeks and months before they have their diploma. The other ones are those who have the courage to go where no practitioner has gone before.

The practitioners who are willing and able to take their skills to smaller cities and towns and who make the effort to connect with the community where they settle seem to do better faster. This does not mean that they have not had to engage in some type of marketing effort. It means that their marketing efforts have been more effective more quickly. Depending upon the situation, we have heard of people with very full practices

PRACTITIONER POINTER

"My advice is, move. This is a tough one for many people who are rooted in the community where their school is based. But it is worth thinking about. I moved to a small to medium-sized community where I am the only one around and I was previously known. My weekly patient load has been consistently high since I opened my practice. This would not have happened had I stayed put after graduating."

—*Daniel Schulman*
Prince Edward Island, Canada

in less than one year. One practitioner we spoke to from a relatively rural area was advertising for a new graduate to come and work for him, his patient load was so large. He had been in practice less than one year. Another, who moved back to his family's small hometown, had an average of 30 patients per week within six months of opening his practice.

In Section 1, Chapter 3, we discussed the need to do demographic research on the town or area in which you think you might like to practice. If possible, we encourage you to include some small cities and towns in your search and to take this medicine to places where there are few, if any, practitioners. There are, at the time of this writing, slightly more than 20,000 practitioners of acupuncture and Chinese medicine in the U.S. There are over 70,000 chiropractors and over 300,000 practicing MDs. With only 3-5% of the American public currently using our services, we have not yet even begun to saturate the market except in cities where there are acupuncture colleges. So do your homework and get out of town!

Think About Specialization | 9

his subject has also come up in several other chapters. However, we feel it is important enough for you to think about it again, and carefully. There are several possible specialties within Chinese medicine that are effective clinically and could bring you success financially. We suggest that you consider the following:

- Gynecology
- Pediatrics
- Dermatology
- Geriatrics
- Sports medicine
- Worker's Compensation injury management
- Oncology
- Assisted reproductive technology
- Diabetology
- Psychiatry
- Chronic pain specialist
- Headache specialist
- Male urologist and sexual dysfunction specialist

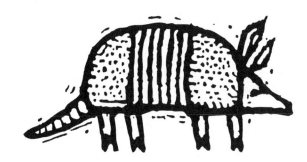

"Specialist"

While it may seem to you that you're limiting the number of patients who come to you if you specialize, consider that there is no lack of people with any given condition. If you become very skilled at treating a specific group of disorders, everyone in your professional community will know of it eventually. I [HW] know one practitioner who specializes in oncology only, especially cancers of the breast. She has almost only women patients and a waiting list of three months to get in to see her! Another friend of ours is well-known for his skill as a gynecologist. He gets calls from women all over the U.S. who want to come to see him.

PRACTITIONER POINTER

"I have recently opened a new and thriving practice, Watsonville Acupuncture. I specialize in the treatment of musculoskeletal conditions and am currently seeing about 70 patients per week. I want to say that nothing I learned in my OM program of study prepared me for what it would take to start a practice of this magnitude: creating a marketing program, establishing referral sources in the medical community, and most of all providing the professional presence that patients want. My goal has been and continues to be to bring OM to all those who have no idea that it exists. This brings me great joy."

—*Eric Meyer-Reed*
Watsonville, CA

You might also consider that being a General Practitioner is the hardest of all "specialties." It requires you to be reasonably competent in the treatment of almost every ailment known to humankind since you never know from day to day what is going to enter your door. It is far easier to become really, really good at treating a smaller, finite group of conditions. In that case, there are only so many symptoms and only so many patterns that are routinely involved. The material you need to have memorized cold is far less. We guarantee that if you specialize, you can get to the point where you know some of the patterns a person will present by the time you shake their hand just by watching them walk in and sit down in your exam room.

Of course, this does not mean that you could not, now and again, take a patient with some ailment outside your specialty. But you might not ever have to. And for those of you who worry that being a specialist is not a "holistic" approach, we say this: Oriental medicine is, by its inherent nature, a holistic approach to diagnosis and treatment no matter what disease or group of diseases you are treating. It is built into the system because we base treatment primarily on pattern discrimination, not on disease diagnosis. Patterns always describe the whole person, taking into account body, mind, and spirit. So we say poo poo to that worry.

POINTS TO PONDER FROM CHAPTER 9

- There are several distinct advantages to specializing.
- There are no drawbacks.

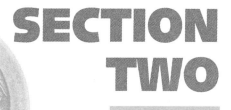

SECTION TWO

Working on Your Own

Business Basics $\big|$ 1

In this chapter, we want to introduce some basic things that you
will need to think about no matter what type of business you
might be starting: your business name, business cards, business
supplies and equipment, software for running your business,
how you keep your records, managing your inventory, paying
your taxes, and more. These are the nuts and bolts of business.
We have covered some of this information in Section 1, Chapter
3 for students. For those of you already in practice, this
information is far more complete.

What's in a Name?

Naming your clinic is, possibly, one of the most important
decisions you will make in the initial stages of your business life.
The name you choose will be your identity. It will represent you
in conversations down at the local diner and from satisfied to
potential patients. It can be a driving force for your business, or
it can fly from the minds of people you meet in a New York
minute. Therefore, when selecting the name of your business,
you will want to keep a few important questions in mind:

- **Does it make my business easy to market?** The more information your business name conveys, clearly and concisely, the
  fewer explanatory words you need in ads, on signs, etc. In
  other words, if the name of your clinic is *Skin Care
  Acupuncture Clinic,* your Yellow Pages or Web ads do not
  need extra lines of type to tell people what you do. It's already
  in the name. Just pay to have it listed in red, get it listed on
  Google Business, and call it good!

- **Is it easy to remember, spell, and pronounce?** *Whole Family Health Center, Boulder Herbal Medicine Clinic,* and *Orange Park Acupuncture Clinic . . .* they are all pretty easy to remember, right? They are short, concise, and can be pronounced by anyone who drives by your clinic. Why is this important? Hundreds, even thousands of people may drive past your clinic sign every day. If the name is weird, hard to pronounce or hard to remember, you may lose that future patient to the guy down the street. We do not suggest that you use Chinese words like *An Shen* (calm spirit) or *Jin Shan* (golden mountain). These sound pretty and may have a meaning for us, but they mean nothing and may even be off-putting to the average American patient.

- **Does it convey a clear understanding of what you do?** *WomenCare Acupuncture Clinic* and *Athletic Edge Acupuncture Services* are good names that communicate to your patient population both that you do acupuncture and that a selected group of people would benefit from your services. Although *Huang Guo Shen Clinic* may sound good, it means nothing to the masses unless you are only treating Chinese people. Look for ways to add words such as "acupuncture," "Oriental medicine," "herbal medicine," etc. to convey your purpose.

- **Does it market you to the specific niche you want to serve?** Again, this is a great way to separate you from the average. Niche marketing can fill your clinic quickly. Every athlete who sees *Athletic Edge Acupuncture Services* will have a pretty good idea what you do!

Once you have your clinic name selected, try it out on friends and family. See what their reactions are. Ask them to spell it without seeing it. You may even try it on the guy at the coffee shop. Who knows? You may just score your first patient!

➤ Check name availability

Now that your mind is brimming with ideas, go to the website for your Secretary of State and search for name availability. Whether you are planning to be a sole proprietor, an LLC, or you are going to go huge and want to incorporate, you will need to choose a business name that no one else has. Most of the Secretary of State websites are either www.sos.XX.us, with XX replaced by the initials of your state, but a few are www.ss.XX.us.

If your chosen name is available, call the number on the website or try to apply for the name online. Find out what the reporting or renewal requirements are for maintaining your business name. Typically, you have to renew your name once per year or once every other year and is not expensive if done online.

➤ Business Cards

Your business card is your daily advertising tool. It is your calling card and your appointment card. You can use them for leaving small messages or for jotting down a telephone number. Whatever your plans, your business card is the second most important marketing tool you will ever design.

Business cards are meant to be handed out like little chocolate morsels to kids on Halloween. Print 1,000 this month and hand them all out next month. If you have the courage to do that, your business will double from where you are right now! This is, of course, assuming that you've got a well designed card! For a thorough checklist, see Section 4, Chapter 5 on the things that must go into a presentation folder. Here's just a short list of things to consider.

Fonts: Keep them simple, easy to read, and no smaller than 11 point type. No more than two font styles on a card.

Phone: The phone number is the most important element on the card, second only to the name of the acupuncturist.

Name: The personal name of the acupuncturist should be in a location that it is quickly and easily distinguishable from the other information on the card.

Business Information: The name and address of the business should be on the card.

Internet Information: If you have a website, place that on the card if you have room. Otherwise, just put your email address.

Logo: If you have a logo already, put that on your card in a location that balances out the information already contained. You may also consider getting the logo done as a watermark in the background underneath the card text. If so, no more density than a 10% screen.

Material: Use a nice quality card stock with some firmness to it. Remember that your business card is your handshake when you meet another business professional or a prospective patient. If you really want to bedazzle people, consider material other than paper. A business card that wows people will not be tossed away.

Color: No neon! It's way too difficult to read. No more than two colors on your card, unless you do a color photo of yourself.

The Back: The back of the card is just as good as the front. Don't let this space go to waste. Use it for your "unique selling proposition," directions to your clinic, or a "next appointment" note. If you live in a small community, print the dates of all of the events for the town . . . "9/25: Pig races." Yearly holidays, the high school soccer team's schedule, an inspirational message, or your mission statement. The point is that the more uses your business card has, the less likely it will be tossed away.

Old Cards: When information changes, such as your phone number, your maiden name, or your website, get new cards. Do not scratch out the old information and handwrite the new. This looks tacky and unprofessional.

Photo: We mean your photo. When someone hands you a card with their picture on it, it becomes much easier to associate that face with a previous conversation or encounter. This makes the card a more powerful marketing tool in the long run. If you are considering putting your smiling face on your business card, then it is highly recommended that you work with a professional photographer! Another option is to order paste-on photos the size of a postage stamp. These can only be made from studio originals, but they are not expensive themselves. Try Photo.Stamps.com or Zazzle.com.

Logo or no Logo?

A company logo is another item, like a USP (see page 96), that will stick deep inside the minds of those who see it. You may decide to start without one and that is also fine. It may take you a while to decide how you want to describe yourself pictorially. Whenever you decide to create this image, a good logo can require some time and effort to produce, and you may want to enlist the help of a professional. One recommendation is to call the art department at the local college and sponsor some sort of competition. Graphic arts students need to assemble a portfolio for potential employers. Getting their designs used by a real business is good for them and can be inexpensive for you. Talk to the graphic arts instructor and see if they have any ideas for a contest or if there is a talented student that would like a side job.

> "Every time I close the door on reality, it comes in through the windows."
> —Jennifer Unlimited

A logo is a visual symbol that should tell a story to your potential patients. It is useful to try and think like a layperson who knows nothing about Oriental medicine, culture, language, or art when you create this design. If a picture is worth 1,000 words, you need to make sure the picture that represents you is worth the words you want it to convey. If you decide to use a

Chinese character, for example, it may be wise to put the English translation in small italic type right below the picture. If you do create a logo, put it on everything you print.

▶ Your USP

"The ultimate driving machine." "It keeps going, and going, and going." "We love to see you smile." It is almost a sure bet that you've already identified the products or companies that these lines represent. These are all good examples of a *unique selling proposition;* a catchy phrase or saying that explains what you have to offer, tells what distinguishes you from your competitors, gives people a reason to do business with you, and makes a claim that you can deliver on.

The best USP is something that appeals to an emotional or personal need (L'Oreal – "Because you're worth it"). As a creature, human beings are need-driven. As much as we may hate to admit it, our emotional needs often outweigh our physical needs. Revlon – "Be unforgettable." State Farm Insurance – "Like a good neighbor, State Farm is there." These all speak to us on an emotional or personal level. Who doesn't want to be unforgettable?

When designing your own USP, try to come up with something that is immediately understood in one and, at the most, two lines. If people have to try to understand what your USP means, then the point is lost. A clear, concise statement that conveys your message of benefit to the masses is an amazing business tool. You can put it on your stationary and letterhead, your business cards and sign, and on your website. Your USP can be your mini-commercial when introducing your clinic.

Here are just a few examples of acupuncture related USPs:
• Athletic Edge Acupuncture Services: "Enhanced performance for every athlete"

- WomenCare Health Center: "Because healthy women make a healthy world"

- Skin Care Acupuncture Clinic: "Because beauty is more than skin deep"

Creating a good USP will take some time and effort. Your best bet is to sit and just throw out ideas one after another without thinking about them too much. The more you come up with, the more creative you will get. If you have the help of a business partner or friend, one of you should write down the good ones, if not all of them. Another option is to record the exercise. When you're finished, go back and listen to some of the ideas. This is a fun exercise that will really get your creative juices flowing.

➤ Software

Welcome to the 21st century. If you want to run an effective business in today's market, you are going to need a computer, and that computer is going to need software to make it run. Not only does good software make the computer easier to use and navigate, but also there are programs out there that you may want in order to operate both the business side and the acupuncture side of your clinic.

For any computer novices that may still be out there, the difference between software and hardware is this: Hardware is the physical stuff that goes inside of the computer, like the hard-drive, the co-processor, the CD drive, and the memory. Software includes any program that operates on the computer to help you use the hardware to operate your business. An example of software is *Windows* or *QuickBooks* or *Adobe Acrobat.*

1. Generic business software:
   Accounting software: Designed to help everyone from the small-business owner to the corporate accountant manage the company books, there are all shapes and sizes of programs out

there. The most well-known is *QuickBooks.* This is a very intuitive, user-friendly bookkeeping program with two versions available: one for professionals and one for the home. The professional version is well worth the money if you are planning to do your own bookkeeping for any number of months or years. Both programs offer help and tutorials, which is a nice feature when establishing your accounts. If you are completely lost after trying to set up your accounting system, it may be worth the small investment to hire an accountant or bookkeeper to set up your *QuickBooks* and give you a short lesson in using the software. This may be a good time to talk trade or barter.

Scheduling: Keeping track of patient appointments on your computer is a nice feature. You can keep a paper copy as well, or you can back up your calendar at the end of each day. The nice thing about having a digital version of your schedule is that you can easily take it with you. If you have a Blackberry or an iPhone you can upload your schedule daily. This is a handy feature when you are just beginning and have to leave your office regularly to do marketing. You can also forward the clinic phone to your cell phone and quickly schedule a calling patient on your Blackberry. When you return to the office, simply sync the portable digital device to your computer and your appointments are instantly updated!

2. **Specific software:**
Medisoft: This program has been around for years and in use by the medical community at large. There are a variety of versions available, each doing more than the last and costing more as well. The top-of-the-line version keeps track of patient appointments, does superbills and electronic billing, can be modified to keep your herbal dispensary inventory, and can bill for multiple practitioners. People who use this software like it, but the price can be a bit steep: $200-1700 depending on how many bells and whistles you want.

Medical Billing Services: If your practice is going to have a large component of insurance patients, you will need to be able to do billing online. That is the direction the insurance industry is taking and will eventually be a requirement. Go to EZclaim.com ($) or OfficeAlly.com (no $) for information if you need something like this now. If you don't get to this point in your practice for a few years, the software may morph and the prices to own it yourself may come down as more competition arises. You can also hire a company to do your online billing for you such as the Healthcare Billing & Management Assoc. (1-877-640-4262, www.hbma.com), OfficeAlly, or a local service in your area. They take a small percentage of each claim, but your billings are not likely to land in the questionable file on an adjuster's desk.

Acupuncture practice software: Very specific to our profession, there are a number of options available. These programs are able to do billing and keep track of herbal inventory. Unlike *Medisoft,* they typically have acupuncture specific info and already loaded in the program. For instance, many of the programs not only offer billing and patient management tools but boast educational information on acupoints, herbs, and herbal formulas. Some programs also come with pre-loaded vendor information for herbs. Prices vary and service contracts. Here is contact information for some acupuncture-office-specific software available (in no particular order):

AcuBase: http://www.trigram.com. Free 30- day trial.

TaoClinic Professional: http://www.taomedic.com/html. Demo available.

ClientTracker: gingkosoftware.com. Free downloadable trial version available.

AcuPartner: www.acupartner.com. Free downloadable demo version available.

Practs.com: Your secure data lives on their server; you pay based on the number of patients you see. Nice idea and you don't waste $$ on buying software..

➤ Business Equipment

There are two types of business equipment that you are looking at here: generic and trade specific. All health service companies have a front desk and a computer but not all of them have needles and TDP lamps! This is a huge section. So, if you need to take a break before reading on, do it now!

1. **Computer:** I [HW] don't know anyone anymore without one, but if you're in that category, you simply need to get one. Not having one makes a person behind the times and out of the loop.

   With endless options available from Dell to Apple, from Hewlett Packard to Toshiba, how is a person supposed to decide? We will tell you one thing and one thing only regarding computer selection and the rest is up to you — *upgrade-ability.* While the life of a new computer is longer now than it was a decade ago, it may still be true that in five years (it used to be 1-2 years!) your system could be outdated and unable to run most of the software being developed. If I were in the market, I'd buy a laptop that is indefinitely as upgradeable if possible and spring for the newest versions of every software you want to use.

2. **Printer:** You'll need one. By having a printer, you can quickly zap out superbills, CMS forms, and invitations to your open house. By having a high-quality color printer, the sky's the limit. This is another area where being too cheap can have you spending money on trips to copy centers like Kinko's that cost you way more in the long run.

   Our recommendation is to get an all-in-one printer-copier-fax-scanner and, if you can find one to make coffee, then get that too! When these machines first came out on the market, they were plagued with problems. Over the past few years quality has gone up and price and size have gone down. Having the ability to copy a list of suggested stretching exercises printed out for a patient on the spot is easy. When you decide to start billing insurance for your patients to increase your patient base and income (see Section 3, Chapter 2), you have to photocopy their insurance card and keep it on file. How will you do this without a copier?

These days, sending a fax is a feature that almost every computer with a phone line can do. But what if what you want to send is not on the computer? If you had a scanner, you could import it or, if your printer was also a fax, you could skip that step and just send it.

Last, if you plan to do any in-house publication of brochures or other marketing tools, then having a scanner is a must. Throw a picture of *Hua Tuo* on your herbal information page on your website or put a picture of your clinic on the flier that you are circulating around town.

For the price of an all-in-one, you get the ability to perform more than the rudimentary functions of a stand-alone printer. Even if you don't see a need for a certain feature today, perhaps in six months you'll get a creative bug and then you'll be happy you can do it all yourself.

3. **Phone:** We all want patients to call us, especially when they are trying to make an appointment! While it's doubtful that we need to talk anyone into buying a phone, there are a few issues to ponder.

It's not clear (yet) that you can run a business from your cell phone. Business landline phones have caller ID, speakerphone, and voicemail. Unless you are going to call a local company and have them outfit you with a professional phone setup, buy the best generic phone you can afford. Although we recommend you have some type of an answering service (many people do not like to leave a message on a machine, especially if it's their first time calling your clinic), an answering machine is the next best thing. If you are not ready to hire a receptionist, set your answering recording on "low" while you are in treating patients with a message that tells people you will call them back in a guaranteed amount of time. You are more likely to get a message that way, rather than a hang-up. More on receptionists in Section 2, Chap.10.

Caller ID is another handy tool and a wonderful creation for the business world. It's hard to count how many times people will call up and leave a message requesting a call back, yet they forget that while you may know lots of things about acupuncture and make the world's best margarita, you cannot call them back if they don't leave their number. Hence, we resort to caller ID.

4. **Office furniture:** Just a small blurb here because we discuss this topic again in Section 2, Chapter 6; The Look and Feel of Your Clinic. Obviously, if you have a computer, a printer, a phone and credit card machine, you are going to need a desk, some chairs, and a work table or counter area. Get a comfortable chair with good back support and cushioning. If you don't have a receptionist, then you will be sitting here thinking, planning, and checking patients out yourself. So invest in a nice place to sit.

Lamps and lighting to go on or around your desk as well as lighting in your treatment rooms and waiting area will make the day's tasks easier than operating in the dark. For more information on lighting and ambience, see Section 2, Chapter 6.

Another office requirement for the HIPAA generation is a locking file cabinet for your patient charts (unless they are all kept in a computer). As we discuss in the chapters listed below, the question is not really *if* you store your patient charts, it is *how* you store them and how you keep them secure. To learn more about HIPAA compliance, please see Section 2, Chapter 9, on HIPAA and Section 1, Chapter 4, on Legal Stuff.

5. **Treatment tables:** A good, sturdy table in each treatment room is a no-brainer. You may be able to find an inexpensive tables by calling massage table companies and ask to buy any of the trade show demo tables they may have around. They are almost always in close-to-perfect condition. They're just worn-in a bit from traveling around the country and having scores of people sit and lie down on them.

Also scour your local paper and eBay for practitioners selling old or unwanted equipment. Whatever you do, make sure the tables you purchase have a decent working weight that will stand the test of time. A colleague of ours and recent graduate from a local massage school thought she got a great deal by getting her massage table at Costco. The price was right, but the patient who was on the table when the leg snapped off did not return for another treatment! Always use equipment tailored for professional and not home use.

➤ Paperwork 💿 http://pointsforprofit.bluepoppy.com

To run your ultra-efficient acupuncture clinic, you will need specific forms. From patient intake and charting, to HIPAA privacy requirements, we've got the forms for you. Included on the companion website is an example of each of the forms listed below that you will need to operate your clinic. Feel free to use the forms as they are or modify them to suit your liking and style. More about forms and their legal ramifications is listed in Section 2, Chapter 8.

Forms on our website:
- intake forms
- patient health history
- liability waiver or permission to treat form
- insurance Assignment of Benefits form
- notice of privacy policy (HIPAA)
- acknowledgment of receipt of privacy policy (HIPAA)

- individual rights for authorization (HIPAA)
- disclosure form (HIPAA)
- informed consent (HIPAA)
- fax log (HIPAA)
- sign-in sheet
- patient private information form
- clinic financial and cancellation policy form
- follow-up care (Report of Findings)
- herb instructions (bulk internal and external, patent)
- referral information sheet

➤ Office Supplies

Day-to-day operation of a clinic rquires basic supplies. Whether you are getting ready to open your business or just creating a stash of supplies in advance of opening, this list will get you started. Ask for these as stocking-stuffers this year!

Stapler and staples: Get a good one. The cheap ones break easily.

Paperclips: You may or may not need these depending on how you take care of your billing notes to the front desk staff.

Paper: Buy it by the box to save money. Office Depot always has a deal on theirs; a box of five reams for the same price as four individual reams. Find them at www.officedepot.com.

Tape: You may not use it often in your clinic, but there are occasions.

CMS 1500 forms: We may all be moving to online billing soon, but you'll want some on hand if you're going to bill insurance. Check online for the best current pricing; we [ES] once got 2,500 for $30 so wait for or find a sale if you can! HIPAA regulations have made that form the standard and we don't foresee it changing any time soon. Lots of companies carry these forms. Do not copy them...they are actually cheaper to purchase and should be all in red, as they come from the printer.

Printer ink and toner: Keep a back-up supply. Nice, sharp forms and super bills say that you are a professional.

Pens: Unless you take patient notes directly into your computer, chart notes must be done in ink (blue or black), and you'll be amazed at how quickly they disappear from the front counter. That fact is a marketing opportunity and there are lots of companies that will put your business name and information onto a decent tube pen for very low prices. Again, do some looking around before you buy.

Postage and envelopes: Even a small office mail can produce a lot of mail. Buy #10 envelopes in boxes of 500, you'll save in the long run. If you have just signed a five-year lease, consider getting some printed with your address, logo, etc. Once in a while you are likely to get well-priced offers for these by mail, but compare with prices you can find online.

Postage you can do one of three ways: 1) Get a postage machine and pay the monthly fee plus postage, 2) go down to the post office and order 100 stamps at a time, or 3) buy postage online or buy mail. The only problem with stamps is that, if you want to send something that is larger or heavier than a regular piece of mail from your office, you won't know how much it costs without a postage meter, which means trips to the post office. Then again, you might do some good one-on-one marketing to your fellow citizens while you are waiting in line. You could probably give away several business cards during a 10-minute wait. If you want to order stamps by mail, the post office will deliver them to your mailbox. Go to http://shop.usps.com.

Tissue and TP: Especially during cold and flu season, but anytime someone puts their head on the face rest for a treatment, it can make them congested. If you are in a building where the bathrooms are not inside your clinic, toilet paper is included in the cost of your rent. If you have bathrooms inside your clinic, then try Costco or your local EcoProducts-type store for TP, paper towels, tissues, and anything else you need for a bathroom such as cleaning supplies.

Ordering Needles

Needles to an acupuncturist are like a wand to a wizard. Some feel good in your hands and others don't. Some practitioners resonate with copper handles, some stainless, and others like the plastic, color-coded handles. By the time you are reading this book, you are likely to know what you do and do not like. So, instead of talking about the style of needles, we will look at inventory, ordering, and ways to get better prices.

Prices: No matter which company you deal with for your acupuncture supplies, there is one common thread to be found: buy more boxes and pay less per box. This is a good incentive to order enough for several months rather than 10 boxes per week.

Most companies will give you a price break per box if you buy 10 or more boxes. If you buy more than 100 boxes, your price break is even greater. On the other hand, some companies won't give you any price break until you hit 50 boxes. Typically, this is only on needles that are less than $6 per box. We have found needles out there for $2.50 per box when ordering 50 or more boxes. Call several distributors of the needles you like and compare pricing.

Another way to get a price break on needles is to become a distributor. Distributorship is not impossible to arrange, although the initial orders required can be substantial. If you have enough money to do that, then perhaps you don't need a price break! Plus, once you get into distributing needles, you may find it difficult to maintain an acupuncture practice as well as a needle-shipping business. Still, if you live far away from either of the coasts, it could be a side business to provide needles in your local area.

Your first order: When you first start out, there's almost no way to know how many boxes of needles you'll go through unless you are buying a pre-existing practice. You can, however, guesstimate how many patients you will see per week in the first month and then multiply that by the average number of needles you typically use. If you are just coming out of school, you should have a good idea of what that number is. Just because you are out on your own doesn't mean that your treatment style is going to change, at least not yet.

Needle companies and distributors are pretty good at getting your order to you in a week and less. Also, if you tell them you just graduated and are looking for a needle company to do business with, you may get an initial order. If you can get a new customer discount, it may be wise to order what you think you will need for a few months just for the sake of the omen.

Our suggestion is to start out ordering a few different lengths of whatever gauge needle you feel most comfortable with. (If you like using 32-34 gauge needles on every patient, we recommend getting a few smaller ones for children, elderly, MS patients, or other very sensitive patients you will undoubtedly be seeing.) Whichever length of needle you use most often should make up the bulk of your order. Then, if you can order enough needles to get a discount, go for that. For instance, an initial needle order might look like this:

34 gauge (0.22) x 1" (25mm) – 16 boxes
34 gauge (0.22) x 2" (50mm) – 9 boxes
34 gauge (0.22) x 3" (75mm) – 5 boxes
34 gauge (0.22) x .5" (13mm) – 4 boxes
36 gauge (0.20) x 1" (25mm) – 6 boxes
36 gauge (0.20) x 1.5" (25mm) – 10 boxes

The total order here is for 50 boxes. Getting a $0.50 price discount per box (from $3 each) this order total is $125, plus shipping and handling, saving you $25.

Some needle and most herb companies require you to register with them or send in a copy of your license. This is even more often the case with ordering supplements and sharps containers from medical companies, however, than in the needle-selling business. Just know that you may run into it.

Inventory: The first thing to do when your needle order comes in is to match up what's inside the box with what's on the invoice and match that up with what you think you ordered. (This is easy if you sent the order in by fax or email.) This is actually something you should do with everything you order, no matter what it is. A word to the wise, the one time you don't check is the one time you'll end up shorted or with something completely different from what you wanted.

So you've checked in your order and, since this is the first order you've ever done, you'll use this to start your inventory sheet. If you have *Excel,* this is an easy task but can also be done with a pen, ruler, and some graph paper. What you are going to do is create a *basic inventory sheet.* "Basic" because you are only doing this to make sure you have enough of whatever the commodity is on hand at all times.

There are five parts to maintaining a basic inventory: 1) date, 2) on-hand, 3) par, 4) balance, and 5) order. The date is only important in so much as you perform an inventory on the same day each week or each month. For this exercise, let's say you decide that every other Friday you will do inventory and place an order if necessary. So, Friday morning you grab your clipboard and go through each room to count the unopened boxes of each size and gauge of needle. Only count the *unopened* boxes because you are only dealing with full boxes here. Then, if you have a storage cabinet where you keep your acupuncture supplies, go there and do the same thing. Count each size and gauge of needle and write those numbers down in the appropriate column. Now, add the numbers across the page for each specific needle. The end result is your total *on-hand.*

Next we come to *par.* Your par is the number of boxes of each variety of needle that you would *like* to have on hand. For instance, if you think that keeping 20 boxes of 34 gauge, 1" needles on hand is necessary, that is your par. This number will change with your practice, so just start somewhere in the middle of what you think you'll use. You'll adjust *par* as needed.

Now subtract what you have on-hand from *par* and the end result is your *balance.* This is what you need to order to bring inventory back up to *par.* With needles taking several dys to get to your office, you will probably never maintain your par levels. That doesn't matter. As long as you don't run out, you're fine. So, your basic inventory sheet could look like the one below:

> **POWER POINT**
>
> Make a few photocopies of both your license and diploma before you have them matted and framed. Keep a clean copy of each in a file. Then, when you apply to an HMO to be certified or when you need to show an herb company that you are who you say you are, you don't have to take them down off the wall and struggle to get another copy made.

Date of inventory:					Friday, August 21st, 2009			
Item	Rm 1	Rm 2	Rm 3	Other	On-hand	Par	Balance	Order
34 x 1	2	3	1	12	18	20	2	2
34 x 2	1	2	2	5	10	10	2	0
34 x 3	etc.							
32 x 1/2								
34 x 1.5								

After you've completed the inventory, send in your order. Then staple your inventory sheet to the back of your copy of the order. If you have a yearly *orders book,* punch your order sheet and file it in the *pending* section. Once the order comes in, check the inventory and contents of the box against your order, staple the inventory sheet to the other two, and re-file that in the *completed orders* section. Keeping track of things like this isn't a requirement, but the information can be useful later on.

Sometime down the road you may start to notice certain trends in patient visits. Maybe your needle orders always go up in March. By keeping track of your ordering, you will be able to better forecast these changes in your spending and can budget accordingly. It can also be helpful to include cotton balls, alcohol wipes, moxa sticks, or any other acupuncture supplies you keep on hand in excess supply.

➤ Hazardous Waste Disposal

Lest we forget, once a needle is inserted into a patient, we need to dispose of it properly, which means appropriate receptacles. Any of the acupuncture supply companies sell "sharps" containers, but it is probaby best to get a contract with one of the many medical waste disposal companies that include a mail-in box for returning full ones. These contracts are quite inexpensive, but check on line and make a couple of phone calls to determine which company has the right program for your needs. What style you like and what kind of space you have in your treatment rooms will dictate the size of containers you order. However, it is best to get containers that somehow mount into a holder on the wall. These will not get knocked over by patient's swinging their coat on or by tiny tots tossing their shoes. A spilled sharps container is not a fun thing. Second best are the large base containers that you can set on a countertop, perhaps in a corner to protect against potential accidental spills. Regardless of the system you choose for sharps disposal, make sure to keep some sort of record of how much you spend in disposal and how often you dispose. There are some managed care networks that like to make sure you do, in fact, use disposable needles and these records are the proof of compliance.

Herbs and Your Dispensary

Herbs are a great asset to any Asian medicine clinic, if not a complete necessity for good patient care. The downside of an herbal dispensary is the initial cash outlay for the herbs, storage space and cost of building that space, inventory systems, and the fact that you will always come up against a specific herb or prepared medicine that you don't have when you want it but which would be great for *this* patient. So, what to do and how to do it?

First of all, I [ES] would not recommend purchasing any herbs (bulk or otherwise) until you are ready to begin dispensing them to actual patients. Although properly packaged dried herbs have a decent shelf-life, you will likely spend more buying herbs in dribs and drabs over time. Storing boxes of herbs in your home, apartment, or clinic will get in the way, may get damaged, or you may find yourself using them for your own needs before you are really ready to open the clinic. Instead, I recommend doing some leg work in the beginning and then making a one-time purchase—often at a nice discount for first-time buyers.

To begin with, create a list of the most necessary herbs or formulas for your style of practice or specialty. Your pharmacy, if you are trained, comfortable, and legally allowed to dispense herbs, can vary drastically in size. Many school dispensaries have a bulk selection numbering in the 300–400 range. While that is very nice, it is not necessary to carry that many herbs when you first open your doors.

A good idea, therefore, is to begin by making a list of herbs and formulas that you used on a fairly consistent basis during your clinical internship. Keep notes of all of the formulas you write and dispense to your patients. See if you can whittle your selection of bulk or granule single herbs down to about 100. The list you come up with will become your initial product order. Just because you have left school does not mean suddenly that you will need *wu gong* (centipede) if you never used it before. You can always add 3-4-5 new singles per week or month as your practice grows.

Another option, and one that we like, is to order the herbs (bulk or granules) of 10-20 base formulas plus some singles to modify those basic formulas. These formulas might include *Si Jun Zi Tang, Si Wu Tang, Ba Zhen Tang, Liu Wei Di Huang Wan, Gui Pi Tang, Xiao Yao San, Jin Gui Shen Qi Wan, Zuo Gui Wan, Er Chen Tang, Ping Wei San, Si Ni San, Xiao Chai Hu Tang, Bu Zhong Yi Qi Tang*, and *Xue Fu Zhu Yu Tang*.

A step up from this solution would be to reference a book on Chinese herbal formulas and order a selection of their recommendations. Blue Poppy, for example, has a couple of books that might help you make these decisions: *The Successful Chinese Herbalist: How to Prescribe Correctly, Gain Patient Compliance, and Operate a Profitable Dispensary* and *Seventy Essential Chinese Herbal Formulas.*

If you are considering prepared herbal medicines, the formulas listed above are a little more difficult to modify, although there are ways. You can buy the granular or bulk herbs to modify these formulas and have the patient swallow down their pills or capsules with the modifying decoction. Also, if you are specializing in gynecology, for example, you will require a different group of formulas than if you are specializing in sports medicine or dermatology.

Storage jars: Bulk herbs can be kept nicely in glass jars. However, purchasing enough jars is a sizable expense. While there are many companies that are more than willing to sell you 100 one-gallon glass jars, there is a less expensive way. Contact local sandwich delis—all of them. Sub shops, sandwich places, local taverns, and restaurants and ask for their empty pickle jars. Aha! What a concept! Most managers are quite happy to dispose of their empty glass jars in the back of your car. Once you begin, though, make sure you keep your word to pick them up.

If you do this, washing the jars a few times will get rid of the vinegar and pickle juice smell—although if you find a way to get the smell out of the car if the jars are left in there too long, let us know! We recommend washing the lids two or three times in a dishwasher. Sometimes the rubber seal on the inside of the lid will not let go of its odor. So you may have to purchase more lids. But, you're still saved tons of setup cash, and that is what the game is all about at this point.

Keeping inventory: Maintaining an herbal pharmacy is a little more labor intensive than your acupuncture supplies due to the number of items that you have to keep track of. There are two ways to keep an herbal inventory. If you merely wish to check your current supply against what you have set as your *par*, then you can set up your herbal inventory exactly the same as your needle inventory. However, if you want to do inventories that flush out any possible theft or freebies, then you have to be a little more detailed.

The setup for both inventories is identical. You begin each inventory by counting the herbs/products you have on-hand

and then comparing that to your *par*. The difference between the numbers is what you need to order to bring your stock back up. Easy, yes? If, however, you work in a facility with more than one practitioner, you will need to do some extra work to be sure that all products are being sold and not given away. The extra step here is that herbs need to be accounted for as they are sold and as replacements are ordered. If you are using a software program that keeps track of products sold and added over the course of a month, this is easy. If you are not using a computer, then you must create a tracking system where you write down each time a certain product is sold or when the last pound of any bulk herb is opened. Likewise any herbs purchased as replacements must be similarly accounted for.

At the end of the month, add up all of your figures. Each herb or formula is compared to its own numbers. For instance, you started off in November with six bottles of *Cold Quell*. You sold four and bought six. So you should have eight on the shelf $(6 - 4 + 6 = 8)$. Right away you know if all of your herbs were sold or if they walked off in some other fashion. If you ended up with only four on the shelf, it's time to either have an office meeting regarding product sales or to re-examine your protective measures for products in the waiting area.

This short section on operating your herbal dispensary is, well, short. For those of you who want a longer exposition about starting and operating a successful pharmacy, see *The Successful Chinese Herbalist: How to Prescribe Correctly, Gain Patient Compliance, and Operate a Profitable Dispensary* which gives you considerable detail on this potentially huge subject.

> ## Paying Taxes

Probably the most common reason for new business failures is that they forget or don't know to pay their taxes. Nobody likes to pay them, of course, but they are an inevitable part of business life regardless of how we feel about it. Even if your state does not require an income tax, you still have to pay federal payroll taxes plus Medicare and Social Security. So how do you figure out when and how much to pay?

Helpful links: For computer users we have listed some very useful links where it comes to discovering your personal tax situation. For state tax information you can go to http://www.irs.gov/businesses/small/article/. Here you'll find a collection of links to all individual state tax organizations. From there you will be able to discern your personal tax requirements and know who to call for help if you need it. The people who work in these departments want you to call if you need them. Their job is to make sure you succeed. Otherwise how do they collect taxes? On the website there is also a listing of each state's tax organization with a phone number for you to contact.

For information on IRS rules and regulations follow the link to the main IRS website, http://www.irs.gov/. At this site you are able to find the most recent tax laws, publications, withholding requirements, and listings of federal schedules and payment guidelines.

Self-employment taxes: Business owners operating as a sole proprietor, a partnership, or an LLC and paying yourself as a partnership need to pay quarterly state and/or federal self-employment taxes as well as estimated income taxes. If you need help with your state taxes, follow the link listed above or contact your state tax organization by phone. The percentage you need to pay depends, of course, on the amount of income you take out of your business.

1. Who needs to pay self-employment taxes? According to IRS rules, a self-employed person who makes over $400 per calendar year must pay self-employment taxes.

2. What are self-employment taxes? These taxes, a combined 15.3% of your income, are the result of Social Security and Medicare benefits (12.4 and 2.9% respectively). We have to pay this, just as if we were working for any other employer. This money has always been deducted from your paycheck anywhere that you have worked in the past. The difference is that when you work for someone else, only half of this money was deducted from your pay and the other 7.65% was paid by the company you worked for. Being self-employed means you are both the employee and company at the same time and, therefore, pay both halves.

3. What are estimated taxes? These are an estimate of what you would have been paying to Uncle Sam in Income Tax if you had been receiving a paycheck from an employer.

4. When are these payments due? All federal self-employment tax and estimated tax are due quarterly on April 15, June 15, September 15, and January 15. You can download the appropriate forms for payment from the IRS website. Look for form 1040 ES. Once you start paying these taxes, the IRS will send you a forms packet with instructions and payment coupons each year.

The good news is that only the first $87,000 of your income is subject to the 12.4% Social Security tax. The not-good-but-not-bad-either news is that you will still be liable for income taxes and the other 2.9% no matter how much you make. So, for federal tax purposes, there are two types that need to be paid. The 15.3%, which accounts for your self-employment tax, and your estimated income tax payment which is what you believe you will owe for your federal income taxes at the end of the year divided up on a quarterly payment system.

Your quarterly self-employment taxes (Social Security and Medicare) are paid using a Schedule SE (Form 1040).

Information regarding the proper use of this form, who needs to use it, and how much to pay is included via a link to the IRS pages on the website—see the form p355.pdf. ⊙

Your estimated taxes are filed with a 1040 ES, estimated tax payments for individuals form. Instructions for this form are at the website link included on the website under p505.pdf. ⊙

➤ What's the best way to keep track of this?

Once you have looked at the formula for figuring out how much you will owe, create a system for setting aside the money that you will owe for these quarterly payments. We then suggest that you create a special savings account and set aside money into that account weekly or monthly based on 15.3% plus whatever you figure that you will owe in estimated tax. If this comes to, say, 30% of your total take home pay of $5,000 per month, you would put $1,500 into that account every month. The money will still be in an account collecting interest and looking good on your credit report, but you have removed it from the business checkbook bottom line and from the temptation to spend money that is really not yours. When the time comes to pay the IRS, the money is there and you have stayed out of trouble.

The other way to handle this, of course, is to create a corporation or an LLC (see Section 1, Chapter 5) and pay yourself a combination of salary (on which all your taxes will already be paid and you will receive a regular W-2 form at the end of the year) and cash dispersals (on which you will not owe Social Security taxes). Again, it is a good idea to discuss the advantages of various business models with a tax accountant to make certain you are keeping track of everything correctly and that you create the business model that works best for you. If you choose to be paid a regular paycheck, we suggest you consider working with a payroll company which, for a very small fee, will handle your paychecks, your payroll, and all related taxes and take this entire issue off your plate, while at the same time making sure your taxes are all paid on time in full.

Is there any way to cut down my tax liability?

One of the great things about being in business in America is that there are many things you can legitimately pay for from your clinic bank account instead of paying yourself and then buying these things from your personal bank account. This practice lowers what you need to pay yourself which in turn lowers your tax liability. We suggest you discuss all this with a tax accountant, but it is possible that everything from magazine and newspaper subscriptions, many travel expenses, certain types of entertainment expenses, even a car including its insurance and repair costs, can be purchased by your business. If you create a corporation, the list of what you can buy for your business may even be longer and more beneficial. There are a couple of book resources that we have included in the Resources for Going Further section in the back which will give you more information about the size of this envelope and how far you can push it and still be within the law. Is this a great country or what?

POINTS TO PONDER FROM CHAPTER 1

- Choose your business name carefully. One that helps you market your services, is easy to pronounce, and explains what you do will serve you best in the long run. Register your business name with the Secretary of State so that no one else can use it.

- Keep your business card simple, clean, and easy to read. No fancy fonts, no small type. If you want to make if fancy, use glossy paper stock and put a nice photo of your smiling face on it!

- Only use a logo if you can design a really good one. Trite symbols of Chinese culture or medicine may not convey much. If a picture is worth 1000 words, make sure the picture you use says the words you want to the market you wish to reach.

- Computers and software are pretty necessary to running a business these days. Get a computer that can be upgraded easily with added memory, video card, bigger hard drive, etc.

- You may want some simple business software such as Quickbooks, some appointment scheduling software, and some medical software, which is available both specifically for acupuncture offices and more generally for any type of medical office.

- Look for deals on office products, furniture, and other equipment that you will need, but make sure you buy treatment tables that will hold all sizes of humans and hold up under the heavy use you are going to make happen in your clinic!

- You can download samples of forms that every acupuncture office needs from our companion website and redesign them for your own use! ⊙

- Keep a careful inventory of your needles to learn how many you use of what sizes over a period of months. Then you can order in larger quantity and get better pricing.

- Herbs. You can make a good profit center here while you help your patients at the same time. If you use them, you must keep track of inventory on these as well. We give you a plan for a starting herb inventory whether you use bulk, powders, or prepared herbals.

- Taxes. Almost everybody pays them. We tell you what, when, how to keep track, and ways to lower your liability.

Setting Your Fees and Managing Your Budget | 2

➤ Setting Your Fees

Setting your fees can be just as important as your location, your business name, and your style of practice. If your fees are too high for your locale, it may deter potential patients from considering your services. On the other hand, if your fees are too low, you will not survive long or at least not thrive in the world as we know it.

So, how do you figure out your rates, especially when opening your first clinic? There are a number of factors you must consider when making this decision: the lifestyle and income level in your area, the going rates of other practitioners in your area, the amount of money you need and want to be comfortable, the type of clinic you are planning to run, and what you think the value of your products and services actually is.

$100 x 50 patients$ 5000

➤ What's the going rate in your area?

First things first. Before you do anything else, find out what the going rate for acupuncture is in your area. In Section 1, Chapter 3, about things you can do to build your practice while you're still in school, we discuss the fact that this task can and probably should be done before you ever get out of acupuncture college. If you are or will be the only acupuncture practitioner in your town, find out the prices in two or three neighboring towns. This is an easy task that can be performed in an afternoon. With pen, paper, and the Yellow Pages (or an Internet connection), jot down a list of all of the practitioners in your neck of the woods. Then, one by one, go down the list and call them.

Introduce yourself as the new acupuncturist in town. Don't be shy. There are more than enough patients out there for all of us to share. One new practitioner only increases the number of potential converts to our wonderful medicine. You should, therefore, be up-front about what you are seeking. Tell them that you are trying to figure out your own fees and ask what they charge. Then ask them how people react to their prices. Are patients easily able to pay and continue with treatment, or do patients sometimes balk at rescheduling for "financial reasons?" If this is too scary, get a significant other or friend to call and simply ask for the rates at each clinic.

Once these calls are made, take some time to digest the information. In general, what is your impression of the numbers? Do they seem too high or too low? Perhaps they only seem that way to you but are the usual and expected fees in your town. Also, are there different rates for different payment types or are people offering a payment at the time of services discount (which may not be legal in all states)?

Other practitioners' numbers may or may not be a factor in how you set your rates, but you need to know this information. If nothing else, you have introduced yourself to everyone else in the area. These practitioners are your colleagues and you may come to rely on them in the future for referrals, for covering your practice when you are out of town, or for a bottle of herbal medicine that you need for a patient but your clinic has run out.

▶ How much is too much? How much is too little?

So what do you feel comfortable charging? What can you bill to your patients and not feel guilty? If you are charging more than what you believe your services are worth, it will come through in your body language and your voice, and patients or potential patients will think them too high as well even if the rates are really quite fair.

Many Oriental medical practitioners tend to undervalue their services from our point of view and that will not serve you or your patients in the long run nor help your practice grow. If you don't feel comfortable charging as much as the other practitioners in town, this may have nothing to do with the real value of your services. There is such a thing as charging too little. If you charge extremely low rates, undercutting all of the local competition, you may find that your patient load slowly decreases into nonexistence. Why is this?

People assign worth and value to things based on what they cost. It is logical to believe that something more expensive must be better. Take, for example, the experience of purchasing a new vacuum cleaner. There you are, standing in the aisle, staring at 15 choices. Some of the vacuums have extension wands, some of them are bagless, while others have a cool little light on the front or hypoallergenic filtration. Of course, the first thing we do is whittle down our choices to include only the ones that have the features we need and believe to be valuable in a vacuum cleaner.

The next step in the process comes down to price. At one end is the least expensive; at the other is the most expensive. At this point, research has shown that most people involved in any buying decision will start discarding choices based on the price. *"Do I really want to buy the cheapest one?" "Why is it so inexpensive?" "Maybe it will break and I will be back here again paying for repair services."* So away go the least expensive choices. Those will be discarded first, before the ones that are too expensive!

At the other end of the spectrum, we have the BMW, Mercedes, and Lamborghinis of the vacuum world. They are sleek and shiny, have huge sucking power, and boast not just one light, but three. *"Do I really need all of those bells and whistles? That red one won't make me vacuum any faster or better. Plus, it's so expensive."* And away go the two or three most expensive choices.

What we are left with now is a realistic selection of comparable items all within a few dollars of each other.

The point here is that, if you are the vacuum at the low end, you may be immediately discarded as *too cheap* or possibly *ineffective.* Of course, there are some who will gladly accept the cheap services you provide. But if a new client who has never heard anything about our industry decides to call around and consider several practitioners, they may decide that your fees are so low there must be something wrong with your services. They may assign less value to you and your services and ultimately choose a higher-priced practitioner because of the perception of value. In the end, most people will make purchasing decisions based on perception of value and trust, not strictly on price.

Consider another example. Most of the people we know are not driving around in the least expensive cars on the road. Otherwise we'd all be driving Yugos and Kias. We buy a car based on a complex set of perceptions and beliefs that include a wide variety of issues. Price may be among those concerns, but not really that high up on the list compared to many other issues. The same is true of how we purchase health care services. People don't necessarily want cheap health care. They want trustworthy, caring, reliable, and effective health care.

There are two other things that you need to consider here. First, it is widely believed that your personal income will be the same as that of your average patient. If your patients all make $25-$40,000 per year, you may as well (the comunity acupuncture model being a possible exception to this). That is one reason why we suggest you check out the financial demographics of any town in which you plan to set up a clinic. It may be wise to pick a town or area where the median annual income is $75-100,000 if that is

PRACTITIONER POINTER

"When working with a local fire department to get my employees CPR certified, I decided to pay for the cost of the training. My thought was that if there was no cost to the employees that they would have no excuse for not getting certified. What happened was a disaster. Of three classes offered at different times on different days only three of 80 employees showed up. The rest called in with stories of car problems, or 'I forgot.'

Two months later I posted sign-up sheets in the employee break-room offering CPR classes for a cost of only $5 per person. As before, the classes filled quickly. To my surprise, I had a 100% employee turnout. Why? Because even though the class was only $5, that money meant something to those employees. They had a stake in their future, and had to reach into their own pocket in order to attend. They had assigned value to the class—monetary value."

—Anonymous

how much you want to take home. Second, it is a proven fact that people who are not charged at all or who are charged very low fees rarely get well as quickly and completely as people who are charged more. That means there is some relationship between placebo effect and money paid for services rendered! If your clinic is lovely, your treatments good, your customer service better than just adequate, and your bedside manner compassionate, you may actually get better clinical results if you are charging a little more for your treatments than if you are charging too little. It bears repeating that *people don't want cheap health care; they want effective, compassionate healthcare from someone they trust.*

➤ How much money do I need?

Have you ever thought about what it would be like to do, mostly, whatever you wanted, whenever you wanted to do it with regards to your finances? Pay all your bills on time, retire your student loans in half the time required, take those weekend trips without four months planning and saving, or repair your clinical equipment without having to forego a monthly paycheck. Who has not dreamed of living the life of the financially well-off or at least financially stable practitioner? So what would it take to get there? We want to take you through an exercise to determine how much money your clinic needs to generate per hour to grant you the paycheck you deserve.

Set aside any of the numbers you have come up with to this point, and now let's look at how much you need to make in order to live the life you want. For this exercise, we are going to use a few worksheets that you can find on the companion website. ● You can see an example of the last page of these work-sheets on the next page, but we suggest you go and print these out and fill them in with pencil as we discuss this information. Better yet, download the thorough Xcel spreadsheet at www.communityacupuncturenetwork.org.

> "O money, money, I'm not necessarily one of those who think thee holy, But I often stop to wonder how thou canst go out so fast when thou comest in so slowly."
>
> —Ogden Nash

We're going to start with the desired end result. How much money do you need for personal expenses per month? Or how much do you want? $4,000? $10,000? What's your number? This has to at least cover your expenses at home, including any student loans, car payments, bills, and the like.

Take your desired income and enter it on the income line for your clinic budget. Now, take a moment and fill in the other budget items: clinic rent or lease amount; building, general liability and malpractice insurance; supplies including needles, herbs, cotton balls, etc; utilities; phone; Internet; and be sure to add in the cost of front desk help.

Budget Summary

1. Money

Total Business	$ _____	
Total Personal	$ _____	
Sum: Business & Personal	$ _____	Total Monthly Budget
Multiply by 12	$ _____	Total Annual Budget
Divide by 50	$ _____	Revised Weekly Budget

2. Time

Hours Per Week [ ]

3. Money/Hour

Revised Weekly Budget Divided by Hours per Week   = Gross $ Per Hour

$_____   /   _____ $ _____

This is what your clinic needs to generate per hour.

If you do not already have a clinic, then use the following figures to help you get started. The going rate for beginning reception help is between $11–14 per hour. For 40 hours per week, then you can expect to pay something between $450–560 per week. On top of this, figure add 7.65% (FICA) and usually around 2-3% unemployment. If you are providing employee benefits, add that in under their salary amount as well.

Now, add up all of your figures (including the front desk wages for a month) and multiply that total by 12 months. The resulting number is your overhead for one year. High, isn't it?

THE COMMUNITY ACUPUNCTURE MOVEMENT

In recent years, a new model of running an acupuncture business has emerged that bears discussion in this book. The community or "working-class" acupuncture clinic model is designed to make our medicine affordable for people who make modest, middle-class incomes but who are not wealthy enough to pay the typical $60-$90-per-treatment fees on a regular basis. These clinics offer basic acupuncture care in a group setting with efficient diagnostic procedures and simple treatment plans. The other important aspect of these clinics is that, because prices are low ($15-$40 per treatment and often based on what a person can afford), people are encouraged to get more treatments closer together, which is closer to the standard of care in China. Undoubtedly, since the median family income in the US is approximately $50,000 for a family of three or even four, this is, perhaps, the only model which realistically allows the vast majority of Americans to experience the benefits of our medicine.

For anyone interested in pursuing this type of clinic model, we highly recommend you join the Community Acupuncture Network at **www.communityacupuncturenetwork.org** and view their video at YouTube. Members receive all types of support for starting a new clinic including guidelines for budget projections, how to organize and market your clinic, and even one-on-one mentoring from older members.

While controversial among some who feel the diagnostic aspect of this practice style in insufficient and among others who believe our practice will be devalued, it is a growing phenomenon in our culture and deserves attention and consideration. We have listed resources on the companion website.

Don't panic yet! We are going to break this down into manageable bites as we go down the form. The next step is to divide your yearly overhead by 50 weeks. We say 50 because you do want some vacation, don't you? If you are planning to take more time off, then use the remaining number of weeks to divide into your yearly overhead.

How many hours per week are you planning to work or do you presently work? Are you a part-time practitioner at 20 hours per week? Or do you work full-time 35–40 hours? Divide your weekly overhead by the number of hours per week. Ta-dah! The number you have before you is the amount of money your clinic *needs* to produce each hour.

Where does this number fit when compared to the results of the previous questions in this chapter? Is this required income per hour higher or lower than the average treatment price of other practitioners in town? Will you have to see two or three patients per hour to get there, or can you meet your overhead with one patient every hour and a half? The answers to these questions will also relate to how many treatment rooms you have available and how you prefer to treat. For example, if you do lots of massage or *tui na,* you may only be able to see one patient per hour. Also, if you have access to only one room, then you are definitely limited in the number of people you can see and your cost per treatment may need to be higher or you may need to consider moving. Remember, however, that your clinic can and should generate income in other ways besides the treatments you give. You may have a room to rent out one or more days per week or during the evening. You should have product lines to sell, whether Chinese herbal medicine, skin care products, nutritional supplements, books, or something else. Just as it is difficult to balance on a chair with only one leg, your budget will be easier to balance with more than one source of income.

➤ Keeping a budget

As your practice grows, we suggest you keep very careful track of where you actually are financially in relationship to where you'd like to be. Keep a log of expenses, income, and net worth each month or each week and compare it to your financial goals. Every day you should have in your mind how many new patients you need to see and how many bottles of whatever you sell in your clinic you need to sell to reach your goals. If you are short by one or two patients per week, take actions to bring

> "By no means run in debt; take thine own measure. Who cannot live on twenty pound a year, cannot on forty."
>
> —George Herbert

them in. Visualize a full patient load. Call your inactive patients to see how they are doing or take some other marketing step to fill in your empty clinic spots. See Section Four below on marketing for other ideas on how to fill up your appointment book. The act of staying conscious of where you are in relationship to your "dream" budget will help you realize that dream.

Any month that you are doing better than your budget, use the extra cash to pay on any debts you have, put the money into savings, hire that person you've been wanting to manage your front desk, or buy something to help you grow your practice, such as a new clinical tool, better treatment table, or new carpet.

Keeping a budget requires some attention to detail, but you will be surprised at the fact that it will actually help you reach your financial goals to know where every cent you make is coming from and where each one you spend is going.

➤ What about a sliding scale?

Many public clinics, like Planned Parenthood or other social service style clinics, base their fees on a sliding scale related to the patient's income. This is usually tied to the federal guidelines ● for what is considered above and below the national poverty line for the size of your family. However, if you bill insurance, you must charge all patients who receive the same service the same fee. Otherwise, you may be prosecuted for insurance fraud. The only exception to this is if you decide to have a formal hardship waiver, which stipulates in writing at what income level a person qualifies for a reduced fee (or if you offer a time of service payment discount of 10-20% for paying right now, which is legal in many states). While this sounds easy and straight-forward, it means that you have to have some way of determining what your prospective patient's income actually is. The point is, if you are going to offer some kind of discounted services due to economic hardship or for any other reason, there have to be written guidelines which are equal and transparent to all. You cannot arbitrarily offer one patient a discount because you feel sorry for them and not offer the same discount to another patient in a similar financial situation. See Section 3, Chapter 2 for more detail about sliding scale fees.

➤ What feels right?

This is the last step. If you have done your research, asked your questions, and added your personal figures. Just by scanning these numbers you will get a feeling for your comfort level with treatment prices. This is extremely important. When you tell a new patient they need to come in twice a week for the next month, they need to sense that you are comfortable with your prices and believe you are worth that amount of their time and money.

If you have checked the local competitors and your pricing is someplace in the middle (not too high nor too low), and it allows you to meet or exceed your clinic's income requirements, you can rest assured that your prices are fair for your market. Being fair means that the people you serve will not feel taken advantage of or gouged. By setting your fees based on a combination of actual facts as well as feelings, you are more likely to feel and behave comfortably with the financial policies of your clinic. The knowledge that your pricing will meet your personal needs without gouging your patients will give you confidence that you are doing what is right, fair, and needful for both yourself and your patients.

POINTS TO PONDER FROM CHAPTER 2

- First find out the going rates for similar services in your town or region.

- Decide how you feel about those rates and whether your services are worth more or less.

- When setting your fees, consider that most people do not want cheap healthcare; they want reliable, trustworthy, compassionate, and effective healthcare.

- Do a realistic budget to decide what you actually need to create in income per hour to make your life work. Remember that you can and should have more than one income stream in your clinic to create the required amount.

- Until your practice is a word-of-mouth-marketing success and you can charge whatever you want, keep a budget so that you know exactly how many patient visits and new patients you need, how many bottles of herbal medicine or other products you need to sell, or what you need to charge another practitioner in part-time rent to make your budget work.

- If you cannot make the numbers work, consider getting professional help from someone who can help you figure out how to make it work. You might contact SCORE, an organization that matches up entrepreneurs with experienced retirees with all types of business knowledge.

- The community acupuncture clinic model is a new and important movement within our industry. New graduates should learn about and consider this model, depending upon where they wish to practice and how they like to work with patients.

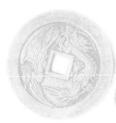

How Much $$ Do You Need to Get Started? | 3

Some people are blessed to graduate from school with very little student loan debt due to savings or family support for their pursuit of a new career. Many, however, are not so lucky. It is estimated that 65–70% of graduates have $50,000–75,000 in debt upon graduation. At 3.5% (the rate at the time of this writing) over 10 years, that's approximately $590 per month for a $70,000 loan! This certainly makes the idea of going out and borrowing another $10–$25K to start up a clinic seem daunting, if not downright depressing. However, there is always more than one way to access capital and, depending upon your personality, an additional $10–20K loan on top of what you had to borrow to go to school may not really make it any harder to sleep at night. In fact, borrowing the money you need may help spur your motivation to work hard and succeed in your practice. In this chapter, we will discuss fixed and variable start-up costs and creative ways to raise the capital you will need during your first years of practice.

➤ **How much cash do you need?**

It is *possible* to start your practice on a shoestring, which we will define as anything less than $10,000 during the first year. Please remember, however, that one of the main reasons for small business failure is undercapitalization. What that means is that a business did not have enough capital for the start-up phase when income is always unpredictable. In such cases, a really bad month or even a bad week can make it impossible to pay the rent unless you have a back-up line of credit or family assistance. In order to determine how much you will need for your new clinic, let's look at some real-world budget scenarios and see what it really costs to start and run a thriving practice.

We will look at start-up budgets for four ways a practice could be run: 1) out of your house, 2) renting space from another practitioner, 3) in a 1,000 square foot clinic space with a partner, and 4) in a 600–750 square foot clinic space by yourself. Figures are based on averages from speaking with practitioners all over the U.S. We have also included costs for equipment and furniture that you may need to purchase at the beginning if you have not collected any of these items during your years as a student. For all scenarios we have assumed a reasonable salary for front desk help.

▶ Practicing from home

Later on in the book we discuss the pros and cons of running your practice out of your house from a professional and logistics point of view. In this chapter, we are only presenting the financial reality for a hypothetical home-based clinic. Please note that this is based on you owning, not renting, the space where you live. We are assuming a clinic with one treatment room and a small waiting/reception/herb area, which seems to be typical for home clinics. This scenario also assumes that the business is being run as a sole proprietorship. So there is no corporation paying rent to you for the space, although that is another possibility to consider. We have figured the costs annually. The cost of buying herbal medicinals is not included in any of our calculations because that is a profit center, not a pure expense, and everyone does it differently. The size of this clinic space is 500 square feet, and we are figuring supply costs based on seeing 30 patients per week. We are also assuming that any practitioner starting this way is buying furniture and equipment for their clinic somewhat on the less expensive side. Also, many people will obviously already have a computer, some extra chairs or an extra coffee table, desk, artwork, carpets, or other accessories that may be pressed into service for a clinic. We understand these numbers will vary. Thus we have made some generalizations that you may add or subtract from your calculations.

Lease cost	$0
Salary for 20-hr./week front desk staff (annual)	$12,000
Share of heat & light (annual)	$600
Clinic supplies (needles, table paper, paper towels, cotton balls, alcohol swabs, moxa)	$750
Malpractice insurance	$850
Student loan payments	$7100
Continuing education	$300
Office and cleaning supplies	$300
Phone/fax/connectivity (assumes two incoming lines at residential rates)	$750
License fees	$150
NCCAOM recertification ($220x2 certs.÷4 yrs.)	$110
Equipment repair or replacement costs (This includes computer breakdowns.)	$500
Marketing expenses	$1500
Bookkeeping and accounting costs	$500
Cleaning costs	$500
Sharps disposal	$25
Total Annual	$26,415

What equipment do you need?

Computer	$500–1000
Inkjet or laser printer	$75–100
Fax machine	$150
Phone equipment	$150
Treatment table	$300
Heat lamp, TDP lamp	$150
Acutron machine?	$1500
New furniture (coffee table, two chairs, carpets, lamps, desk, office accessories)	$2500

All this means that your annual costs in your first year if you are practicing at home might come to $20,000–27,000 or between $1,500 and $2,200 per month depending upon what things you have accumulated before graduation, what services you hire out, such as cleaning and book-keeping, how many hours per week you hire someone to answer the phone, and the size of your student loan payment per month. If you have graduated with some shiny new equipment for your clinic, then your first year will be a few thousand dollars cheaper than those who have not. But these figures will give you a place to start, and you can assume that in any scenario we create in this chapter, we are including a student loan payment of $600 per month, which seems to be about average.

POWER POINT

If you wanted to take home $3,000 per month in your first year and your home-based practice is costing you an average of $1,700 per month to operate for a total of $4,700, you would need to see 21 patients per week at $55 per patient visit to get there. That's only 4.2 patients per day, five days per week at a very reasonable rate! (Note: these numbers do not include any product sales in your clinic.)

Renting space from another practitioner

Your annual costs in this type of scenario will obviously vary depending upon a number of factors, how much space and time you use, how much equipment you do or don't need. If the clinic is fully equipped and you are just coming in with your black bag of practice supplies, you may pay a little *more* in rent, but it may cost you far *less* than if you are renting and equip-ping an entire room or two for full-time practice. No matter what sort of deal you work out, you will still have some fixed costs such as CEUs, insurance, practice supplies, license fees, marketing expenses, and possibly student loan repayment as well as whatever you are paying for rent. Let's talk about rent costs.

The average cost around the U.S. for professional rental space is between $14–$20 per square foot per year. Depending upon what part of the country you live in, how much of the shared clinic space you have access to, and how many hours per week you are using space, a 200 square foot room (12.5X16') used three days per week plus receptionist services and storage for your files could cost you $300–500 per month. You will have to sort out issues such as how your appointments will be made, access to herbal medicines in the clinic, use of common areas, receptionist services, and storage of your patient files. Access to the phone and fax, heat and light, cleaning service, sharps disposal, or other upkeep costs may also be included in your rent depending upon what you can negotiate.

If you are using someone else's completely equipped rooms and front desk services, you should probably expect to pay higher per hour or per day rent than if you are supplying all the furniture and fixtures, but such an arrangement can be helpful in your first year or so because it lowers your variable costs. In such cases, make sure you have something in your contract for what happens if something breaks, you drop burning moxa on the carpet or the table and cause a burn, or for any other possible source of friction that may arise when someone is renting someone else's property in addition to the space.

POWER POINT

If you rent space three days per week and pay $600 in rent monthly, your *average* cost to run your practice will be around $16,000 per year. If you can see an *average* of 20 patients per week at $55 per visit your first year for 48 weeks of the year, your take home pay for *those three days* per week will be $36,000 before taxes. If you can see an average of 20 patients per week at $60 per visit, your take home pay will be $44,000 before taxes. (Note: these numbers do not include income from sales of any products and $55-60 is a quite modest price per treatment around the country.)

▷ A shared clinic

So you're graduating and two of your friends from school want to go in on a clinic space with you. Once you have agreed upon a location, name for the clinic, ideas about clinic décor, designs for letterhead, business cards, and any other decisions that must be shared, you will have also to decide on how the space, time, and costs will be shared. Our first suggestion is not to get too small of a space. The universe will not let your shared practice grow and expand as easily if there is nowhere for it to expand into. Our feeling is that 850–1,000 square feet is the minimum size that would be workable depending upon the layout of the space and whether everyone wants to practice full time. That will allow three generous or four-five small treatment rooms, a waiting-reception area, a storage closet, and a small pharmacy area. If the space costs $16 per square feet per year, that's $1,200 per month split three ways if everyone is paying an equal share. There will also be a damage deposit and possibly last month's rent to come up with in advance. In such cases, we suggest that you either create a limited liability company [LLC] (see Section 1, Chapter 5) or that everyone in the clinic form their own professional corporation [PC] in order that each of you is protected from the others' potential clinical errors.

Whatever business structure you choose, you will still need some sort of contract drawn up. You may think that you are great friends and will never have disagreements. Don't believe it. In our mutual experience, a good contract protects friendships. It is worth hiring a lawyer to do this for you. To keep the legal fees to a minimum, sit down together and create a list of the things you want the contract to do or to prevent. Even if you create an LLC or a partnership contract, there are all sorts of things that need to be decided and agreed upon in order for all of you to be happy and feel secure. This will include items such as what expenses will be shared and which will not, whose name(s) will be on the lease, what lines of herbal medicine or other products will be carried in the clinic and how the profits from those sales will be tracked and shared, how disputes will be handled, who will be in charge of hiring and firing employees, how someone gets out of the contract, under what circumstances others may join your practice, and what to do if one person's practice gets off the ground faster than the others and he or she needs more space and time. This list could go on and on.

Still, it can be a wonderful experience to practice with others (see Section 1, Chapter 6). You can lend each other moral support, refer patients to each other, cover each other's practices during vacations, share creative marketing and décor ideas, and even help each other with clinical issues. And it will cost you less than opening your practice alone, no doubt! Your costs in this situation are likely to be similar to those of someone who is renting space from another practitioner or perhaps a little higher. See page 135 above for a list of other common expenses.

▶ Your own private clinic

This situation is the most expensive in both start-up cost and continued operation cost. However, if you are moving somewhere you don't know anyone or you are not excited about renting space or sharing space, you"ll need to consider the costs of doing it all by yourself. What we hear from around the country is that the average cost of running a clinic is $27–40K annually or about $2,500–$3,250 per month. This will be higher or lower depending upon what sort of space you rent, where you live, and what amenities you offer. As we said above, you may be able to control some of the variable costs of running a clinic, but the fixed costs are just that, fixed. See Section 2, Chapter 4, on negotiating a lease to help you get the best deal you can. We also suggest that in order to thrive, you need two treatment rooms in addition to your reception/pharmacy area. You may be able to get by with 650–700 square feet, but probably not a lot less than 600 unless the second treatment room is really tiny. Also, you want your clinic to look professional and comfortable, not cramped and dingy. And you cannot chop your marketing budget down to zero, although in the marketing chapters of this book we give you lots of ideas that will cost you more in time than money.

In any case, based on a practice cost of $30,000 and a take home pay of about $50,000 before taxes your first year, you will need to see 28 patients per week at $58 per patient visit to get there. To just break even and cover your clinic costs, you will need to see about 12 patients per week at $58 per visit. That, of course, does not account for product sales, renting out space, or anything else you might do to earn a living in your clinic.

"If you are going to worry, don't do it. If you do it, don't worry."
—Michael Nolan

How to generate working capital

If you are lucky enough to have a working spouse, you may be able to start with the "break even" numbers listed above in all the scenarios we have discussed, not that you want to hang out there for very long. If you *have* to make a living, however, in addition to paying back your loans, you'll need to get your patient visits up to 20–30 per week pretty quickly. See the marketing chapters (Section Four) for ideas on how to do that. In the meantime, if you have no money at all to start your practice, you will need to generate a few thousand in working capital and do it quickly. So what are the cheapest sources of money you can find?

- **Home equity**
  If you have not done so already, it might not be a bad time to refinance your house. If you are paying more than 6.5% in mortgage interest, you could get several thousand dollars out from a refinance and still be paying the same amount in monthly mortgage payments. (If interest rates rise, this may

not be a viable cheap money source). Put it in an interest-bearing money market account and only use what you need. If your practice grows really quickly, you can use the money you borrowed from yourself for your monthly mortgage payments! Or, if you are really gutsy, sell your house in the city and move to a smaller town where life is less expensive. Use the money you have left over after buying a new, less expensive house to capitalize your start-up years. A third method might be to ask for a line of credit based on the equity in your home. Such credit lines can be quite inexpensive. Again, only use what you need and pay your minimums and as much more as you can each month promptly.

- **Join a credit union**
  Credit union loan rates are often an entire percentage point or more less than a regular bank. If you have a family member that is already a credit union member, you should look into the rules for joining as well as their loan and line-of-credit rates.

- **Borrow from family**
  This, of course, is one of the best ways to borrow money because there is often very low or no interest on the loan. There may, however, be other more complex "strings" attached to such cash, but depending upon your relationship with your family, it *is* a source of funding to consider. If you are worried about the potential effect on your relationship, write a simply contract for repayment and stick to it.

- **Moonlighting**
  When I started my first business [HW], I had several house-cleaning jobs that I used in order to pay my bills while I got the new business off the ground. I made enough to pay my rent and modest living expenses. So the new business did not have to support me for the first year. This is a tough row to hoe in terms of personal time, but, if you are young and healthy, it can work.

- **Life insurance loans**

  If you have a life insurance policy, you can often borrow from the cash surrender value without any business plan or other qualifications. These loans also have very attractive interest rates in many cases. The same may be true with some types of retirement accounts.

- **An acupuncture birthday gift**

  This is for anyone with a large family. Write your friends and family just before your birthday during the last year of acupuncture school. Tell them that you will need $7K, $9K, or $10K to start your practice and you are looking for pledges which can be paid back over the next three years or can be taken in free treatments. You may find that your family supports what you have been doing in school over the last 3–4 years and will pledge their support quite generously.

- **Look for an angel**

  Private venture capital is not out of the question. If you are dreaming big and want to start something truly special in the way of a clinic, we suggest you get a book called *Finding Private Venture Capital for Your Firm* by Robert Gaston. He estimates that over 700,000 people commit nearly $56 billion in venture capital annually in this country. Ask around to your banker, lawyer, accountants, or other business people you know if they know anyone in this category, or look online at places like www.findthatmoney.com or www.ventureworthy.com. You might have to go and give a speech explaining and supporting what you want to create, but, if you have a big dream and a *good* business plan, you never know. You could also find an investor by posting a classified ad in the "Business Opportunities" section of your local paper or business publication. Remember that such people are looking for a good return on their money, not a gift. That means your plan must be well-organized and designed to turn a solid profit within five years or less.

- **Contact the U.S. Dept. of Agriculture**
  This branch of the federal government oversees about 29 money programs. Their Business and Industrial Loan Program can help start almost any kind of business as long as it is in a town of fewer than 50,000 people. They want to foster economic growth in rural America. They will not loan you the money directly, but they will guarantee up to 90% of the principal for the local bank that does the lending. You can check out their website at http://www.rurdev.usda.gov

- **SBA micro-loans**
  The Small Business Administration has a new program designed especially to help part-time or home-based businesses. These loans can be a few hundred to several thousand dollars and have very reasonable interest rates. Call 800-827-5722 for more information.

- **Traditional bank line-of-credit**
  If you have a good credit history, it is not difficult to get a line-of-credit from most banks. You can often get credit for up to $50,000 which, of course, you don't have to use if you don't need it, but it's there if you do. With interest rates at reasonable levels in recent years, this may be easier than a traditional loan. A business plan and application may be required.

- **Get grant money to fund a research project**
  If you are a good writer and have a specific area of interest or you plan to serve a very small niche market, you might be able to find grant money to fund a research project using acupuncture or Chinese herbal medicine. This would be a way to see lots of patients and get experience in a specific area in which you will become an expert. It might limit the

type of patients you can see for a while, but it could be a very good way to get a clinic started and get a reputation in a specific field of interest. Your public library should have some listings of foundations and corporations and the type of research they find interesting. Or, for more information on grant-writing, contact the Grantsmanship Center in Los Angeles. Ask for their article called "Program Planning and Proposal Writing" which is just for the novice grant-writer. This can be hard work, but if you can find a project that gets some foundation's interest, it would be a huge feather in your cap and a great item on your resumé. You can start planning for this type of funding before you ever get out of school.

➤ Conclusion

You *can* find, create, borrow, receive, or earn the money you need to start your business. That is one of the things our country has always been about . . . new business growth. You'll even be surprised at who might help you. First you need to think about how and where you want to practice and do your homework about how much you will need over the first 6–12 months of your life as a practitioner. Once you know exactly what you need to generate, it is easier to figure out how you are going to do it. Also, consider that if you are in a certain amount of debt already, don't choke as you are rounding third base. If you do borrow money, 1) *do* create a business plan and a careful budget and 2) *don't* be wasteful or fritter away your capital on things that are not necessary.

POINTS TO PONDER FROM CHAPTER 3

- The typical private practice costs somewhere between $2,500–4,000 per month if you are practicing out of your own private office. Home-based practices cost somewhat less.

- We have given you some average fixed cost figures to use to tally up what you will need and how soon after graduation you will need it.

- You may not need all the money immediately, but it will be difficult to start up with less than $10,000 in seed money during the first year.

- If you start your practice out of your house, renting space from another practitioner, or sharing a clinic with one or more other practitioners, your start-up costs will be less than if you start by opening your own private clinic in a commercial or professional leased space.

- There are lots of possible sources of funding including personal bank loans, private family loans and grants, loans against your home equity, your life insurance policy, and your retirement accounts.

Finding Space and Negotiating a Lease | 4

There are several factors that go into negotiating a lease for your practice space. With a little luck you will be dealing with a reputable, trustworthy person who is not out to cheat you. That being said, good contracts make for good relationships because everything is clear and down on paper. It is good to know who is responsible for what so that if a problem or question arises, there are no gray areas that may lead to arguments or even legal action on one side or the other. Here are the things you need to at least consider when negotiating a lease.

What does the ideal space for you look like?
I suggest you write down in advance what your ideal clinic space will have. Will the street be quiet or a high traffic and visibility area? Will there be public transportation nearby or a large parking lot? Will it already be zoned for business or medical office space? What build-out needs, such as sinks, railings, shelving, or extra treatment spaces, will you ask for? Do you require DSL or digital cable connections for your computer? What square footage do you want? How many sinks or bathrooms do you want to have? If it is a multiple-use office building, who else is in the building and will they be sympathetic to what you do? Is the building ADA (Americans with Disabilities Act) compliant? What about using moxibustion?

Do you need broker representation?
A professional broker service is a nice option if you are busy and want spaces previewed according to your specifications before

you take the time to look. Such services will also help insure that your lease is fair and they will be your negotiating agent for anything you want to request from the landlord, such as build-outs, new carpets, and annual rent increase percentages. It is usually the person who is renting space who pays the broker's fees. However, if you use a broker, make sure that they have done some representation for people in some type of private medical or allied health practice so they have some idea what your needs are. If they have specialized in negotiating for manufacturing firms, they may be excellent at that but may not really have a clue what your needs are.

What is rentable vs. usable space?

Be sure you know how the space is being measured by the landlord. Rentable space means that the landlord is including that space in the square footage for which you are being charged. Usable space means it is the actual space you can use for your work. Rentable space for which you may be charged is common area space such as hallways, lobbies, public area bathrooms, elevators, or crawl spaces. This is often split on a percentage basis between all the tenants in the building and can be substantial. If you are to be charged for any rentable but not usable space, try to get a cap on how much these expenses may be raised during each year of the lease.

Is the building in good shape physically and legally?

Make sure you take a look at the age and condition of things such as elevators, stairwells, and ramps for disabled people. If the building is old, for example, try to get a clause in the lease that excludes you completely from paying for improvements that may be mandated by city or federal codes. Such extraordinary items could cost you thousands in unexpected expense, such as replacing an old elevator or adding ADA required ramps. As a lessee, these should not be part of your financial responsibility.

Is the lease gross or triple-net (NNN)?

What do these terms mean? A gross lease is great, but getting more and more rare. It means that all the taxes, insurance, and maintenance of space is included in the total amount of the lease. Triple-net means that, over-and-above the square foot per year cost of the space, you will be charged a portion of 1) taxes, 2) insurance, and 3) CAM (common area maintenance, discussed above as rentable space). This can include repairs, gardening, lighting, snow removal, depreciation of machinery, security, resurfacing, and other expenses. Make sure you get in writing what is included in the triple-net and get a cap on your annual NNN fees.

What is included in the term of the lease?

The term of the lease includes how long it is and describes your renewal options. It is a good idea to make sure you have the right to extend or renew the lease and that you are clear about the required timing of giving notice to stay or go at the end of the lease.

Are you allowed to alter the space?

Unless you are walking into someone else's acupuncture clinic, it is likely that you will need to alter some things about the space. You need to know whether you are required to get permission for things like putting up paintings or shelving, making holes in the wall, moving walls or doors, or anything else you may want to do to the space. Also, be clear in the lease about how major repairs will be handled during the last year of the lease. You don't want to repair something major on your nickel during the last year you are there.

Who is responsible for rebuilding after a casualty?

If there were a fire, flood, or terrorist attack, can you negotiate a "no rent to be paid" arrangement while repairs and rebuilding are being done? If not, you need to make sure you have an insurance policy for this and a "plan B" for where you would practice in such a case.

What is escalation of costs?

Most leases will increase by a small percentage per year over the life of the lease. If you can, try to negotiate this as an exact figure or percentage not tied to the consumer price index or the current lease values in your area. This allows you to plan in advance what your costs are and what your income requirements are. As a new practitioner, try to start as low as possible even if it means a higher amount at the other end.

What is meant by breach/cure?

Breach/cure is a legal term describing what happens when you do something (on purpose or inadvertent) that is expressly a break in your lease. The most important example of this is that you be sure how your landlord handles lapses in payment and eviction notices. For example, what if your check gets lost in the mail? Will he or she call you after X number of days instead of serving you with an eviction notice? This sounds like it should be simple good human communication skills. However, it is important to have it spelled out in your lease so that no misunderstandings arise.

What are your insurance requirements?

It is important to include in a lease what sorts of insurance your landlord requires. Make sure that, if he or she requires double coverage for liability insurance, that the companies have a mutual waiver of subrogation between them. That means that they will not be arguing instead of getting the job done for you if there is a suit against the building for any reason. Try to negotiate this down to a simple Renters Property Insurance policy. These are usually quite inexpensive unless you are using deadly chemicals or something. Also, get more than one quote; they can vary enormously. And be careful what your insurance liability really is as a renter. If someone falls down in the parking lot, is that your responsibility or the landlord's and how much coverage should be required of you for various types of incidents?

What is your exit strategy?

Be sure you are clear about under what circumstances you may get out of the lease. For example, do you need to sublet but keep the lease remaining in your name? Or can you transfer the lease to another party? Or will the landlord require a completely new lease? Be sure you understand this clause.

➤ Renting Space in Someone Else's Clinic

Above are the basic items that you need to consider when you are signing a lease for your own clinic. If you are signing a rental agreement with another practitioner to use all or part of his/her clinic for some part of each week, there are other things you need to negotiate.

How will your rent be figured?

If you are just starting out as a practitioner, you may wish to try negotiating an arrangement whereby you only pay a percentage per patient. Such agreements do exist and are fine. However, we see a motivational problem with this type of deal. If you have to pay a flat fee per month for one or two or three days per week in rent, you are more likely to do what needs to be done to fill up those hours with patients than if you only have to pay rent by the patient. Your mental "space" about your practice is hugely important, and we encourage you, even at the beginning, not to operate from a position of fear.

The important thing as a sub-lessee to avoid is any responsibility for the specific items in the lease-holder's agreement with the landlord. That is to say, your rent should be a flat fee with no clauses regarding insurance, no responsibility for building up-keep, snow removal, etc. You should have a clause regarding an exit strategy just to keep things clear as well as specifics about when your rent is due, hours of access to the clinic, keys, management of HIPAA privacy rules for your patients and other practitioners' patients, any financial obligations concerning clinic-wide marketing campaigns such as open-houses, website costs, or Yellow Pages ads, and guidelines regarding the clinic pharmacy usage and profits.

Who owns the herbs?

It is extremely inconvenient for you to have to bring your own herbs with you if you are renting space in someone else's clinic. On the other hand, it is also inconvenient for your patients to have to write two checks on each visit (one for the treatment and another for the herbs). This is even more complex if the clinic allows credit card payments. Then there is the issue of who gets what part of the profits on the herbs sold if they are not specifically yours and how inventory is managed. Who decides what lines of product will be sold?

One clinic that I know about has a credit card payment log with a section for each person who rents space in that clinic. When the renting practitioner sells a bottle of herbs and a treatment using the clinic credit card service, he or she writes down on the log sheet the total for the treatment and the total for the herbs and the date sold. At the end of the week, it is the front desk person's responsibility to total up each renter's treatment and herb payments and check the log against the credit card receipts. The total paid for treatments for each practitioner who is a renter plus 10% of the herb sales are subtracted from that renter's next month's rent payment. This is double-checked against the card services report that comes each month. If the credit card payments for the month total more than the renting practitioner's rent, the clinic cuts a check back to the renting practitioner once per month. This is equitable, if cumbersome, and does give the renting practitioner a small amount of the profits on any herbs or other products sold out of the clinic. The clinic lease-holder pays the 2% credit card fees out of the herb profits. If the patient is paying with a check, two separate checks must be written: one to the practitioner for the treatment and one to the clinic for products. The 10% cut is added in to the credit card proceeds described above. In this same clinic, there is an inventory sheet where any product that is sold is written down. This way, the person in charge of ordering can have that product replaced as necessary.

This may seem quite cumbersome, and there are other ways to handle this situation. One practitioner I [HW] know prefers a different product line from the ones that are carried where she rents space. Her method of dealing with this is to have all herbal products drop-shipped directly to the patients from the herb distributor on the same day as they come in for treatment. That way the product reaches the patient within 48 hours of the visit. She has the patient pay her for the product in advance. Then she pays the bills to the distributor once per month. Another practitioner pays to rent her own shelves within the clinic so that she can have her own preferred product lines on hand all the time. You have to see what arrangement will work best for you and the person from whom you are renting.

> ### PRACTITIONER POINTER
>
> "Hire an attorney to check your contracts if you plan on renting space from another healthcare practitioner. Everyone says, 'It's just a formality, I just trust everyone.' But, if things go south, a little investment in the front end can save you thousands in dollars and headaches down the road. Take care of the details up front and avoid any costly errors down the road. Good luck!"
>
> —*Geoffrey Hudson*
> *Springfield, MO*

However you work out such arrangements for herbal product sales, it is always better to have your specific deal in writing so that everyone knows what to expect.

Creating a Business Plan for Your Clinic | 5

Wait! Don't skip this chapter! We know you don't want to do this, but we will hold your hand (see the website) and try our best to convince you that this is A) doable, B) important, and C) fun. Yes, really! So, give this a look and you will see why it will help you be more successful. OK, here goes nothing.

According to David M. Anderson in an article titled "7 Deadly Sins of Start-up" published in the August 2001 issue of *Entrepreneur,* the number one deadly sin of a start-up is *no business plan.* If you plan on opening your own private practice or clinic, we've got news for you: You are a start-up. As Anderson says, "There is no single omission that bodes worse for a start-up's future than the lack of a comprehensive business plan."

Having a written, comprehensive business plan means that you've done your homework and you've carefully thought out how you are going to open and run your clinic and make a profit. *It is your own self-created road map to success.* It is a goal-setting document. It is a reference tool. It is, at the end of the day, a very encouraging piece of work that actually shows you how you are going to get from here to there, who your allies are, where any stumbling blocks or potholes in the road may be, and what you need to do to realize your professional dreams.

It is up to you whether you develop this plan for your own use or to share with others. But, if you plan to borrow money from a bank or other professional lender, they're going to want to see a written business plan. Why do lenders require a business plan? Maybe because they know that anyone with the energy and focus to do the work required here is more likely to be able to do what they say they will and pay back their loan! It means you are a grown-up who has thought about what running a small business really takes. Think about it. If this feels too complicated and difficult, do you really think you are cut out to be in business for yourself?

It is our feeling that even if you're going to fund your new business from your own savings, it's imperative that you write out a business plan to insure the likelihood of your success. If you are lending money to yourself, you need to be able to answer the question, 'Would I lend money to this person?' with an emphatic "Yes!"

A good business plan is a working document that helps keep you on track for success. It is both a planning tool and a reference that you can look at weekly or even daily to help guide you when you can't remember what you were going to do next. A good plan should focus on the following key issues:

- your capital (money) requirements
- your cash expenditures
- your market opportunity
- a marketing plan
- a competition analysis
- an operating plan
- projected earnings
- and an execution schedule.

Although we have not been able to find hard data on this, contemporary wisdom suggests that up to 50% of graduates of American acupuncture schools are not in full time practice five years after graduation. While there are many possible reasons for this, one common reason is inability of many acupuncturists to earn an income that allows them to do what they love to do full time. One of the main reasons for this inability is not carefully thinking about the economics of what they are going to do before jumping into practice. Depending on how you write your business plan and then follow through on its execution, you can guarantee yourself an income of $100,000 per year or more *if that's what you really would like to do.*

No matter what you are trying to accomplish, the process of planning, setting goals, and then successfully following through on those plans are the same. The difference between a dream and a goal is a step-by-step plan which leads you to that goal. If you use the forms we have put in the companion website as a workbook, you will have many of the elements of a successful business plan. If you want to present that plan to a bank or other lender, all you have to do is print out the information you have written into the forms to have a finished business plan. If you fill in all of the forms and go through the exercises putting them directly onto your computer, you are very close to fleshing out the bones of a solid business plan and you will have basic information about any sections that we have not covered in depth. In the Resources for Going Further section at the back of this book, we also suggest several books and pieces of software that you may wish to use to help you further.

As you go through this information, you will note that we typically talk about customers as opposed to patients. We also use such other standard business jargon as sales, marketing, publicity, competition, competitive advantage, etc. These terms may sound strange at first when applied to a healing art. However, we have used them on purpose in order to drive home the point that, no matter how good an acupuncturist you are, if you want to succeed in private practice, you also have to be a good businessperson, and that means thinking like a businessperson. Hopefully, you will be able to separate and keep these two hats straight, but, if you're not willing to put on the hat of the businessperson when it comes to running your practice or clinic, you should consider being someone else's employee.

> "Begin each day as it if were on purpose."
>
> —Mary Anne Radmacher

➤ What is included in a typical business plan?

Business plans typically follow a pretty standard outline, especially if you plan on showing this plan to a bank or other professional lender. Business plans are meant to provide specific information about the starting up and running of your business. The business may be exciting and spiritually meaningful to you, but the writing of your business plan should reflect the audience for which it is intended. Remember, this plan is going to be read by bean-counters. It is not summer reading at the beach, a Hollywood screenplay, or a spiritual essay. The following outline is based on *Adams Streetwise: Complete Business Plan* by Bob Adams published by Adams Media Corporation, 1998; *Business Plans for Dummies* by Paul Tiffany and Stephen D. Peterson published by IDG Books, 1997, and information provided by the U.S. Small Business Administration. This outline has been expanded on the website with explanations and samples of what each of these might say.

1. Front matter
>   Cover letter
>   Nondisclosure statement
>   Title page
>   Table of contents

2. Summary
>   Business concept
>   Current situation
>   Key success factors
>   Current financial needs

3. Vision
> Vision statement
> Milestones

4. Marketing analysis
> The overall market
> Changes in the market
> Market segments
> Target market
> Customer characteristics
> Customer needs

5. Competitive analysis
> Industry overview
> Nature of competition
> Changes in the industry
> Primary competitors
> Opportunities
> Threats & risks

6. Strategic planning
> Key competitive capabilities
> Key competitive weaknesses
> Strategy
> Implementing the strategy

7. Services (& products)
> Services (& products) description
> Competitive evaluation of services (& products)
> Future services (& products)

8. Sales & marketing
> Marketing strategy
> Sales tactics
> Advertising
> Promotions & incentives
> Publicity

9. Operations
  Service & product delivery
  Customer service & support
  Facilities
  Insurance
  Licenses

10. Financial management plan
  Equipment & supply list (start-up costs)
  Pro forma income projections (profit & loss statements)
    Detail by month, first and second year
    Detail by quarters, third years
    Assumptions upon which projections are based
  Pro forma cash flow
  Breakeven analysis
  Balance sheet

11. Supporting documents
  Tax returns of principals for the last three years
  Personal financial statement (available from your bank)
  Copy of proposed lease or purchase agreement for office
    space
  Copy of licenses & other legal documents
  Copy of resumes of all principals
  Copies of letters of intent from suppliers, etc.

Simply by thinking about each of the above things and then describing them or your plans for them on paper, you will have *radically* differentiated yourself from the majority of American acupuncturists. You will now have a much better idea of what you are getting into and how you are going to make a success of it, however you describe success.

We have included samples of every single one of the above outline items on the companion website! You can download any or all of these letters, statements, and forms, changing them as you need to reflect your situation. If you want to present that plan to a bank or other lender, all you have to do is reformat and print what you have written to have a finished business plan. As business people ourselves, we absolutely encourage you, with pom-poms, bull horns, and 76 trombones, to complete this project, even if you've been in business for a while. You won't be sorry; we guarantee it!

POINTS TO PONDER FROM CHAPTER 5

What's in a Business Plan and why should I do one?

- It is an important planning tool that makes you really think about what you are doing.

- It helps you realistically focus on your current position, forces you to state your short- and long-term goals, and make decisions about how you will go about reaching your goals.

- It gives you an action plan against which you can check your progress.

- It helps you in borrowing money and/or finding investors.

- It radically improves your chances of success because you have done your homework and are not just winging it.

The Look and Feel of Your Clinic | 6

In the world of medical research, it is believed that placebo effect accounts for up to 40% of any clinical interchange. If that is true, then every sensory impression inside your clinic, including the sights, sounds, smells, and smiles, is hugely important! When the first-time patient walks through your door, what they take in through their five senses will imprint on their brain and form their first, very difficult to change, impression. Thus, the design elements you choose may either help you stay afloat or sink your dreams of being quickly successful.

As with the clinical aspects of our medicine, interior (and exterior) clinic design will vary widely from person to person. And, no matter how good you think your clinic looks, the opinions that matter will ultimately rest with your patient population. The purpose of this chapter is not to tell you what is right or wrong. It is to help guide you through some of the more rudimentary decisions, prod you to think about your choices of color and ambiance, and to offer suggestions for cool possibilities.

▶ Choose a Feeling

Being an alternative care provider means you have many options when it comes to creating the 'feel' of your clinic. While the choice is up to you, choose something that vibes well with the community you practice in. Whether you decide on a more 'Western medical' feel, a 'New-Agey-yoga-and-tofu' feel, or a 'you've-just-stepped-into-the-Orient' feel, make sure the feeling does not alienate anyone. Going too far in any one direction is rarely a good thing.

From the Outside In

Other than possibly your business card or flyer, the very first thing a new patient will see is the exterior of your clinic and, in some cases, your signage. If your clinic property contains more than just the brick exterior of a professional building, such as a lawn or some other green space, you have to take this into account. Some yard maintenance or creative design will help to increase not only your curb appeal but can be a talking/selling point for people who drive or walk by. Nice shrubs, flowers, or even a labeled Chinese herb garden can all work in such cases, but make sure it is weeded and watered.

Make sure your building, outdoor signs, the walkways, the porch, or entrance areas are all clean. Mark one day on your calendar each week to take a brief trip around the edifice and check for dirty walls, cobwebs, hornet nests, paper, or anything that may have blown into the yard. These things can and will occur naturally and spontaneously. Keeping them at bay can be managed with only a once per week, 30 minute effort.

Each morning you should check the main entrance area for debris and garbage that may have collected from the previous day's traffic. This is easy to do on your way into the clinic each day, unless you enter through another door than your patients do. In our clinic [ES], the practitioners and staff typically enter through the rear of the clinic, and we have had to make it a priority each morning to go into the front yard, check for garbage, pick up the morning newspaper, and ensure there are no defects in the walkway or ramp which may interrupt the flow of people coming into the clinic.

Color

Walls, ceilings, carpeting, desk and furniture, all have to be in some color or another. Consciously or unconsciously, the colors you choose can and will affect each patient you welcome into your clinic. Just based on your own experience, you know that there are some colors that are more welcoming than others. Some colors may invoke emotions like anger or sadness, and some are generally soothing and calming. The trick is to stay with a reasonably neutral scheme, while not being boring. Bright or rich colors can be beautiful in moderation. Art on the walls can be attractive or even stunning. What you want is a happy medium of inviting, rich, and interesting, without being garish or busy.

If you are like me [ES] and know nothing about color combinations, themes, or interior design, then one recommendation is to take a trip to your local paint store or home improvement center. Aside from being staffed with usually helpful people, you will find paint cards that contain a combination of colors that all go together in blissful harmony. By narrowing your primary colors for walls to one or two, you can pick up any number of accessory colors to accentuate or blend for ceilings, floors, furniture, and accent walls.

Most practitioners choose a very basic color for walls and ceilings. This is done as much for ease in selecting furnishings and artwork as it is for patient relaxation. A white ceiling, satin latex, will blend nicely with any other wall color and floor covering. The ultimate goal is to create a clinic in which the patient feels both at ease as well as a sense of professionalism. Keeping that in mind, use your creativity and heart to create a beautiful, healing space in which you will enjoy working many hours per week and which you feel will enhance your patients' health as well as encourage them to talk to their friends.

▶ The Waiting Area

All medical facilities have a waiting area. Why? First of all, a waiting room can be a marketing tool in two ways. One, a full waiting room signals new patients that you and your colleagues are in demand. Two, any information that you want to share in terms of products, classes, new services, or special events can be advertised in your waiting area. (This is discussed in detail in the marketing chapters.) Finally, no matter how good you are with scheduling and running on time, there will be days when you cannot keep strictly to your schedule or you may have to add an acute pain patient into an already busy day. When this happens, one key to keeping people happy is to have a nice waiting area.

There are three elements to a good waiting room: comfortable seating, pleasant lighting, and interesting or professionally relevant reading material. Anything else you add, such as artwork, toys for children, piped in music, or medical information, is gravy. So, whatever size space you have for your waiting area, make sure to use comfortable chairs that are not difficult for older patients to get out of. Small stackable chairs are acceptable but make sure to get ones with ample padding on the seat. Chairs with arms are always a nice touch. If you cannot afford them at first, put them on your wish list for the not too distant future. Make sure to include a small table for magazines, plants, or a water feature. You may also want to have a sideboard or shelving for educational information, product displays, a lending library, or children's toys.

After seating and tables are taken care of, turn your attention to the lighting in the room. The amount of light should be appropriate for light reading but not so bright as to hurt the patients' eyes as they depart the treatment room. If you have good natural light, take advantage of it, but plan for clouds and dusk by adding a desk or pedestal lamp. The key here is to have the lighting just right—neither too bright nor too dark.

Reading material is the last piece of the puzzle for a good waiting area. When people show up to their appointment early or if you are running behind, then having something for them to thumb through is like a consolation prize on a game show. You don't really have to do it, but it's a nice gesture. Plus, if you are really on the ball, you will use this thirst for reading material to your advantage by filling a rack on the wall with books about Chinese medicine for sale and brochures about your services. This not only increases patient awareness about your services but can be a nice extra income. A corkboard display of your community involvement is also a very nice touch in this space.

When you do bring in magazines, don't get stuck in the traditional trap that many in our profession do. Yes, patients do like to sit and look through *Acupuncture Today* while awaiting their turn for acu-land. However, the most frequently read, number one magazine in the country is *People.* Other popular periodicals are *Newsweek, US Weekly,* and *Entertainment*

PRACTITIONER POINTER

"The waiting room in my clinic is large enough to seat nine people comfortably. It has two large windows for natural sunlight and two pedestal lamps for evening visitors. There is a broad oak coffee table with current magazines as well as a magazine rack with older issues and less frequently read periodicals. In one corner there is a box of wooden train track with trains and Hot Wheel cars, in the other a running water feature. Against one wall is a smaller table with a rack containing books for sale, books to check-out, and brochures on our services. I often have patients show up 10-20 minutes early just to sit, relax, and read before their session. On cold days we also offer hot tea.

—Doug Grootveld, Canby, OR

Weekly. It is more than okay to array your office with all sorts of reading material concerning our medicine, but you may also carry those things that many people really want to read as well. Whatever you do provide, make sure it is current. Put a little money and effort into your lobby and get a subscription or two. Once the magazine is a few weeks old, donate a stack of them to a low income medical facility, a homeless shelter, or the like.

Treatment Rooms

How plain are your treatment rooms? Obviously there are a number of items that you require in each room, *i.e.,* table, needles, sharps containers, and cotton balls. By adding just a few extra touches, you can bring the patient into an experience, not just a treatment.

Music

Music is a very nice touch in each room, not to mention in the lobby. It cuts down on background noise or overhearing private conversations in the next room and also serves as a mental distraction while the patient is 'cooking.' When selecting the music, be sure to choose something that cannot be considered offensive to the masses. While some of us may appreciate *U2* and others *Enya,* there are just as many who cannot. Music should not be so loud that you have to speak over it. Instead, it should be just background enough to be heard but not to be distracting.

If you are not comfortable with choosing appropriate music, then there are music services out there who will come in and install the speakers, wiring, and other equipment. You have to sign up for their service, which is not a bad deal. It is typically a one year service agreement, and the music is broadcast by satellite into your receiver. The number of options is mind-boggling. From pop to disco, from *The Beatles* to *Beethoven,* the selections are endless. When you start shopping for music, make sure to ask a few questions:

1. **How long is the service contract?** You don't want to be required to pay some extra fee just for dropping the service. If the contract is more than a year, try to find another service.

2. **Can each room be fitted with a volume or on/off switch?** While many patients will enjoy the soft, soothing sounds of Yanni, others may get nauseous or angry. It's a nice touch to be able to turn off the music in each area of the clinic separately. Second to this is to have a volume control in or for each room. Maybe that guy really likes Yanni and would like it a little louder while he cooks.

3. **Does your service have music without words?** This is a difficult issue. While nobody truly likes elevator music, sometimes the words to a song can be distracting. You should also ask if the service provides natural sounds, such as rainfall or white noise (very popular), or classical music from the Orient. Be careful with the Chinese plunking music, however. You don't want to paint yourself into a stereotyped corner (more on this later).

At our clinic, [ES] we purchase CDs of current music that is acceptable to the masses and pick songs from each one to mix onto a CD for clinic use. This is not illegal as we are not selling the music, nor did we acquire it without cost. We maintain all of the CDs in the basement of our clinic. All together, we now have 20 different clinic mix CDs that we change daily in a five disk CD-changer. Each morning, we just set the player to 'random' and away the day goes.

➤ Aromas

Other than the ubiquitous smell of moxibustion, which may be controlled to some extent by air filtration, there are other smells that often pervade an Oriental medicine clinic that you may not be able to control. For example, if you treat a lot of pain patients, such things as ointments and liniments have definite aromas, and, if you have a bulk pharmacy, the smells of the herbs will also permeate the air. Many patients will like all these smells, but some may find any or all of the smells worrisome due to them being unusual. Also, allergy patients may have a real problem with either moxa or bulk herb dust. If you decide to do air filtration, Consumer Reports Online rates air filters. The highest rated that we have heard of include the Freiderich C-90A, the Holmes HAP675, and the Whirlpool AP45030HO. These will cost you between $200-500 but can keep your air both sweeter smelling and healthier if you are making either dust or smoke. You might also consider some aromatherapy in the way of oils, candles, plug-ins, or even cut flowers in season to give your clinic the olfactory flavor that suits you and will make your patients comfortable.

On the Walls

Treatment rooms are a great place to hang acupuncture charts. Channels, points, auricular, and dermatome-man are all very good 'wall coverings' as well as educational pieces. If you specialize in working with children, perhaps a few *Harry Potter* or *Dr. Seuss* pictures would be a nice touch. If you treat athletes, then frame and hang your autograph from Michael Jordan or put inspirational (framed) posters on the wall. Whomever your audience, try to speak to them through the types of images you place in each treatment room. A fun decorating idea is to have a different theme in each room. Outdoors, adventure, medical, or kids things. Your patients will appreciate the effort and you will appreciate the escape from monotony.

A Place to Sit

Each room should include two chairs if there is room: one for you, the practitioner, and one for the patient. In the honeymoon stage of the relationship with a new patient, many times they feel more comfortable sitting in a chair and discussing their chief complaint and life history, rather than sitting on your treatment table. Providing a second chair is also nice when the patient brings a friend or relative and to avoid any issues of sexual misconduct with new female patients. For example, if you happen to have a younger female who comes in after hours and your receptionist has gone home, ask the parent to join you in the treatment room. Mom can sit and read her *People* comfortably while you work on her daughter, comfortable in your skin.

To Write and to Store

A desk or small cupboard with a writing surface is another handy item for your treatment room. A cupboard may do double duty here because it allows you to keep a day's worth of sheets, fresh towels, and treatment gowns dust-free and out of sight and gives you a writing surface at the same time. This is far better than having clean laundry items stacked up on the floor under the treatment table. If you use table paper over sheets, then you can use this space for extra boxes of needles and cotton balls. Also try to keep a day's worth of treatment items in each room. This prevents running out of your favorite length needles halfway through a treatment.

A writing surface of some kind to set charts on is a huge bonus. If you have a smaller treatment room with no space for a cabinet or small desk, then perhaps you can install a corner shelf. Another option is to purchase a drop-down desktop from a medical supply company. Those are very nice and sturdy and add a touch of professionalism to the room.

Lighting

Lighting is extremely important in your treatment rooms. Like the waiting area, there is a 'too dark' and a 'too bright.' The ideal setting is to have adjustable lighting. Overhead lights on the ceiling can be put on a dimmer switch if they are not florescent. If you do decide to go with florescent lights, use the full-spectrum ones so that the room does not have a 'cold' feel to it. Then, add either a pedestal lamp in a corner or use a wall sconce that plugs in and has a power switch on the cord. We're shooting for mood-lighting here, but you also need to have adequate light for a clear view of the tongue, the patient's skin color, careful point location, and any other features that you may need to see during treatment.

➤ Flooring

Carpet, carpet, carpet. Hardwood floors are nice and pretty, but they get dirty quickly, are difficult to keep warm, add to the noise level, and can lead to splinters if it's real wood. *Pergo* or some other type of laminate wood is easier to maintain than real wood floors. However, like real wood, they will be noisier than carpet and can feel cold on bare little piggies. If you like hardwood or laminate flooring, use nice area rugs and hallway runners for warmth and quiet.

By using carpeting, you cut down on room noise, give the patient something soft and warm to step on in their bare feet, and you relieve yourself of the need to dust every day! When choosing carpeting, it's best to go with something commercial. Regular carpet may wear out quickly with the amount of foot traffic you are expecting. Spending a little extra now will get you another 3-5 years out of the carpet, if not longer.

Also, commercial carpeting comes in just as many colors as home carpeting and will go with whatever colors you've selected for the walls. Commercial carpets are typically short fiber carpets, have some level of water and stain resistance, and have padding already attached to them. When you are ready to get carpeting, take another trip to your local home remodeling store. They can help you choose something that will match the color scheme you've already chosen, and then they can either install it for you or show you how.

Another idea is to look for a carpet remnant store or look in the newspaper for hotels that are getting remodeled and giving away their old carpets. These are good low-money options, but your color choices will be severely decreased.

➤ Feng Shui

Once you have chosen a particular feeling for your work space, some colors, carpets, and furniture, you might consider hiring a feng shui specialist for an hour or two to give their opinion about placement of objects and any other problems with the flow of qi in your space. Whether you go in for the more esoteric aspects of feng shui, some of the suggestions that may be made will be very practical. You may be pleasantly surprised at the impact that just moving a lamp or a picture, addir plant or a mirror, or changing a wall color can have. It is something to give some serious considerat the cost may be much less than you think.

➤ A Final Note

The best part of interior design is: That which you do today, you can easily change tomorrow. Unless you are tearing out walls and plumbing, the things you do to the inside of your clinic can be corrected or updated with little effort. If the paint you put on the walls in room number three now looks too pink when seen in contrast to the new blue carpet, then you can repaint next weekend. Our final suggestion for your clinic decor is to be as creative as you can. Try new things often, fix them when they don't work out, and have fun. If you don't do anything at all in terms of decor, the most important thing is to keep your clinic clean, clean, clean, especially the bathrooms. We simply cannot emphasize that point enough.

Beyond how your clinic looks and smells, the way it feels to people will be based on the human element. How every patient is greeted, the tone of voice, dress, demeanor, and 'scripts' used by your front desk staff, as well as the last words they hear when they leave, play an important role in the feel and, ultimately, the placebo effect of your treatments.

POINTS TO PONDER FROM CHAPTER 6

- The impact of your treatments can be improved or diminished by the look, feel, and smell of your clinic.

- Make sure the outside of your clinic is as clean as the inside. Bathrooms must be spotless every day.

- Pick a complementary color scheme for your clinic rooms. Start with a neutral base color for ceilings and some walls.

- Your waiting room needs comfortable chairs, pleasant reading light, and fun or interesting things for people to read.

- Your treatment rooms need carpeting or area rugs to keep people's feet warm!

- You can get advice on color schemes and almost anything else to do with decorating from home improvement and paint stores.

- Consider a feng shui consultation to make sure the qi of your clinic space flows optimally.

- Remember that your clinic staff and what they say and how they say it is part of your overall clinic "feel."

- Be creative, have fun, make it beautiful.

Outside the Doc-in-a-Box | 7

here are many ways and places to establish your dream clinic. The purpose of this chapter is not to define all of the possibilities *ad nauseam* but to help you determine if either of the two most popular out-of-the-box options might work for you. Both home-based clinics and mobile practices are intriguing options, each with their own positive and negative aspects. Before you travel down either path, make sure you do your homework and stay within legal guidelines.

➤ Welcome Home

Working out of your home *can* be very beneficial. Low overhead and zero travel time are big temptations for anyone first starting their own business. However, there are also many reasons *not* to practice from home, such as

business liability insurance issues, separation of work and social/personal life, zoning/parking conflict, and the effect on your neighborhood. Just as everything has yin and yang sides, so there are *pro's* and *con's* for every business decision.

➤ The Pro's

Working from home is a very European concept. The baker gets up before anyone else in town, dresses, and has her morning coffee. Once the cup is half empty and beginning to get cold, she sighs, slips on her shoes, and walks downstairs to begin baking and preparing her wares for the day.

The baker has a very *cake* job—at least in terms of location. Setting up camp in your house keeps your overhead at a minimum, especially in terms of rent, lease, or other loan payments, and there are tax deductions for a home office. Your mortgage will not go up one dollar just because you are practicing out of your house. This appears to be an ideal setup for a beginning practice. The lower your overhead is and stays over the life of your practice, the more profits there are for you at the end of the day.

PRACTITIONER POINTER

"It seems that many clinics are NOT places in which I feel relaxed enough to do healing work on myself. There are the phones, the noisy patients, the tired or impersonal acupuncturist, the music, the lighting, the colors, which combined, make for an experience that's too much like being in an allopath's office. So, having worked in other people's clinics and having had to tolerate the environment, I decided to create my healing space in a clinic that's in the first floor of my house and has its own entrance.

I have created a place that soothes the person the moment he walks in. At least, this has been the feedback I've received from many people."

—Maria MacKnight
Arlington, VA

Other pluses with a home-practice are that you will never be late getting to work (unless you oversleep!), you may get a break on your car insurance because you have no commute, you save on gasoline as well, you will be around while your children grow up, the bills for your clinic almost disappear when you leave on vacation, and you can write off a portion of your mortgage or rent payment to lower your tax bill.

➤ The Con's

Working out of your house means that you will never truly be able to separate business and everything else in your life. Your office is just downstairs. You may have to walk through it several times a day, even if there are no patients. Is it likely that you will be able to resist the urge to flip on the computer and wrap up some billing issues or draft a brochure, do some research, whatever? Maybe you will, or maybe you won't.

Patients in your house is another thing to contend with. Every person on your patient roster will know where you live and will have spent time in your house. If you aren't able to establish a separate entrance into the clinic portion, patients will walk through your house to reach the treatment area. Many of us have had this very personal experience with our massage therapist, aroma-therapist, or what have you. Issues like cleanliness, pets, noisy kids, and even the color of your carpeting will make an impression on those who walk into your world. No matter how immaculate your clinic office, treatment, and waiting areas are, your personal space will become a major part of a patient's view of you *and* your clinic.

With all your patients knowing where you live, you also open yourself up to the possibility of harassment. If you are in practice any time at all, we can guarantee you will have an occasional patient who ia a little on the scary side. Having those people in your clinic 20 minutes away from your house is much more comfortable than having them in your living room!

The personal nature of going to the practitioner's home may also bring patients to ask for late or early treatment appointments. How do you say no to the person who asks you to see them after your normal business hours? It isn't like you won't be close to the office. The obvious way around this is to just say no, but you may feel sorry for someone or make the exception just that once. Then what? It's bad for your health and your relationships to be seeing patients until nine o'clock at night and not to take time for yourself. Setting definitive hours of operation is extremely important in these situations, or you may not get the down time you need.

Last, there is the issue of liability. Treating patients in your home will definitely increase the amount of your general home owner's liability policy, and you will be more than likely encouraged by any good business lawyer to carry $1 million/3 million malpractice insurance as well as business liability. We could 'what if' this issue until pigs fly. However, while the chances may be highly unlikely, if you are ever involved in a liability law suit and your clinic *is* your house, you could lose both unless your business legal form is set up very carefully.

➤ Is it legal?

The first step in setting up a practice in your house is determining if it is legal to do so. Unlike many European countries where people often live and work in the same building, we have zoning laws. These laws determine what types of buildings, services, and production can go on in any given area. Zoning is what keeps a paper mill from setting up shop right next door to your vacation condo and forbids a huge apartment building from plopping down on a nice, cobble-stone outdoor mall.

Regardless of the size of clinic you intend to establish, you need to check the zoning of your house and neighborhood. To do this, call your city or county planning department if there is one. They will be able to look up your zoning by your address. After asking about the zone, you can ask the city planners or call the business licensing department to inquire about practicing out of your house. They will want to know that this is a business that requires people to come to your location—and that it is a health facility (business type: Health and Allied Services, SIC 8909). Once you know the zone you are in, you will have three options.

Assuming you reside in either a commercial or mixed residential/commercial area, you will run into little, if any, legal obstacles in setting up your dream clinic in your house. If, however, you are in a residential-only zone, you have two choices: 1) decide to set up your clinic elsewhere (maybe next to a Starbuck's with great visibility and superior foot-traffic), or 2) try to get a special use permit from the city.

While it is possible to simply bypass all of this and open your clinic without anyone's permission in spite of the zoning laws, you run the risk of unhappy neighbors who will rat on you because of the traffic and parking issues. If you get caught, you may only get your wrist slapped (via a cease and desist order), or you may get a fine. You may also lose several potential referring friends, neighbors, and city employees and get some unfortunate publicity in the paper added to the bargain!

➤ Special use permits

A *conditional land-use permit* is what you will need to acquire if you are setting up an acupuncture clinic in a residential area. These are not easy to come by since your business will create at least some traffic and congestion. The rules and methods of obtaining a special use permit may be different from city to city, but the basic procedure is as follows:

- Call City Hall (planning department) and tell them what you would like to do (set up an acupuncture clinic in your house). They will tell you the area is not zoned for that. Tell them you would like to apply for a *conditional land-use permit*. They will either mail you an application or you can go down and pick one up. Fill out the application form, and be prepared to wait.

- The planning department will send people out to investigate the feasibility of your proposal. Assuming the city is unopposed to a residential clinic, they will place a sign in your front yard inviting everyone in the area to comment on the proposed business. Typically there is a wait of 60-90 days, after which there is a public hearing. Assuming no opposition and the city sees no problem with your business in a residential area, you can be given a *conditional land-use permit*.

There are some things you can do to make this go more smoothly. First of all, be nice to your neighbors. Mow someone's lawn or dog-sit for them while they are in Maui for Christmas. Of course there's no guarantee with this, but it may sway public opinion in your favor when the time comes! The second thing you'll want to have handy is a guesstimate of how many cars per hour or per day will be traveling through the neighborhood just to see you. This is especially important for those neighbors who have children and may be information you will be asked for on the application for special land use.

> If you want to work from home, look into buying in the many new "mixed-use" projects that are springing up all over the US. This may improve your odds of practicing from home legally.

Except in very small towns, it can be *extremely* difficult to obtain such a permit when you are trying to set up a business that requires people to come to you. If you wanted to build furniture and mail it off to website customers, that would be fine. But if you are zoned residential, there is little chance of the city allowing a restaurant in a neighbor's house or a clinic in yours.

Another note regarding conditional land-use—this title stays with the property so granted. It does not move with the practitioner, nor does it stay in effect once the previous occupant relocates. In other words, if you buy a house currently operating as a business under a conditional land-use permit, that permit expires the moment the previous occupant leaves *unless* the business will be exactly the same type of business. Should you happen to take over an already established acupuncture clinic, then you will be fine!

The best scenario for establishing a clinic out of your house is to purchase a property to live in that is already in the correct zone for a commercial business. When I [ES] purchased the building for my clinic, I had done my research. The 1,800 square foot home was already in an expanded commercial zone and was flanked by an engineering firm on one side and a medical software company on the other. All I needed to do was apply for a change of occupancy, converting the one-time single-family abode into the commercial clinic of my dreams.

Accessibility

Just like setting up a clinic in an office building downtown, people will need access to your clinic. This means that not only will your patients need a place to park their vehicles, they will need clear, unobstructed access to your work area and treatment rooms and an available restroom, all of which may need to be in compliance with the Americans with Disabilities Act. For complete information about ADA law and how it applies to you, see the link on the website.

The planning department will also be able to assist you with ADA requirements. Some of these, however, are universal. All entrance and exit doors and hallways must be 36 inches wide. You may need to install an ADA toilet, which is taller than your average commode, and needs to be centered 18 inches from any wall. This may require some plumbing work. So make friends with a plumber while you're in school! You will also have to install hand rails around the toilet, the height and length of which is ADA-law specific. If you have steps leading up to your office, you will also need to install an incline ramp. The general rule of thumb for ramps is 1 over 12, or 1 inch of rise for each 12 inches of length. For example, if you have two steps leading up to your front door and that door is the primary entrance for the business, and assuming the stairs are a standard seven inch rise, you will need a 14 foot ramp (two steps at seven inches tall each is 14 inches—equals 14 feet).

The amount of parking required will vary depending on your city. Your local planning department will be able to tell you this information. The number of slots or spaces will depend solely on the square footage of the working space. It will not matter that you only have one treatment room. If that room is 600 square feet, you will need enough parking to comply with the rules for that size of a space.

Again, these guidelines may vary by area of the country and some may be omitted depending on the age of the building and tone of the planning department in your town. However, if you have bitten the bullet and are going to set up this beautiful clinic in your home, make sure to ask all of the questions of the planning department, code enforcement, and the business-licensing office. You do not want to do anything that you don't have to, and you don't want to leave anything out.

➤ The Mobile Clinic

There is a *huge* market out there for those practitioners who are ready, willing, and able to travel to the homes of those in need and treat them in the surroundings where they are the most comfortable. The practice of home visitation was largely abandoned by the Western medical community after the advent of the American Medical Association. Now the predominant in-home therapeutic care is provided by the massage industry or home-care nurses. If you are thinking of setting up a mobile acupuncture clinic, then, similarly to practicing out of your home, there are pro's and con's to consider.

▶ The Pro's

Low overhead—the mantra of the small business owner. The lower your expenses are, the higher your profits will be. If your only expenses are supplies, malpractice insurance, and your car expenses, then your overhead will be extremely low. Assuming that you are able to charge what you need for your treatments *and travel time,* then you could be very successful.

Also, if you have to purchase a new vehicle in order to start up your soon-to-be successful practice, you may be able to reduce your taxable income quite a bit. There are two options for your auto expenses. One, you may consider the vehicle a business expense. This allows you to deduct the entire price of the vehicle as a deduction divided up over a 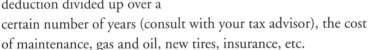 certain number of years (consult with your tax advisor), the cost of maintenance, gas and oil, new tires, insurance, etc.

The other option is that you can consider the vehicle a personal expense that you use occasionally for business. This enables you to write off a specific amount per mile for the number of miles you drive *for the purposes of completing your work.* Regardless of which path you take, you will be required to keep a very precise log of the miles you drive the vehicle. If the vehicle is a business expense, you will have to note any and all miles it is driven for personal use. The miles will be added up at the end of the year and you will have to reduce the mileage from the deduction. If the vehicle is your personal car, you will have to keep track of the mileage for work use. This will be added up at the end of the year, and you will take this as a deduction.

Another benefit is that your vehicle can be your traveling advertising banner. A nicely-done painted sign with an easy to remember name, number, and web address could be seen by hundreds of people every time you get in your car. Of course, you can do this in any case, even if your clinic is not mobile!

➤ The Con's

Treatment price

If you are doing in-home care for your patients, you will not have the ability to stack multiple patients in multiple rooms. Therefore you will need to increase the price of your treatments significantly. On top of the standard treatment price in your area, you need and deserve to bill for the convenience and ease your patients experience by not having to go anywhere to receive your care. However, this may be a limiting factor for your client base.

Travel time and expenses

When you are on the road, you are not seeing patients. Although you may be heading from patient to patient, the time in between patients is just as precious. Therefore, you need to become a very precise planner. Set certain appointment times and days aside for specific areas of town. Traveling 50 miles from one patient to another is a waste of time, unless you also bill for travel time.

Also, the expenses you incur while traveling will only come back to you in the following tax year as a deduction. You will not physically get that money back. So, all of your fuel and maintenance costs, insurance, etc. need to come out of your pocket now.

Liability

Treating under the roof of your own clinic implies a certain amount of liability. Working under the roof of your patient implies another. If you are going to set up a mobile practice, contact a lawyer and make sure you are completely protected.

Malpractice insurance is a must in these instances. You want to make sure your acupuncture services are completely covered. In terms of general liability, trips and falls by the patient at the patient's home should be covered by their home-owner's insurance. However you may want to make sure that you have coverage if *you* fall. Find a good insurance agent with whom you can discuss all these issues.

Advertising

A mobile clinic has, as stated above, good advertising that can go with you every time you drive your car. Watch your driving though. A clinic name and phone number is easily remembered when you cut someone off in traffic or speed past them because you haven't left yourself enough time to get to the next appointment. This could cause your advertising to work against you.

In terms of Yellow Pages advertising, make the most of the fact that you offer in-home visitation service. You may be the only one in your area doing this and you should use that as an advertising advantage. Also, make sure you have a mobile phone with you at all times, with the best possible service so it does not cut out in the middle of making an appointment with a new patient! Even if it is set on vibrate when you are treating a patient, you need it on your person and charged every day. You don't have the advantage of being in an office to pick up the phone when it rings. Another option is to refer all calls to a professional answering service and check in at scheduled times or after every appointment. If you are a mobile acupuncture service, fast response time could be an important part of your marketing plan and you want to be available as close to instantly as possible.

➤ A Last Note

One last note regarding treating patients in their own home or office, and this is definitely more of a concern to mobile practitioners than to those working in a clinic setting. What we are speaking of here is personal interactions with patients in their home, especially contact with those of the opposite sex. These must be monitored very carefully if you wish to protect yourself. Unless you are driving around with an extra person in your car to be present during each treatment as a witness, you can easily leave yourself open to any and all claims of impropriety.

We suggest that you make certain to always gown and drape properly, use towels for coverage of appropriate body parts, and if you are unable to bring someone to act as witness, ask the patient to have a friend or family member in the room for the treatment and any physical exam that you perform. If you are feeling uncomfortable about a treatment situation, then consider using distal acupuncture for her sciatica or his pelvic pain—nothing local at all. Finally, make sure that you are dressed appropriately at all times. Your white clinic coat is perhaps even more important as a mobile clinician than for those working in a clinic or hospital setting.

Women practitioners, if you feel that a call from a new male client is shady or not on the up-and-up, you are better off to tell the man that your practice is full and refer them to someone else than to put yourself into any jeopardy from a weirdo whose intentions have little to do with treatment.

So, if you can work with all these opportunities and limitations to your happiness and advantage, we wish you the best. Call us and let us know how it's going.

POINTS TO PONDER FROM CHAPTER 7

- Working from home may be a good solution for you if you have a separate entrance and an easy to find location.

- You may need a zoning variance or special use permit allowing you to practice at home.

- Don't make people walk through your "life" to get to your clinic. It is very unprofessional.

- People may think you should be able to treat them just any time at all because you are at home anyway.

- There may be patients whom you would prefer not to know where you live.

- If you decide to have a traveling practice, remember that you must charge extra for your travel time and expenses.

- Make sure there are no possible implications of sexual impropriety if you are practicing in your patient's homes.

Files and Recordkeeping | 8

very clinic has to maintain a certain amount of paperwork on their patients and Chinese medicine clinics are no exception. Also, with the new requirements of the Health Insurance Portability and Accountability Act (HIPAA), some forms and paperwork are no longer optional. In this chapter and the next, we discuss the records that you must keep and others that you may want to keep on every patient you treat. We have included samples of most of these records on the companion website. ● We encourage you to download these and "tweak" them for your own use.

Basic Intake/Medical History Form

This is the form that a patient fills out to explain all their major and minor symptoms and medical history. Many practitioners use this form as the basis for the questioning phase of the four examinations. Use of a written intake form can help you save time, looks professional, and can protect you from certain legal liabilities. For instance, it can help prove that you did or did not know about certain signs, symptoms, pre- or coexisting conditions, or medications. You can have new patients fill out the intake form on their first visit while they are sitting in the waiting room, make forms available to be downloaded from your website, or you can mail forms to them before their first visit. This latter option is particularly professional looking. At the same time, you can send the patient written directions to your clinic or any other appropriate pamphlets or brochures.

➤ Educational/Professional Disclosure Form

This form is required in some states and tells the patient what your educational background is, who has licensed you to practice, what examinations you have passed, etc. It allows the patient to decide if your education and professional history are adequate for the treatment they seek. You may also include your fee schedule and cancellation policy on this form.

➤ Informed Consent Form

This required form is how the patient gives you specific, written permission to treat. It is a short statement of the risks involved with acupuncture and has a statement declaring that the patient understands those risks and is requesting treatment.

➤ Patient Confidential Information Form

This form is useful especially if you will be billing any type of medical insurance and if you do mailings or other marketing directly to your patients. It gives you a great deal of demographic information about your patients, their family, their insurance coverage, their contact information, social security number, etc.

➤ SOAP Notes Form (Optional)

This is a form you use to record subjective, objective, assessment, and treatment plan information. Subjective means the patient's report of what they feel, *i.e.*, their symptoms. Objective means the signs that you observe in your examination, such as tongue and pulse signs, colors, smells, sounds, etc. Assessment means what you believe is happening based on the combination of the subjective and objective information. Plan is obviously what you decide to do to treat the patient. The information on this form can be very helpful if you ever need to give a deposition, support your treatment plan in a lawsuit, or for remembering why you did what you did when the patient goes away for several months and then returns.

➤ Report of Findings Form (Optional)

This can also be a PARQ form, which is short for procedure, alternatives, risks, and questions. This form is used to help you explain to the patient what you plan to do for them and why, what alternative therapies they might investigate, what the risks of the procedures might be, and then gives the patient a chance to ask any questions. You can give this form to the patient and keep a copy in the patient's file.

➤ Assignment of Benefits for Insurance Form (Optional)

This form is used for insurance patients and tells the insurance company that you and your clinic are to be reimbursed directly for medical services provided instead of reimbursements going to the patient or any other third party. This form will go to the insurance company being billed and a copy will remain in the patient's file.

➤ Financial Policy Form

This form discloses to the patient how your clinic operates financially. It tells them your fees for various services, your cancellation policy, whether and how you bill for insurance, what happens if the insurance does not pay, and, in general, what will be expected of them financially.

➤ Follow-up Care Form (Optional)

This optional form is where you write down what was done during each office visit and why. It is a short version of your SOAP form.

➤ Request for Release of Patient Information Form

If your patients want you to have access to their current or past healthcare information from other practitioners of any type, you need to use a release form that is sent to the practitioner in question with the patient's signature and information about where the information is to be sent.

➤ Consent to the Use & Disclosure of Health Information for Treatment, Payment, or Healthcare Operations Form

This form is a HIPAA requirement explaining to the patient that their personal healthcare information may be used to plan their care, for financial and billing purposes, and other routine operations and information processing within your clinic. It also explains to the patient that they have the right to object to their private information being used in any published directory, to your sharing any information about HIV/AIDS, drug or alcohol abuse, or mental health conditions, and that they may give you permission and later revoke it, which revocation must be done in writing.

Below is a checklist that you may use to be sure that you are keeping your records in accordance with good risk management procedures. Remember, if a patient sues you for any reason, your chart notes are your only defense and will be the first thing your malpractice insurance agent or the lawyers on either side of any case will subpoena. If you are doing all the things on this list, your charts will be relatively unimpeachable, unless you are simply doing things that are outside your scope of practice or are, for some other reason, indefensible.

➤ Clinic Recordkeeping Checklist for Each Patient

❐ The patient name must be on all pages in your files.

❐ All pages should be secured into the treatment folder.

❐ All notes organized chronologically (most recent date on top)

❐ Always write legibly, be consistent, clear and concise.

❐ Maintain records in ink, use the same pen for each entry on the same day.

❐ Do not alter the records after the fact, do not erase or use correction fluid.

❐ Fill in all blanks, do not skip lines or leave spaces, or line through large blocks of empty space

❐ Do not "squeeze in" notes at a later date and do not indent on any line.

❐ Make additions and changes appropriately on a different line. You may reference the line on any specific page that you need to change and give a reason for that change.

❐ Record all patient contact.
   a. Missed appointments documented
   b. Telephone messages documented
   c. Entries dated, timed and initialed
   d. Patient noncompliance documented

❐ Initial all reports from an external source (X-ray, lab, diagnostic, consultant) before filing them.

❐ Dictation, correspondence, and reports to insurance companies or other practitioners should be proofread and initialed before filing.

❐ Maintain a legend for any abbreviations used if needed for later reference.

❐ Document the reason for the visit, any unusual events and avoid or explain contradictions.

❐ All clinical findings (positive or negative) should be documented and the problem or complaint list kept current.

❐ Treatment plan documented and updated with each visit.

❐ Entries are objective and do not criticize other providers or their treatment methods.

❐ Properly identify the record, the record keeper, the technique employed, the table and/or room used and the details of each treatment.

❐ Any patient instructions are documented.

☐ Informed consent is in the chart.

☐ Be certain that the "Release of Records Authorization" form in the chart is correct and valid.

☐ Referral letters or prescriptions are in the chart.

☐ Herb list is current, when due to refill, reactions or allergies.

☐ Patient education materials given to patient is documented.

☐ Customize the forms you use.

☐ Keep financial and clinical information separate.

☐ Retain the records forever because of the statue of limitations on malpractice cases.

☐ Signature of the provider of services.

Keep your patient records forever. A patient has, in some cases, up to two years from the discovery of a problem to sue you. While it is unlikely that a patient's problem would arise 10 years from your treatment and be traceable to you and a specific clinical event, it is not impossible. Basically, that means that you should keep all files in storage or on a CD or tape memory drive forever.

POINTS TO PONDER FROM CHAPTER 8

- There are many forms that are required by law in your patient interactions.

- There are other forms that are optional but can streamline patient care and make your clinic feel professional, caring, and organized.

- If you take nothing else from this chapter, read and follow the recordkeeping checklist.

The Wonderful World of HIPAA | 9

> ## Health Insurance Portability and Accountability Act

This act, also known as the Kennedy-Kassebaum bill, was passed in 1996 and became law in April 2003. It was originally designed to help workers take their insurance coverage from employer to employer without any gap in health insurance coverage and for employees leaving the workforce who wanted to maintain their health insurance. It has been expanded significantly into other areas of compliance that clinics must do to keep their patients' records private as well as limiting the ways in which this private information may be communicated to anyone else. With regard to that, there are a few pieces of paperwork that you must present to your patient or that you must maintain in case of legal auditing. Also, there are rules about how you keep your patients' records private as well as codes that you use for insurance billing.

P O W E R   P O I N T

Interesting facts about health care information

1. Twenty percent of the consumers in the U.S. believe that their health information has been used or disclosed inappropriately.
2. Seventeen percent of Americans report that they have taken action to avoid the inappropriate use of their information, including providing inaccurate information to health care providers, changing physicians, or avoiding health care altogether.
3. The Association of American Physicians and Surgeons report that 78% of it's members have withheld information from a patient's record due to privacy concerns and 87% of its members have had a patient request that information be withheld.

There is some confusion in our profession about who must comply with the HIPAA regulations and rumors that you must comply only if you bill electronically. This is incorrect. Even if you do not bill electronically for your insurance patients, any insurance billing must still comply with the guidelines in the Transaction Code Set section of HIPAA (Electronic billing is not yet required but may be in the future). Furthermore, the Privacy Regulations and Security Standards of HIPAA apply to anyone that has gathered personally identifiable health information from any patient, whether you bill their insurance company or not. All patients have the right to privacy and security of their information whether the clinic does electronic insurance billing or not. Details about these compliance requirements are discussed below.

P O W E R P O I N T

Are You a Covered Entity Under HIPAA?
Covered Entities are defined as any healthcare provider who:
- Transmits any patient information electronically, whether by fax, electronic transmission, or by email.
- Has oral communication with a patient.
- Gathers health information and writes it in a chart.

Any health information that is gathered, whether stored on paper or in a computer or is orally transmitted is Protected Health Information. Acupuncture clinics are covered entities by virtue of the above definitions.

▶ **What do you need to do to comply?**

There are several things you must do for your clinic to be in full HIPAA compliance. These things are not really that complex for most small clinics, but you could get into trouble if you do not understand and implement these few requirements.

1. Appoint a Privacy Officer

Who is a Privacy Officer?

You may be your clinic's Privacy Officer, or someone on your front desk staff may be the Privacy Officer if you are in a larger or multi-person clinic. You can simply create a "To Whom It May Concern" letter for your Compliance Manual (discussed later on) that states the name of your Privacy Officer.

What does a Privacy Officer have to do?

- Understand all the privacy and security requirements under HIPAA (Health Insurance Portability and Accountability Act) as well as the business aspects and the technology information systems in the practice.

- Can appoint additional people to assist and oversee the compliance of the privacy policies and procedures in the office if need be. If others are appointed then each person must have clearly written instructions about the policies and procedures.

- Train newly hired personnel. Each office worker has to be trained, within 30 days of their hire date, in all privacy regulations and security standards.

- Create and maintain an office policies and procedures Compliance Manual. This can be as simple as a three-ring binder in which you keep all the required HIPAA forms.

- Revise all forms in current use in the clinic as necessary. Updated forms should be kept in your compliance manual.

- Maintain and monitor keys to entrance and exit doors. Make sure you know who has all keys. Keep a list of who has keys and when they received them or turned them back in to you in your manual.

2. Maintain a fax log

This should include the date and time of all incoming and outgoing faxes, who sent the fax and who received it.

3. **Create Business Associate Agreements with any appropriate company**

   Who is a business associate?

   Any legal/attorney firm, accountant, consultant, accreditation group, or any group for which the acupuncturist is a provider, any billing service, any interns or volunteers, or janitorial services are considered *business associates.* You need an agreement that assures the privacy of your patient healthcare information with each business associate. These agreements with each company or individual go in your compliance manual.

4. **Make sure all patients have signed any form required by HIPAA in conjunction with their private healthcare information. Keep these forms in each patient's file.**

   What forms will you need to keep your office compliant?

   - Consent form. Each patient (or legal guardian for minors) must sign a form showing that they understand that their Protected Health Information can be used for treatment, payment, and healthcare operations in your clinic.

   - Privacy notice. Each patient must be informed of your privacy policies and must sign a form stating that they have read and discussed the policies with someone in your clinic. This form is kept in each patient's chart.

   - Authorization form for release of protected health information. The patient has to sign this form for the release of any and all health information. This form is limited to use for a specific period of time or a specific incident (such as a car accident). The patient has the right to tell you that they do *not* give you authorization to release any information regarding HIV/AIDS, substance abuse including drug or alcohol abuse, or mental health information.

- Patient must sign an Individual Rights Relating to Authorization form which shows that they understand their rights concerning what can and cannot be released. ●

5. Create a Compliance Manual

What items need to be logged and kept for compliance?

- Privacy Regulations Checklist. ● This checklist shows all the HIPAA requirements and when you began implementing them.

- Requests for Restriction of PHI (protected health information) from any patient.

- Patient communication list. Any patient who has asked you to limit your communication to them or about them in any way should be on a list in your compliance manual. Before any communications are sent out from your office or any protected health information is sent to another party (lawyer, insurance company, medical doctor, other), this list must always be checked.

- A description of your office security measures with regards to computers, faxes, email and paper files needs to be in your compliance manual.

- Trading partners and vendors list

- Fax log (listing of all faxes in and out) ●

- Computer log of who used any computer where you maintain your patient information on with date and time.

- Business Associates Agreements

- Complaint log: A record of complaints from any patient with dates, main substance of the complaint, and who spoke to the patient.

- Access Codes for your computer

➤ Review of the Areas of HIPAA Compliance

1. **Background:** Where are you and your office in relation to the *privacy requirements and security standards?* In other words, are you keeping your patients' private healthcare information private and secure? This is the baseline or starting point. If you are not keeping this information private and secure, make corrections and implement compliance requirements.

2. **Privacy:** This means limiting the availability and use of *individual patient identifiable health information* within and from your office. This describes the "what" that is to be kept private.

3. **Security:** This is the system used to maintain privacy. Whether it is physical, as in paper and charts, or electronically maintained information, your method of limiting access to individual patient identifiable health information is what this means. This is the "how" of keeping your patients' information confidential. For example, you keep all file cabinets locked or you maintain password-protected computer files, etc.

4. **Transaction Code Sets and Unique National Health Identifiers:** This is the code used for transmission of information between two parties to carry out the financial or administrative activities related to health care. Codes now in use for these purposes are the International Classification of Diagnosis (ICD-9 or ICD-10) codes and Current Procedural Terminology (CPT) codes commonly used on the standard Health Care Financing Administration (HCFA or CMS) form. Secondly, each healthcare provider is now issued a unique national provider identifier number to be used in all billing. See Appendix A on how to get your NPI.

As you can see, there are a few things your office needs to keep track of for basic HIPAA compliance. Once you have the necessary compliance forms and notebook created, this is not impossible to do and will become just another part of your office procedures. Privacy of communications and records is really the important thing to consider and control. There are samples of many of these forms on the companion website and several websites listed in the Resources section if you need further detail about HIPAA and its impact on professional practitioners.

POINTS TO PONDER FROM CHAPTER 9

- If you collect personal information from your patients, you must comply with the privacy compliance sections of HIPAA.

- We give you lists of the minimal things your clinic must do to comply.

- If you bill insurance companies for your patients, you need to use ICD-9/10 codes and CPT codes for your billings. Eventually, you or your clinic will have a unique identifier number . . . but not yet.

- HIPAA is a minor pain in the ***. However, don't lose sleep about this stuff. Just do these few things and you are protected.

Hiring and Keeping People to Work for You | 10

As we have said in other chapters, we believe that making the commitment to hire front desk help is essential to your overall business success. While this may feel scary (will my cash flow handle it?), it is absolutely necessary for your practice to grow and be successful. Without adequate help, you are always being pulled in too many different directions. This means you are not practicing the best medicine you can or providing your patients with the best customer service. In an age where good customer service is a huge part of your marketing, this one change in your business can have more impact than almost anything else you could do for your professional life.

What should you look for in an employee to work the front desk? How much should you pay them? Can you hire someone as contract labor? What are the rules for being able to fire someone? We get asked about this subject a lot and it really is pretty important stuff with many potential pitfalls. While there are no magic bullets here, we will give you the best guidelines we can.

Having had many, many employees myself [HW], I can absolutely promise you that this is and always will be one of the most difficult and mysterious parts of running a business. When you hire someone into a very small business, they become a part of your extended family very quickly. That means you get all of the craziness of anyone's life along with whatever wonderful things they may bring to your business. The problem is that, as a prospective employer, you are not allowed to ask questions like, "Do you have a girlfriend or boyfriend that drinks too much?"

"Does your husband beat you?" or, "Has your teenage son ever been in jail?" Other than the general impression you get when you interview prospective employees, it can be difficult to ferret out the details of someone's life that will become a problem for them and, by extension, for you later on. That being said, there are great employees to be had, and we are convinced that you can make a better living and help more people with front desk help than without it.

POWER POINT

Before starting to look, do your homework!

We suggest you start by making a list of what you are looking for in an employee.

For example:
- How many hours per week do you want someone?
- How much can you afford to pay per hour?
- Can you offer any benefits besides an hourly wage?
- How long do you want them to commit to working in your clinic?
- Do you want someone in a certain age range?
- If your clinic grows and they don't want more hours or more responsibility, how will you handle that?

There are many other questions you (and any clinic partners) may want to ask yourselves. The point is that the clearer you are about what you are looking for, the easier it will be to recognize the person who fits the bill when you meet them.

➤ How to find potential candidates

1. Consider looking within your circle of acquaintance or your client base. If you know lots of people in the town where you practice, you might consider putting out the word that you are looking for an employee. This has both advantages and

disadvantages. It may save you money on advertising and time doing interviews, which are a huge drain on your time and energy at best, and confusing and frustrating at worst. The major disadvantage is that you may damage a friendship because you don't want to hire someone's favorite niece who is looking for a job but doesn't fit your description of the perfect employee.

2. Write a specific job description. Once you have decided what your new employee will be responsible for, put it on paper—the more detailed the better. This document will become the basis for your advertisement and for your interviews. When well written, this tells everybody what is expected. An effective job description should include:
   a. the job title
   b. the job summary
   c. the job qualifications
   d. the job duties and responsibilities

3. If you only want part-time help and live in a city with an acupuncture college, consider hiring an acupuncture student. Now that there are close to 50 acupuncture schools around the U.S., you might find the perfect candidate within the student body of the local school. Especially if the school has mostly evening or weekend classes, a 24-hour per week job in your clinic could give the student valuable experience and solve your receptionist problem for a couple of years. Given the fact that few people in such jobs last longer than 2–3 years, this may not be a bad solution, especially if you are still in the early phase of growing your practice.

4. Consider retiree organizations. Older workers are mature, reliable, and have no child care issues. If you only want part-time help, they often have very flexible schedules.

5. If you do have to put an ad in the paper or on CraigsList, make your description of what you are looking for as clear as possible. Don't scrimp on words in your ad to save money. A

clear description of the person you want to hire and what you want to hire them for can weed out lots of job seekers who aren't right for you and will save you time in the interview process. Something like, "Alternative health clinic with two acupuncture practitioners seeks full time, reliable, mature front desk receptionist. Basic computer and good people skills a must. Medical office experience helpful. Position starts immediately. Fax resume to 333-3333."

It is illegal to put age or sex preferences in a job ad. However, if you put only a fax number or a P.O. Box number, you can weed out many of the people who are not going to be appropriate candidates for whatever reason. You are not required to contact anyone with whom you are not requesting an interview.

If you get 25 faxes, you may only want interviews with 8–9 of them. Some will be overqualified, some with the wrong type of background, and some will be too young. Call the candidates that seem to fit and pay attention to their phone voice and language skills. Would you want this person answering your phone? Have a script for yourself with one or two questions about something specific from their resume. Tell each person that you are doing a short phone interview with many applicants before scheduling anything in person. If you can immediately tell that they are not right for the job, thank them for the resume and say you'll get back in touch with them by the end of that day if you want to schedule an interview. That way you don't string them along for more than a few hours and you don't have to take the time to call them back if you don't choose to do so. When you speak with someone who sounds great on the phone, schedule the in-person interview immediately.

This phone process will whittle down your list by one or two more, at least. You can manage five or six interviews in one afternoon or evening, if you are efficient. Don't schedule an initial interview for longer than 1/2 hour. Make a list of specific questions and try not to ramble. A possible list is included below.

➤ What to look for during an interview

In a way, interviewing a potential employee is similar to doing a patient interview. You want to know what this person's "diagnosis" is, because that is who they are. Their patterns will have a tremendous impact on your business! Of course, you cannot ask to take their pulse or look at their tongue, but you can get lots of information about them by the other types of examination in Oriental medicine: looking, listening, and questioning. Here are some things to think about during an interview and some questions to ask:

1. Reference one or two items of interest on their resume. Ask them to describe the job, educational experience, or volunteer position that you are referencing and what they liked or did not like about it.

2. Find out why they left their last job.

3. Perhaps give them a short tour of your clinic and tell them in a few sentences about you and your services, but let them do most of the talking.

4. Notice if their nails are clean and shoes are polished.

5. Do a visual pattern discrimination from their face, skin, body type, carriage, and movement style. For example, if they have serious liver lines between their brows, they might be very efficient but could they also be irritable with your patients? Do they have a reasonable amount of qi? If they are excessively overweight, will the phlegm and dampness affect their memory? What types of diseases do you think they might manifest and how might that impact their work? This may not be fair, but it is a reality, and it's also your money and reputation they will be managing.

6. Did they show up on time? If they will be unlocking for you in the morning, you cannot have someone who is chronically late working for you.

7. Look at their clothing, purse, or backpack. Do they seem organized or scattered?

8. Ask about long term goals and aspirations. What do they want to be doing in five years, for example. You may not expect to keep them for 10 years, but you don't want someone who will disappear in six months.

9. Find out what they think is a lot of money. If they think $100 is a lot, for example, they may have a difficult time asking your patients to pay what you are worth.

10. Ask if they have had experience with difficult customers (sick people can be difficult) and what they do or say in such situations.

11. If they are clearly not a people person, end the interview as quickly as you politely can because they are not what you need.

12. Give them a timeline of when you will have made this decision. It's unkind to keep people hanging on for days and weeks.

Once you have narrowed it down to two candidates, you might want to schedule a second interview with more pointed questions about compensation, working conditions, and your needs and expectations. You may want to do an online background check for police records and, since they will be handling your money, their personal financial history. You have to get permission from them in writing to do these checks. The costs vary but will be $35–75 depending on how much information you want to find out.

You should have decided in advance how much you can afford per hour, what other perks you may be able to offer, a schedule for raises, a dress code, what types of behaviors are grounds for dismissal, acceptable personal telephone usage, vacation policy, holiday policies, whether you will use mediation for disputes, or anything else that needs to be discussed. For all office policies concerning the above subjects, it is absolutely essential to have it all written out as an "Employee Manual" which can be given to the employee for reading and signing. That way, there are no "he said, she said" issues to come up later because policies are in writing.

Contact everyone you interviewed, out of courtesy, within the next 24 hours. You can say something very simple, such as, "Thank you so much for coming in. We had many fine candidates for this job and we chose someone else at this time. We wish you the best of luck in finding a position soon."

If this is your first real employee, make sure you check both state and federal labor laws. To be in full labor law compliance, you will need a few posters from the government concerning Worker's Comp rules that must be posted somewhere visible. You can find these on the Internet from several companies; we have a list on the website. We suggest that you read them before you post them so you know what promises the government has made to employees on your behalf!

If you decide to have a payroll company handle your payroll, which we do encourage you to consider, you may want to have this set up before your new employee starts working. See Section 2, Chapter 1 for a longer discussion of taxes and payroll in general and Section 1, Chapter 5 for more information on the tax structures of various styles of business.

Managing employees

This is a huge subject. There are entire books and weekend seminars that you can take on employee management, motivation, and reward structures. None of us is a human resources or

POWER POINT

Things Your Employee Can Do When the Phone is Not Ringing

- Inventory your needles and herbal medicinals
- Sort and prioritize the mail that is still sitting on your desk
- Call insurance companies to check on patient benefits
- Clean the bathrooms
- Vacuum and dust all the treatment rooms
- Call patients to reschedule missed appointments
- Do out-bound calls to patients who have not been in for several months
- Do appointment reminder calls to people who have appointments tomorrow
- Make copies of forms that are running low
- Pull all the files for tomorrow's patients and organize them by time
- Write checks for bills to be paid and for you to sign; enter the data into QuickBooks
- Dust the herb shelves and product display shelves
- Fill out CMS 1500 insurance forms and address envelopes to mail them
- Order needles and herbals
- Fill brochure holders; move different ones to different rooms
- Update your waiting area scrapbook
- Clean and maintain your water/tea/coffee service for patients

employee management expert (even after many, many years in business), but we can give you a few general guidelines.

To begin with, arrange to spend an hour or so each day for the first several days training your new employee. You both need to feel comfortable that all the tasks involved with the job are understood. Keep training sessions to no more than one or so hours of new material. Most people cannot manage more than that in their brain at one time. Perhaps they will only work 1/2 days for the first week and only on tasks for which you have trained them. The exception to this will be people with a great deal of medical office, computer, or phone experience.

Make sure your new employee has read, understood, had a chance to ask questions about, and signed their employee manual *the very first day.* If you have a contract of any kind, that should be signed as well. If you do use a contract, make sure it is read over by an employment law attorney if not written by one in the first place.

We suggest that you use a simple form stating that there is a 90-day probation period and that there will be two reviews of the employee's performance during that time. The first will be after 30 days to discuss your employee's progress and to answer questions they might have. The second will be after the 90-day probation period is completed to determine if they move into regular employment (non-probationary) status. This gives you the chance to fire the person within that period without being liable for unemployment compensation, for which your state and federal accounts will be assessed. If you make the mistake of keeping the wrong person because you don't have the courage to fire them when the first signs of trouble occur, you can end up paying a lot of unemployment compensation for someone who only caused you trouble when they were on your staff.

My belief [HW], learned the hard way, is that if something does not feel right with an employee, you are better off to cut your losses and let them go as soon as possible. The longer you maintain a dysfunctional relationship with an employee out of fear, misplaced compassion, or simple laziness, the worse off you will be both emotionally and financially in the end. Believe me, you will end up firing them sooner or later, and sooner means less complexity, less unemployment compensation liability, and less potential issues for a lawsuit. The more grown-up you can be about this the better.

P O W E R   P O I N T

What to Do When You Are Having Trouble with an Employee

- Give them a first warning that the behavior is not acceptable. Give them a specific demand about what needs to change, with a deadline if appropriate. Put a note in their employee file with the date, the infraction, the conversation, and your specific request/demand. Tell them that this note has been made.

- If there is a repeat of this infraction, give them a final warning. Document this conversation similarly to the first one. This documentation gives you what is called "cause" or grounds for dismissal. It is this "cause" that keeps you from having to pay unemployment if you do have to fire them.

- If the specific behavior does not improve, fire them after the final warning. If the very first infraction is totally unacceptable (theft, showing up drunk, absence with no phone call, abusive behavior to your patients, etc.), you can fire them on the spot. Make sure you have a list in your employee manual of unacceptable behaviors for which people will be dismissed immediately.

- Remember that good documentation of all these situations is your legal protection against lawsuits or unfair unemployment compensation requests.

If the front desk person will be collecting money for you, make certain they understand what your fees are for various services, or, better yet, fill out the "charges" part of the chart and hand it to them as the person is leaving so there is no guesswork. There should be a daily income sheet or computer "form" on which the name of the patient and what was collected from them is entered. At the end of each day, you should check receipts against this form. This must then balance against bank deposit slips, credit card machine tallies, etc. At least for the first several months of any new employee's tenure, you probably want to do all the bank deposits yourself.

➤ Long term employee maintenance

Treat good employees as well as you can afford. It is our belief that if you take care of your employees, they will take care of you and your patients. Remember that your staff is a huge part of your customer service and can be either a wonderful asset or a terrible liability. Small gifts to recognize jobs well done, extra days off here and there, movie tickets, birthday remembrances, and a simple "thank you" when called for, all these things are important in the long-term health of your employee/employer relationship. There are several good books on the subject and we urge you to read one or more. See the Going Further section in the back of this book.

By the way, before we get to the end of this chapter, the answer to the question about hiring front desk staff as contract laborers is *no.* The federal government has very specific rules about the definition of someone working as contract labor and there is no way that a front desk person working for you can fit within that definition. If you get caught doing this, you will owe huge amounts in back taxes! There are websites you can look at the rules to confirm this for yourself, including www.IRS.gov, but I promise you we are telling you the truth.

Every practitioner we have spoken to about the advantages of having the right someone to take care of their front desk has stated, *unequivocally,* that this person makes their life easier and allows them to make more money with less stress. So take the time to find the right person with the right fit for your clinic. Train them well and treat them well, and this "could be the beginning of a beautiful relationship."

POINTS TO PONDER FROM CHAPTER 10

- A good employee is one of your clinic's most valuable assets. Take time to find the right person.

- Decide what you will require your new employee to do and write a very specific job description. This should include the job title, general description of the overall functions, qualifications, and a list of specific duties and responsibilities.

- Consider alternative methods of finding an employee such as canvassing your patients, notices at the local acupuncture college, retiree organizations.

- If you do put an ad in the paper, don't scrimp on the text. A clear and well-written ad can save you a great deal of time. Put a P.O. Box or fax number only and collect resumes. Do not put your phone number on the ad!

- Following our guidelines for the interviewing process can save you lots of time. During the interview process, remember what you know about Oriental medicine. Don't hire someone whom you suspect to have serious health issues.

- Write a short, clear employee manual with your policies for vacations, holidays, personal phone use,

"Points to Ponder" continues on the next page

grounds for dismissal, and anything else of importance to you. Your new staff person must read and sign that they understand this information.

- Train your new hire carefully; give them a 30-day review and a 90-day "yes-you-are-now-really-an-employee" review. If you think it's not a good fit or are at all uncomfortable, fire them sooner rather than later.

- Document any conversation about a problem or infraction of employee rules. Good documentation with employee issues, just like good documentation with your patients, is your best protection if a legal situation arises.

- With the right person answering your phone, you can make more money, have less stress, and run a more successful and professional clinic.

Patient Management, or, How Do You Keep Them Coming Back Happy? | 11

Communication and confidence are the most important tools you can have when it comes to patient management, but there is quite a bit more to consider here. This aspect of running your clinic is, possibly, the most important function you undertake, second only to managing your finances. Oftentimes, you will find that getting new patients is easier than maintaining them and keeping them on your active roster for years to come. When you *can* do this, however, you will also be welcoming their referrals to your clinic on a regular basis.

We wish there were magic bullets for this skill. There are not. Like most things in life, it is a group of cofactors that make you successful at managing your patients' feelings about you and their interactions with your clinic. In Section 2, Chapter 6, we discussed the importance of the look and feel of your clinic. In addition to these relatively subconscious responses, there are many other aspects of clinic interaction where you may "guide" your patients' feelings into the most positive zone possible.

Initial responses

Remember that patient management begins before the person walks through your door. It starts with the first phone contact, how prospective patient questions are answered by your front desk staff, what it's like to find a parking space near your office, even the response to your brochure that they picked up at the health food store. Assuming you have done a good job with all these preliminary pieces, the next part of your work in this area includes the appearance of your clinic and lobby, the professionalism of your front desk staff, and even the quality and appearance of your initial paperwork. These things can have that potential lifelong patient thinking either that you are a good addition to their medical toolbox or that you are a quack. Since keeping patients is essential to the survival of your clinic, you need to think about these initial prospective patient interactions that will happen long before they've seen the inside of your treatment room or experienced the insertion of a needle.

▶ Close encounters of the telephone kind

Whether referred by a business colleague, a free lecture at the library, or a business card picked up at the climbing gym, most of the time people's initial contact with your clinic will be on the telephone. Whether you are the one handling phone communications or you have a front desk staff, this contact needs to be scripted, at least to some extent. You can write down several ways that your phone could be answered and allow your front desk person(s) to choose the option they like best. Whatever you have them say, it is most important that:

- They (or you) don't mumble or speak too quickly. This is a common problem with Asian receptionists speaking in English because Chinese and other Asian languages are spoken at a much faster tempo than English. This can be a difficult issue for Chinese coming to the U.S. to understand and is a common experience with Chinese product suppliers (*i.e.*, you-call-them-but-you-are-not-sure-what-company-you-called-because-the-person-answering-the-phone-speaks-too-quickly-to-be-understood).

- They sound upbeat and helpful, not bored, preoccupied, or surly.

- There is actually someone to answer the phone during normal clinic hours, such as 8-to-4 or 9-to-5. Would you expect any doctor's office to have only an answering machine with music in the background that says, "I'll get back in touch with you within one working day"? If we wish to be perceived as professional medical care providers, we have to act, at least in some ways, like other care providers in our culture. That means having normal business phone hours during which people can reach a real person, even if that person is not you.

- They have some scripted answers to commonly asked questions so that they sound competent and professional.

- They have some idea what to do with people calling about a problem or complaint.

- They know approximately how long various procedures require, what initial paperwork needs to be completed and signed, and if there is any other information you need from a new patient prior to their first visit.

POWER POINT

What are the most commonly asked questions at an Oriental medical clinic?

Here are some common questions from prospective patients. Write some scripted answers for yourself and especially for any front desk person working for you.

- How long do your appointments take?
- What do treatments cost?
- What kinds of things can your clinic treat besides pain?
- Does acupuncture hurt?
- How many treatments will I need?

When writing the short scripts to answer these and other questions, remember that you want each answer given by your front desk person speaking to a prospective patient to lead to: "We could see you at 2 PM on Friday or at 10 AM on Monday. Would either of those work for you?"

▶ Forms and paperwork

Your new patient has just arrived, grabs a clipboard stuffed with paper and sits in your comfortable lobby to read, check, circle, and sign. Everyone in this country who has ever seen a medical practitioner in their life is used to going through this process. Don't apologize for it and don't cheapen it with homemade-looking forms that leave large gaps in a necessary medical history. As well as gathering information from your patient, this process is designed to tell your patient how you do business, how their account with you is to be handled, what your rates are, and any other information that you wish to give them. An informed patient is a keeper. Remember that people don't like to feel confused.

> ## PRACTITIONER POINTER
>
> "If an initial appointment has been made at least a few days ahead, I like to mail people's paperwork to be filled out in advance so that I can include a small packet of information and directions to my clinic. I do this both because it looks professional and gives the person confidence in my services before they even get inside the door, and because it gives us time to get patient records from other providers if necessary."
>
> *—Gary Klepper, DC*
> *Paonia, CO*

Forms you need for an initial exam and visit: ⦿

• Patient information—Name, address, phone number, email, emergency contact, etc. How do you get in touch with this patient? What do they prefer to be called? Who referred them?

• Health history—Chief complaint, secondary and other more minor complaints, medical history, prescription drug and supplement use, last medical exam and reason, recent surgeries. This form is designed to flesh out why the person is there, what they have done about it in the past, gives you a social and family history, and points to any communicable or life-threatening disease or disorder they may suffer concomitantly.

- Financial policies—What you offer, how much it costs, and accepted forms of payment. If you have a sliding scale, describe the process here and how they must prove hardship if requesting lower fees. If you bill insurance yet want patients to know they are responsible for any unpaid balance, tell them here. If you offer a payment at time of services discount, describe it in detail here. It is very important that you have people sign this page signifying they understand your policies. Some clinics take an imprint of a credit card in the case of nonpayment; if this is your policy, describe it here. The more you tell people on this form, the less difficulty you will have in getting paid later.

- Office policies—Do you have observers or interns from the local acupuncture college? Do you have a required cancellation window of 24 hours, or 12? How should changes in appointments be handled and with what notice?

- Privacy policy—If you are abiding by HIPAA rules, you are required to tell patients *how* you will protect and use their Personal Health Information. Please see Section 2, Chapter 9 for more details on this.

- Insurance form—If the patient presents you with an insurance card, make a copy of it and then present them with a form designed to gather all of the necessary information for you to bill said insurance company. Make sure to include information such as the insured's name, date of birth, address, and Social Security number. Do you accept assignment of benefits? Even if you are compliant with HIPAA, add a release of information block so that there is no misunderstanding that you will share information with the insurance company.

- Consent to treatment—If you do not have malpractice insurance that requires the use of a certain form, make one up. Consent to Treatment form is designed to tell people what the risks associated with your services are: acupuncture, herbs, tuina, cupping, guasha, moxibustion, and the like. This is not meant to scare people. However, if you list that a possible side effect of acupuncture is bruising, and they read and signed the form telling them this, then they will be less likely to be upset about getting a bruise.

- Arbitration agreement—Although a touchy subject, some malpractice companies will cut you a break on pricing if you have patients sign an arbitration agreement. This form waives the patient's right to a jury trial, saying that they can sue you if they want, but they will arbitrate instead of going to trial. More and more professionals are using this type of form, including medical practitioners and even real estate brokers.

The more information you give to your patient, the less reason they have to claim ignorance or, worse, to be ignorant. Tell your patients up front everything about how you expect the exchange of your services for their green qi is to take place. Tell them their information with you is safe. Tell them, without saying it, that you are a well-trained medical professional.

➤ Intakes that WOW

Your initial intake is like a first date. This is where you can possibly make up for the cramped lobby and poor lighting conditions in the bathroom. You have a chance here to really impress this person who has possibly never had an acupuncture experience. Dimes to dollars, however, they have seen a doctor at some point in their life. It is for this reason that doing an intake that *wows,* something that really knocks their socks off, is crucial. How about a silk brocade cushion to take patients' pulses? (Remember your fascination the first time a good practitioner took your pulses?)

Being that we are performing a medical service, we all know that asking all about the chief complaint is one of the first steps in this process. Next, the nature of our medicine stipulates that some of the questions we ask are those that no person has ever had asked of them before, unless they are suffering from some sort of bowel or sexual disorder. Just by this alone, we are already spending more time face-to-face with our patients than most physicians spend in a day with all of their patients combined—a definite plus.

Take their blood pressure. Obviously, in some cases, this is called for (such as headaches and dizziness). But take it on the first visit no matter what. (In some states this is a requirement before every treatment.) This is also a great tie-in to what patients are used to from their previous life in the Western medical system. Does the blood pressure fit into your Chinese medical diagnosis? Probably not. Does it convey a sense of professionalism and show that your medical techniques have some feeling of being grounded in a reality they are comfortable with? Definitely. A thorough exam on a patient's first visit to your office will go a long way into wowing them back again. You may also consider weighing them and doing a simple urinalysis to check for sugar content if you feel comfortable with that.

Let the patient talk, but control the flow of the conversation. When you begin your intake, you may start with some open-ended questions that allow you to get some general information, some of which the patient does not even know they are giving (such as general energy level, tone and strength of voice, and body language). Then, as you whittle your choices of pattern discrimination down, ask more "yes/no" questions that leave little room for explanation but give you the specifics you need ("Is the nasal mucus clear and thin or yellow and thick?"). If and when the patient veers off course into some story about their brother George who choked on a hamburger at the family reunion last summer, pull them back gently to the process at hand. Remind them again of the question you require an answer for and give them another chance.

Be an active listener. Don't just stare at your chart and make notes as they talk. Make eye contact and *look* as though you are listening as well as actually hearing them. Repeat their statements to them when you are looking for confirmation. Patients really appreciate knowing that you have heard them. "So, Mr. Johnson, you're complaining of left lower quadrant abdominal pain that eases once you have a bowel movement. Is that correct?" Once the intake is over, you have another chance to really shine.

Explain your actions. That's something that you rarely get in a doctor's office. What are you doing and why? Why do you need to touch me there? My pain is over here. Why are you looking at my tongue? What do you feel when you take my pulse? By telling a patient, in simple terms, what you are looking for during a physical exam or what you are trying to accomplish with your treatment, you give them more power over their own body. Remember, we like smart patients, and most patients like to feel that they are participants, not passive receivers of care. The more you tell them, the more educated about their own body and health they become, which only makes your job easier.

Allow the patient to ask questions. While you may want to control the flow of the intake, allow your patients the opportunity to fulfill their need to learn about what it is you think is going on, what you think you can do about it, and how many needles you are going to stick into them! Again, knowledge is power. Answer whatever questions you feel comfortable with, especially about the needles. It seems everyone has a question about those. Keep metaphors as simple and straightforward as possible. It is easy for people to understand analogies from the natural world, but Chinese or quasi-spiritual jargon may turn them off or scare them away.

Finally, be sure to explain to your patient any side effects they may expect after the treatment and then give them some treatment options from which to choose. Some practitioners prefer to simply tell people to come back X number of times in the next X number of weeks, but it can work better to give the patient the option to choose from a couple of treatment plans. Another form you may want to use is a written assessment of the patient's condition and how you think you can help. List a few treatment options such as "Band-Aid," "good," and "best." Who in their right mind doesn't go for the *best* treatment plan when it comes to their health?

➤ Communication

Most of the section above has a common thread— communication. Talk to your patients about everything you are doing. Let them know where you think you can make a difference and even let them know when you've made a mistake. If you really botch something up, take care of the problem and see it through to satisfactory resolution. Don't let someone walk out your door angry, upset, or frustrated. It may come back to haunt you in court.

I [ES] have a perfect example of this. I know an acupuncturist (who shall remain unnamed) who was doing some cupping on a brand-spanking new patient. The patient had read his forms and disclaimers and signed all of his paperwork, but what happened was not covered on that form. He lit the patient's inordinate amount of back hair (slathered in Tiger Balm) on fire. Not just a little singe of hair—three foot flames licking him in the face. The practitioner and the student observer from the acupuncture school quickly extinguished the flames. The patient was not harmed, but it was more excitement than any practitioner really wants! After the treatment was over, the practitioner explained what went wrong but did not apologize excessively. The patient rescheduled for the next week. He was fine and his back pain was *much* better even if his back hair is a little less thick.

This situation could have been a nightmare. In fact, when I first heard of the encounter, I got out my Rolodex of attorneys to give him a referral. However, after speaking with the practitioner and getting a good feel for how the situation was dealt with, I felt relieved. It also helped the next week when our hapless practitioner put a fire extinguisher in the treatment room just as that patient was arriving. Laughter is still the best medicine, you know!

➤ Getting the second appointment

It is important to remember that most patients need several appointments to get well. When you read Chinese journal articles, you virtually never see a protocol that was successfully completed in only one treatment. Most of us will, rightly, suggest a plan involving 4–8 visits for an initial course of treatment. It is up to you to help your patient follow through with this plan. Advise the patient that you really believe you can help them (unless you don't believe you can) but that, to restore the dynamic balance in their body, they will require a course of therapy that is sensible and manageable. Make them aware that they can get appointment times more suitable to their schedule if they make them in advance. Some practitioners sell an appointment "package" at slightly reduced pricing. While it is technically illegal to do this in some states, it is encouraged in others, and it works well to motivate patients to come in for a series of treatments. Check with a lawyer or your state board about this type of practice before you leap into territory that may be illegal.

220

POWER POINT

The Bonding Call

We suggest that you *always* call every patient within 24 hours after the first treatment. This is called a *bonding call* and it tells the patient that you really care about what happens to them and how they are doing. Make sure you have their chart in front of you when you make the call and can ask one or two specific questions about their response to treatment. If they have not made a second appointment already, this is your opportunity to suggest it.

Secondly, you should simply assume that patients will be coming in for a series of appointments because that is what they need to get well. Explain to each patient that this is how acupuncture works and that they can expect improvement in their problem only with several treatments. Otherwise, you are probably short-changing yourself and your medicine and not meeting your patients' needs either. If you have internal questions about whether a patient will ever come back to see you again, your patients will subconsciously pick up on this lack of confidence and you probably won't see them again. Don't even go there in your mind. Either take courses to improve your Oriental medical skills (and thereby your confidence in yourself) or find a mantra or affirmation to help yourself get past this imaginary monster in the closet.

As a course of treatment is coming to an end, you should have a short consultation, either on the phone or, better, in person, to decide whether treatment is completed or, if not, how much and in what way it will continue. While it is important not to string people along unnecessarily, it does not serve a patient to give them fewer treatments than they need. If you have done 10 or more acupuncture treatments, it may be useful to let the patient rest for 2–3 weeks before continuing therapy.

If you are largely an herbal practitioner, you should explain initially to your patient that you are giving them a one-week supply of medicine after which time they will need to come in for a short appointment for you to take their pulse, ask a few questions, and adjust their formula. After that, they can call in to have their formula refilled for up to one month without a re-visit, unless there is some problem or change in their situation that arises. You may have to change these parameters depending upon what type of patient you are treating or the nature of their problem (for example, infertility patients may need a different formula each of the four weeks of the menstrual cycle). If you are doing largely herbal medicine, it is assumed that you are managing many patients and that a good portion of your income is coming from filling your patients' prescriptions.

Another pointer for the largely herbal practitioner is the issue of dosage. Just as acupuncture usually requires adequate numbers of treatments closely enough spaced to have the needed effect, herbal medicine requires adequate doses to do what it is meant to do. I [HW] can't tell you how often I have seen patients who were properly diagnosed and the proper medicine prescribed but treated with such low doses that they came to believe that, "Chinese herbs don't work." This is useless for the patient. Think carefully about how much medicine a patient would be getting with a standard decocted formula *in China*. If you are not doing bulk herb decoctions, take a look at the type of medicine you are giving the patient (whether pills, powders, tinctures) and the concentration ratio of that medicine. If you don't know the concentration ratios from the bottle, call your supplier and find out. While powders or pills may be easier for your patients, you need to make sure you are getting something close to a daily dose that would match the standards of care *in China* down your patient's throat. Otherwise they may be wasting their money and not getting better. This will do nothing for your reputation or the reputation of our medicine.

This is especially true in the case of acute or serious disorders. So remember, good patient management with Chinese herbs means giving the right dose.

PRACTITIONER POINTER

"I have noticed an interesting phenomenon when a patient is getting ready to leave the office. I have found it makes a difference whether I say, 'Do you want to call, or do you want to schedule now?' versus, 'Do you want to schedule, or do you want to call?' They have a greater tendency to pick whatever I say second."

—*Valerie DeLaune, L.Ac.*
Juneau, Alaska

What to do about the disappearing patient

If a patient comes in once or twice and then never makes another appointment or does not show up for one that is already scheduled, it may be that you "cured" them in one or two sessions, but it is more likely that something in your new-patient procedure needs improvement. You must try to reach that patient and learn from them what you could be doing better. This may be difficult in that they may be embarrassed to tell you what was wrong with their experience or they may not really be able to articulate it. They may not return your messages or, if they do, you may not get honest answers to your questions. However, if you can get them on the phone, we suggest the following approach that may disarm them enough to actually try and tell you about their experience of your clinic and your care. Hopefully, you already did a standard bonding call with the patient. So you know how they seem to have responded to the first visit to your office. If not, this may be the first thing you need to add to your procedures.

In any case, first ask them how they are doing. Ask them if they would like to reschedule or if they have any questions about your exam or treatment. Tell them you are sorry if their experience was not everything they expected it to be and that you'd be happy to assist them in finding another practitioner or another type of service to solve their health problem. That should disarm any "armor" to some extent. Explain to them that, as a health care practitioner, it is your responsibility to close their file with some "release from care" and you need to know that they are better or have determined another way to manage their problem. Depending upon how they respond to this, ask them if they have any advice about what you or your clinic staff could have done better or differently that would have allowed them to make the decision to return for further treatment. Thank them for trying Oriental medical or acupuncture care and assure them that, should they have further problems or questions about their health, you would be most happy to help them if you can. This is a class act, and anyone that you'd really want to associate with will recognize it. Some may even reschedule on the spot. If not, tell them that you will put them in your inactive files and consider their record closed for the present time but that any other practitioner of any discipline may request a copy of their files if it would be helpful in their future care.

If you get advice or a complaint, don't be defensive if you can help it. Listen carefully, take notes, and decide if their statement is valid and if there is anything you can do to improve in whatever area(s) they bring up. Discuss what they tell you with your staff or partners and try to find a way to respond that is workable for you. If you do this phone call *with every dropped patient* and listen carefully to any advice you receive, the numbers of "disappearers" will decrease with time.

➤ **Staying in touch with your patients**

When a patient terminates care, even for all the right reasons, you will probably want to stay in touch with them from time to time. In the marketing chapters, we discuss various ways to keep in touch with your patients at great length. See Section 4, Chapters 2 and 4 for lots of ideas.

➤ **Confidence**

As a practitioner of anything, there is, arguably, nothing as important as confidence. Trusting in what you believe, think, and say goes a long way toward patients having confidence in you. If you are wishy-washy about your treatments, patients will know it. If you lack assurance about their follow-up care, they will too and may not show up at all. Choose a point and treat it. Write a treatment plan and follow it. If, today, you can only think to needle St 36, do it with presence and a confident heart! Your patients *want* to trust in your judgment and experience. Don't try pulling wool over their eyes; but know that you have learned and can do this work, so do it!

Conveying a sense of confidence when you walk into the treatment room puts the patient at ease that their healthcare is in your hands. They are going to pay you hard-earned money for your attention and expertise. Concomitantly, while your patients want to feel at ease, they also want to feel in control of their lives, which brings us back to communication.

Confidence and communication—these are your two greatest allies in the skills of patient management. Give a patient knowledge about her body and an understanding of how you and Oriental medicine are going to help her and you empower her to better health. Do it with confidence, and you win your clinic an educated patient who cares about their health and who will, in turn, have the confidence to send you their friends and family members. That is how you grow your practice.

POINTS TO PONDER FROM CHAPTER 11

- Communication and confidence are the two most important attributes for managing your patients.

- Make sure to follow the recommendations in Section 2, Chapter 6 because patient management includes a lot more than paperwork and phone calls.

- Consider writing standard "scripts" to answering basic phone questions. These scripts should always lead to the appointment-making phase of the initial phone conversation.

- In order to serve your patients well, you need to help them follow through with the treatment plan you create. Make sure they know that, in order to work with you, a certain number of treatments or a certain amount of herbal medicine will simply be what happens in your clinic.

- Don't under-dose with Chinese herbal medicine; not giving enough medicine for the person to experience relief from their symptoms is a waste of that patient's money.

- Your clinic forms should be thorough, clean, not a xerox-of-a-xerox, typo free, and easy to understand.

- Use a bonding call within the first 24 hours of a first treatment to find out how a patient responded and to answer their questions.

- If you lose a patient before the treatment plan is complete, find out why and how you could change your clinic procedures, phone practices, décor, or whatever is necessary so that you would not lose another patient for those same reasons.

- If you don't have enough confidence in your skills as a practitioner, decide what you need to do to change that feeling and go do it. When you have confidence as a clinician, it is contagious and growing your practice is much easier.

Using the Services of Other Professionals | 12

Sometimes the difference between success and failure is asking for help. The key is knowing who to ask and when to ask for it. The misconception among many small business owners is that doing things yourself will save you lots of money so you can become more profitable. This is actually not true in many cases. In fact, using the resources of other business and trade professionals can not only free up your valuable time, but also can end up saving or even making you money.

Many of the professional services included in this chapter are ones that you may not need right away. They are things you actually can do until you get busy enough with patients that you are no longer able to do them yourself. Others it's better to start with a profession from the beginning. The main idea here is to find the help you need when you need it, and to not let a gap in service, cleanliness, or general business operations slow you down in your quest to run your clinic as well as you possibly can. For some of these you may be able to work out a barter arrangement. This can be great if you don't have a full practice. But, however you pay for these services, most of us in business will need help from some of these at some point in time. Below is a list of professionals whose help you may need at one time or another.

Accountants and bookkeepers

Number crunchers are inexpensive depending on the services you are looking for. In return they can relieve you of some of the headaches of your financial issues from the day-to-day bill paying and deposits to preparing your taxes and doing your payroll. The size of your clinic and the number of employees you have will determine the type of professional you need.

A bookkeeper is someone who takes care of recording the daily business transactions that occur during any given accounting cycle. They can perform routine calculations, checkbook reconciliation and bank transactions, ensure that all transactions are recorded properly, and keep copies supporting documents. Bookkeeping services are usually not hugely expensive and, if you are really bad at or bored by this type of work, we suggest you find one with whom you are comfortable working.

An accountant, on the other hand, is usually quite a bit more expensive but is a professional manager who can develop and maintain an entire accounting system if that is your need. A good full service accounting firm can collect data and prepare reports, supervise accounting employees such as bookkeepers, and prepare and file taxes for your company and for you personally. You may not need an accountant immediately, but by the time you have three employees, own an extra rental property, take care of 500 patients, have a three year clinic lease and a child in college, you will probably want at least the occasional advice of a good accountant.

➤ Tax preparation

As a business owner you owe it to yourself to have your taxes prepared and filed by a professional. Just as you have invested thousands of hours to education for your profession, professional tax preparers are very well trained and informed. Tax laws, breaks, rebates and incentives change yearly and staying abreast of these can save you hundreds of dollars. However, unless you are planning to spend days reading over the yearly changes, the task of doing your business taxes is best left to the paid professional. Save all of your receipts, track your expenses and hand these over to someone trained to prepare your taxes. This may be the one time each year that you use the services of an accountant and it is an excellent time to do so.

That being said, some small companies find it very useful to have an accountant look over the books in October or November and give end-of-year advice for things that you need to do before December 31st to lower your tax bill.

➤ Lawyers

Contracts, disputes, waivers, and leases. These all fall within the realm of a legal advisor. While many of the forms and waivers used in our profession are standard, it never hurts to have a lawyer verify the legality of any publications you produce, especially if they are going to be signed by a patient or sent to insurance companies to verify your relationship with a patient.

Also, whether you are establishing a corporation, a partnership, or an LLC, a lawyer will be able to draft your articles of incorporation and bylaws and set up and advise you about your corporate structure. Also, if you are entering into a lease agreement, or purchasing a piece of property on contract, running your paperwork, contracts or agreements under the eyes of your attorney can protect you from making very unfortunate, very expensive mistakes.

Many businesses keep a lawyer on retainer. This is a monthly payment made to a lawyer or law firm in case you require legal aid. It's sort of like healthcare insurance—it's there for emergencies. However, while this arrangement does get you access to an attorney if you should find yourself needing one, in the beginning of your practice your legitimate legal needs are probably too minimal to justify this cost. A better idea is to find a government supported legal aid office or a low cost walk-in legal office that hires young lawyers to read documents and make suggestions on how to protect yourself legally. Most towns and cities have such services. If you cannot find anything else, try contacting the local Small Business Administration office and see if they can make a referral or have an on-staff legal advisor who could read the form or letter in question. If you live in a university town with a law school, you could try contacting them to see if they have a low cost legal clinic. For simple document checks and other minor legal questions, you may also want to try the services of a paralegal (see below).

If all else fails, try barter. When I [HW] was starting my first business, I traded my services for a lawyer's services for the first year. I had to give or arrange for a massage for him every week for a year, but his advice was invaluable and, at 26, I had more time and creativity than money. This may not be your situation, but it is worth investigating if you have family or friends in the world of law. Also, if a lawyer likes your work he or she may refer their clients or law partners, so a barter arrangement may have some marketing value as well.

The times that you really want help from an attorney are if and when you hire anyone for whom you want to create a contract, when you are creating a corporation, partnership, or LLC, when you have questions about firing employees, if you have serious trouble with anyone with whom you have already entered into a contract, when you are offered a contract by another employer (hospital, MD, DC, school, publishing company), or when any legal document or possibly-could-be-legal document gets created by you.

It is a statistical fact that MDs can expect to be sued by a patient or their family once every seven or eight years, whether they did anything wrong or not. Acupuncturists are, so far, doing much better than that, but should you get into trouble of some kind with a patient and you have purchased malpractice insurance, the insurance company lawyers will usually be responsible for representing you. If you get into trouble with any other entity such as your state acupuncture board or the state board of medical examiners, you probably want to hire your own private legal representation and pay them as well as you can afford.

POWER POINT

A word about retainers . . . If you are seriously considering hiring a lawyer on retainer, make sure that the majority of what you are paying for is *preparation.* These are the hours your attorney will spend in advance of any case trying to win, lose or get it thrown out and can sometimes number in the hundreds. Unlike the glorification of television shows, very little of most cases consist of trial hours. If you have a good attorney, they will do enough homework to resolve the issue before it ever gets near a judge's chambers.

➤ Paralegal

Unlike a lawyer, a paralegal cannot steer you one way or the other when it comes to legal advice. They can, however, draft your articles of incorporation or other business or personal legal paperwork. For the price, a paralegal is a good choice for your company's paperwork in the beginning. If you do need a lawyer, the paralegal will tell you.

➤ Building contractor

A good contractor can do anything. From remodels to new construction, the contractor is a valuable asset, especially when it comes time to start, or change your existing clinic. Having been in the contracting business in the past, I [ES] can tell you that asking for references is a must. Although contractors must be licensed in most states, there are very few repercussions for contractors whose work is slow to the point of negligent. Shoddy workmanship is also not a punishable offense. Therefore, when you first interview your perspective contractor, we recommend the following:

1. Ask for three references from other businesses in town, or specifically regarding the type of work you are looking to get done. Contact those people and find out:

a. was the work completed on time?

b. was the work completed to satisfaction?

c. if there were any problems, were they addressed to satisfaction?

Keep in mind that the contractor will only be providing you with names of references where everything turned out on the positive side. An important question of references, therefore, is *when was the work performed?* If the three references were all three years apart, go back to the contractor and ask instead for the last three jobs at businesses in the area. Having such time between referenced jobs can mean either very few people want to be references, or only that many jobs turned out okay. If the contractor is good there should be no shortage of people wanting to gush about their services.

2. Verify the contractor is licensed, bonded, and insured.

Here's another tip on contractors. Depending on the project you have ahead of you, the contractor may need to call in a specialist, such as an electrician or plumber. This is called a sub-contractor; a professional working under the direction of a contractor. If this is the case, make sure the contractor is not adding on unnecessary fees for this. While the electrician and plumber need to be paid, the contractor does not need to take a profit on their work as well.

Also, no matter the size of the project your contractor is going to undertake for you, make sure that all necessary permits are drawn, and that all local codes are being followed. There is nothing more gut-wrenching than watching your contractor drive down the road with your money as the building inspector walks through your front door and says it's all got to come down. Of course the contractor has some liability, but ultimately this is your clinic, your money, and your lost time.

➤ Electricians and plumbers

While a contractor can do most things, if you need a toilet moved or pipes repaired, call a plumber. If you are moving switches and outlets, adding new or updating old electrical systems then call an electrician. The right person for the job is more likely to help you stay out of trouble by making sure the job is done the way it should be according to your city codes.

➤ HVAC

Heating, ventilation and air conditioning is a specialty you do not want to even touch unless you are planning a career change. If you are leasing professional space then most likely your HVAC needs are taken care of. However, if you are purchasing a property to renovate into an office you will need to acquire the services of someone in this field.

Offices need to have adequate ventilation, for starters. Proper ventilation in both treatment areas and offices will prevent that afternoon stuffy feeling. Also, you want to ensure the proper temperature for practicing acupuncture. Appropriate heating and cooling will provide a comfortable environment for your patients.

Most modern properties already have adequate heating and cooling systems. Then all you need to add is a little ventilation (fans or air purifiers for moxibustion) and you are ready to roll.

➤ Answering services

If you want to capture more patients on the first call to your clinic you've got two options: hire a receptionist or pay an answering service. When we first opened our clinic [ES] there was no money to afford a receptionist to answer patient calls. The result was that two-thirds of our first month's incoming calls ended in a hang-up. The only people who left messages on our trusty machine were patients we already had!

If you cannot hire help from the get go, invest in an answering service. People want to talk to a real person. Let's say someone is in intense pain or has the incredible urge to quit smoking NOW and they decide to actually pick up the phone and ask for help from the friendly neighborhood acupuncturist, even though they don't know you. When that prospective patient calls on a whim they will have all sorts of questions, but mostly they will want to talk to a living being on the other end of the phone. If no one answers, they may lose the impetus.

Saying this, you must also realize that the answering service will not have information regarding the benefits of acupuncture. However, you can give them a short script if they are willing to use it. You should also faithfully check your messages on an hourly basis (or wear your cell kept on vibrate mode) when you are in the office and on a daily basis when you are not.

Receptionist or office manager
Whether you think so or not, a receptionist or office manager is another professional that you need if you are a serious practitioner and will absolutely love having in your life! A good

---

POWER POINT

It is important when you go on vacation to have another practitioner to whom you can refer your patients if they need care. This practitioner's contact information should be left with your answering service and/or on your phone message machine. This relationship should, of course, be mutual and is very valuable. Leaving town without coverage for your active patients is, in some states, legally actionable as patient abandonment. Furthermore, shouldn't we all have someone with whom we regularly trade acupuncture and Chinese herbal care for ourselves?

---

receptionist is like having your mom at work. The phone is answered, the patients are greeted, forms are filled out, and databases kept up. If you are really lucky and you can pay a good salary, they will do your insurance billing, keep your herbal shelves stocked, clean the restrooms, and turn your treatment rooms between patients as well!

Nothing says "professional medical practitioner" like having a skilled receptionist. How many times in your life have you had the experience of the doctor herself picking up the phone when you call to make an appointment? Your grandfather may have some stories like that, but no one else in this country! The fact is that all medical offices have receptionists or other office help. This is not a luxury. It is a requirement if you want to dedicate yourself to the work you were trained to do: aiding in the health and welfare of your patients.

The day we hired our first receptionist [ES] we knew we couldn't afford to pay her. In fact, we hired her knowing that it could mean that we might forego a paycheck for one to two months. The result, however, was quite the opposite. She not only paid for herself, she ended up increasing our profits almost immediately.

By having someone else collecting for services, scheduling follow-up visits, and answering the phones we were, for the first time, allowed to just be practitioners. Not only did it not feel weird to treat someone with an illness and ask for money, but there was no problem telling them that only with XX number of follow-up sessions would they get better! The difference was amazing, and well worth the investment.

Not only do we have a receptionist, but we have what everyone needs . . . an advocate around town singing the praises of acupuncture. To this end, you want to ensure that you hire the right person for the job. Now this is not a book on conducting employment interviews, although I've done hundreds and would welcome any questions, so I will keep the following short and to the point [ES]. Also, we have an entire chapter on this subject elsewhere in this book (see Section 2, Chapter 10).

A receptionist should be able to fill the following requirements:
- A warm, friendly disposition
- Good phone etiquette and communication skills
- Computer literate
- Able to multi-task
- Trustworthy

Here's a final note on finding the right person. No matter how well someone may fit the bill of reception-type duties, you need to ask one very important question; "What is a lot of money to you?" We say this because if your perfect receptionist thinks that $60 is big money, then asking patients to pay $70–$100 for your examinations and treatments will seem like highway robbery to them. And, it will show on their face and in their voice. By finding a person, your representative, who thinks that your services are well worth the money asked in exchange, you will have a very valuable asset indeed.

When you are ready to hire this type of help in your clinic (read *as soon as possible*), either check online or call around to other medical practitioners or acupuncturists and see what the going rate is for reception pay. In the beginning you may only be able to offer a set amount with no benefits other than some holiday pay and free acupuncture. But as your company grows, so too must the benefit package. Don't be greedy. Share the wealth of your clinic (or any business venture) with those that help you make it great. Health benefits, life insurance, vacations and 401K's are how we take care of our employees. And, if you take care of them, they will always take care of your clinic and your patients. A well-run clinic and happy patients is what takes care of you. Again, for more detail on the subject of employees, see Section 2, Chapter 10 for the full report.

Janitorial

It goes without saying that a medical office of any type needs to be clean . . . really clean. Janitorial services, if not a part of your lease agreement, are quite inexpensive for the results. Unless you have the time to vacuum each treatment room, empty garbage, mop bare floors, dust all the flat surfaces, and clean the windows and bathrooms, you may want to consider hiring a janitorial service. Many companies offer a reasonable monthly rate for once a week cleaning. The more professional companies are also bonded and insured.

Yard maintenance

Many offices will not need this type of service because it is included in the lease agreement. However, if your clinic is in a freestanding building or you own the building yourself, then though it may seem trivial, ignoring it can eventually leave you in the weeds. There are many specific jobs you may want done depending upon your yard and any good company

> **POWER POINT**
>
> Remember that HIPAA law requires you to have a business associate agreement form on file for any service provider who is in your space on a regular basis and may have required or inadvertent access to your patient's medical records.

can help you with choosing what is appropriate. If you like to get out yourself and mow the lawn once a week, great! Then you can schedule a yard maintenance company to come out once per quarter to fertilize, trim, clean up, aerate, or whatever else needs to be done depending upon the season. Remember that leaving your yard neglected because you do not have time to pull the weeds will not help you pull in new business from those driving by!

➤ Snow removal services

This may never be a problem on the southern tip of Florida or in Hawaii or if your clinic is in a high-rise building with a covered garage. But if you are responsible for snow removal, don't wait until the first heavy snow to find someone to clear your parking lot. We recommend taking a few moments before the season begins to contact a few companies and get prices if you don't have your own snowplow. Your yard maintenance person may actually do this in winter but find out what they charge before the snow starts to fall. Also, find out how they prioritize their service. Do they send out crews to businesses first or is this one guy with a shovel or a plow? Using the services of an individual over a company might pay off with reduced rates, but the timing may not work if you open your clinic at 8 AM.

➤ Laundry service

This is another nice addition to save some time, energy, and water. If you have towels, sheets, gowns and the like, a laundry service can be the way to go. Imagine the amount of laundry required if you see 8–10 patients a day, and each uses a gown, towel, and sheet. That's potentially 30 pieces of laundry in just a day. If you have a laundry facility in your clinic, the situation may be manageable, but that is rare indeed. And, if you have two or more practitioners, this can quickly become a headache.

A laundry service will not only pick up and delivery, but your whites will gleam, and everything will be folded neatly and ready to be shelved. Once you grow to a point where laundry is crawling up and out of its bins in the closet, it's time to hire this out. Prices vary from service to service, and there are usually minimums, so check around.

➤ Medical transcription

Something to consider when you are experiencing rapid growth is a transcription service. Usually there is ample time in a day to complete charts as the patients are being seen, however there are some days when this is very difficult. A medical transcription service is a person or company who will take your recorded medical notes and transcribe them into written form to be placed into patient charts (paper or digital).

This service is not only for the very busy, it is also handy for the very messy or illegible writer. If you see many insurance patients requiring chart notes to be sent with billings, you may want to consider adding this service to your roster of business partners. Their services will make your charting cleaner, more professional, and definitely easier to read.

If this is something you decide to do, ensure that the company you are dealing with signs appropriate HIPAA nondisclosure forms. They will have full access to the patients' protected health information, including their disorders. To this end, you also want to make sure that you hire a professional company for this service and not Betsy from down the street who has fast keyboard skills. First of all, medical records must usually be written and presented in a very specific way for insurance companies and besides, Betsy probably knows everyone in town!

Billing service and clearinghouse

Even if you decide to hire a receptionist, at some point your accounts receivable can grow to such a size that you need to use a billing service. A billing service is an organization designed to handle everything related to billing and receiving payment for the services you provide. Be it billing patients directly for their visit or herbs or billing an insurance company, a billing service is built around the needs of the medical community. They are also required to be fully HIPAA compliant.

A clearing house is something that is more and more widely used now in the world of medical insurance billing. Many allopathic practitioners have been using these systems for years and, in fact, it was the advent of electronic billing and the billing clearing house that prompted the creation of HIPAA. When you bill electronically, you must use such a clearing house, which takes all of your insurance billing through an electronic submission called a batch and submits electronic CMS-1500 forms to the necessary insurance company.

Both billing services and clearing houses cost money. Some companies charge a flat rate by volume, others a flat rate plus a percentage of collected amounts. Be wary of any company that wants a percentage of the *billed* amount as this is usually a different rate than what is actually reimbursed to you by the insurance company. Also the percentages charged should be very small . . . certainly no more than 5%. One of the largest clearing houses is HBMA (Healthcare Billing & Management Association), online at www.hbma.com for more information. Another, with very inexpensive services, is Office Ally, online at www.officeally.com.

➤ Computer geek

Remember that kid in high school that everyone made fun of? The one that never had a girlfriend and instead sat at home on Saturday nights rewriting the code for *Space Invaders?* Well now you need that guy. Your resident computer techie, nerd, or geek is now a well-loved asset to almost every business. He (or she) is going to be your savior time and again, unless you are among the Neo-Luddites who refuse to accept the computer age in any form. Ours [HW] is practically a staff member at Blue Poppy because we have 14 computers!

You may never have 14 computers, but even one hard drive crash is all it takes to prove that it's good to know someone who can effectively communicate with computers and is not intimidated by their peculiarities. Not only will a computer tech be able to help with crashes and more minor computer disasters, they are also able to keep your system up-to-date with new and better hardware and technology as it is released, keep your equipment protected from viral infections, and help you with most computer-related problems or questions that arise. So, unless you plan on using an abacus to tally your cash receipts, you may wish to find a good techie before you need one.

Web designer

Web sites are either a powerful tool for your business or a fruitless waste of money. We won't get into all the purposes of a web site here (see Section 4, Chapter 7), but simply say that if you have a site and it is not well-designed and well-optimized, you will not capture the interest of potential patients. There are many ways to design the site yourself (or much of it), but making sure that someone will see it could require some assistance.

If you are going to invest in a website, I'd at least interview a web designer or two. You may be able to find a student that is learning HTML or Dreamweaver. Our first website in 1997 [HW] was done by a university student in a web design class. She was eager to learn and wanted a good grade in the class, so we got lots of work from her in a short period of time and even some minimal training on how to maintain the site ourselves. So, if you plan to have a website, protect your time and cash investment by bringing in at least a semipro-web designer to help you, even if you do some of the work yourself.

Marketing firm or specialist

Unless you are an expert in the field or have not yet read our chapters on marketing, you may find the services of a marketing firm useful. Not only do such firms develop ads, brochures, signs, press releases, and other tools tailored specifically to your needs, they can also put together and send out promotional mailings and press releases to specific mailing lists for you.

Marketing firms also usually maintain their own bulk mailing license, reducing the cost of targeted mailings.

That being said, you will see that in our chapters on marketing, we have not suggested anywhere the use of such services. It is more important for you to create a great clinic experience for your patients, request and reward their referrals, and to get out and get to know your community than to pay for fancy ads and brochures. Also, once you are seeing so many patients that you have no time to develop new marketing strategies or written materials, you can probably keep your marketing activities to a minimum, at least for a while if not permanently. Marketing firms are great, however, for those who have very little confidence in their own marketing abilities or for those who have no time at all due to family or other commitments. Even with the help of a marketing agency, however, you cannot avoid the need to create a wonderful clinic, keep your skills sharp, and network within your community.

➤ Graphic designer or artist

When it comes time to spice up your business cards, brochures, web site or the sign out front of your clinic, you are ready for a graphic designer. Different from an artist, a person in graphic design has a specialty in making logos, effective text, pictures, and visual effects on the computer. Having your "artwork" in a graphic file on computer allows you access to it for your everyday publishing needs.

An artist, on the other hand, is someone skilled in one or more media formats, often including computer graphics. An artist may not only be able to help you design the logo or brochure art that you seek, but may also provide you with art to decorate your clinic. Patients always like seeing original artwork, especially by someone local. Why not offer local artists a place to do showings that you rotate quarterly or semiannually? If you live in an "artsy" community, this is a great way to become more widely known as a team player and supporter of the arts.

Printers

With the exception of business cards, in the early days of your practice you may be able to do most of your printing in-house by purchasing a decent printer. However, like most of the services included in this chapter, there are always reasons to use a professional and sooner than you might think it will become more cost and time efficient not to be doing forms, brochures, and other printed materials yourself.

Shop around as prices vary. However, professional printing is actually quite affordable. Plus, ordering a few reams of your clinic intake forms, patient health history and the like will prevent you from running out at inopportune moments and may look far more professional. Also, many printers now use environmentally friendly papers and inks and will keep you from replacing so many plastic print cartridges, not to mention a burnt out printer. Finally, your printed pieces will look and feel professional and not home-made . . . unless homemade is the look and feel you want.

As publishers who have printed more typographical errors than we would care to remember, we can only say proofread, proofread, proofread. It is extremely disheartening to have 1,000 copies of something that looks really beautiful only to find two or three nasty typos that no one noticed. Hire a professional proofreader if you can, or have two or three people read your printed pieces backwards and forwards (we mean that literally) before you send them to the printer!!!

Banks

This is a no-brainer. The minute you open your doors for business you will no doubt be bringing in money, hopefully hand over fist, and much of it in the form of credit cards and checks. Once this trend begins we are hoping that it continues for you. However, you will need a place to put your money and that is usually a bank.

Check out banks in your local area first; it's always nice doing business with local people when you can. The key is finding out what a business account costs and what the benefits are at each institution. Most business accounts have some sort of service fee, unless you can get it waived by keeping a certain balance in the account. There may also be a limited number of checks you can write or deposits you can make before the bank will start assessing fees. Make sure to get all of this information.

Once you've made the rounds with all of the banks in town, sit back with a nice cup of tea and start comparing apples to apples. You are obviously looking for the best deal. It is sad to say, but you may find that you get better deals after you have been around for a year or so. Banks like to let you start with someone else and then try to capture your business after you are established. It's interesting how that big corporation will try to woo you away from the mom-and-pop bank later, when they wouldn't do anything much to help you on day one.

In most cases, what we say to you is this. Base your banking decisions on business, not personal loyalty. Unless, and this is a large unless, there is marketing value involved (for example the bank president refers you several new patients per year)! If you live in a small town and have a close personal relationship with people at the town's main bank, an extra $50–100 per year in banking expenses is worth it for the communitarian value. Otherwise, look for the best price for the best service. If you are getting that now, then don't switch banks. If the larger bank is going to cut you a deal, how long does it last? Make sure you get this all in writing before you change . . . but sometimes change is good. If you really like working with the bank that you use even though their financial deals and services are less attractive, go and talk to them. See how close they are willing to come to matching the offer of the larger bank.

➤ Bulk herb preparation services

If you live in a large city, especially one with a decent sized China Town or lots of Chinese medical clinics, you may want to farm out bulk herb prescriptions to one of them. This may change as you grow your practice and, who knows, you could become a bulk herb prep service yourself at a later date. In any case, you can at least check out who's out there and what their

---

POWER POINT

Checklist for Choosing a Business Bank

1. Can you get a personal banker to call whenever you have a question or problem? This relationship can be very helpful in a variety of ways.
2. Do they charge per check that you write? Under what circumstances will they waive that fee?
3. Do they offer free online banking for businesses?
4. Do they charge per check deposited? Under what circumstances will they waive those fees?
5. Can you use any credit card processing service you like (Costco for example)?
6. Are there minimum balance requirements?
7. Are there new customer perks and how long do they last?
8. What are the ATM card charges?
9. Are there any perks for small businesses such as yours that will save you time or money?
10. Is the bank friendly and do they seem enthusiastic about having your business?
11. Do they offer reasonably priced lines of credit to help you manage cash flow? What else will they do to help you grow your business?

service entails in prices, timing, and delivery service. In addition to whatever is local, at least one major U.S. distributor and several of the powder herb companies will do custom prescriptions and drop ship them directly to the patient using overnight shipping service.

Insurance

There are two types of insurance that you definitely want to carry as a business in the medical world. One is medical malpractice insurance, and the other is general liability. Insurance is usually not a happy word for people because, when you need to use it, usually something bad has happened. Looked at another way, however, insurance is a safety net for your practice and for all the patients that you are able to help. If an accident or an inadvertent mistake forced you out of business, many people would lose your services.

General liability insurance is something most businesses carry. It protects you in case a patient gets injured on your property due to your negligence, their lapse in attention, or mere happen-stance. Trust us, this is not a cost you ever wish to incur out of your own pocket. Nor, in fact, is liability insurance usually optional. It will cost you something, yes, but you are remiss if you do not carry it and often it will be required in any lease that you sign for business space. Many companies provide this type of insurance, it is usually not expensive, and you just call around to see who provides the best coverage for the lowest cost.

As for malpractice insurance, we find it a bit scary how many acupuncturists out there do not feel it is necessary. Arguments against carrying it usually center on a state's not requiring it or that no one ever gets hurt with acupuncture. But that is not true. In 2008, there were approximately 500 legal actions against acupuncturists in the U.S! And, in the world of MDs, the average is one lawsuit per doctor every 7–8 years, whether they did anything wrong or not! And even if you believe that you practice safely and conservatively, it does not mean that no one will sue you, claiming that they were hurt or injured, or that you were negligent in your needling practices, or your gowning techniques, or your use of moxibustion or herbal medicine. Malpractice insurance covers more than the injury to the patient, it also covers the cost of your defense.

I must admit [ES] that for some time we did not carry malpractice insurance in my clinic in Oregon. The list of "why-nots" was not very long... we just didn't want to spend the money on it. However, once we got into billing insurance for auto accidents and decided to get on a few of the major medical insurance panels around town, we had to change our position. In order to be paneled by any major insurance carrier you've got to have malpractice coverage. The minimum coverage acceptable by most panels was one million/three million dollars, so that's what we carry. And I have to say, now that I am on some 15 panels, all of which send me patients, the insurance is definitely worth it.

POINTS TO PONDER FROM CHAPTER 12

- There are many professionals in a variety of fields whose services will benefit you, save you time, and lower your stress level. This chapter gives you a long, if not comprehensive list.

- The belief that you have to be able to do everything in and for your clinic in order to save money is not true.

- If you don't have enough money right away, work out a barter system with some of these much-needed pros.

- Remember that in order to be paneled by any of the major insurance carriers, you must have malpractice insurance.

SECTION THREE

GETTING PAID

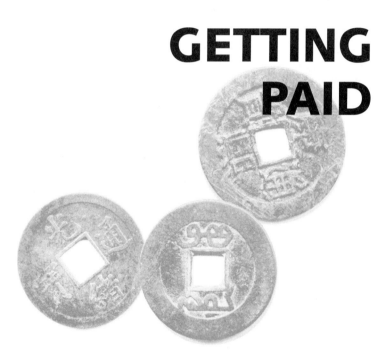

Attitudes About Money | 1

Few of us grow up without some issues where money is concerned. Add to that the fears that a new practitioner may have about the level of their skills compared to someone down the street who's been in practice for 5–10 years, and you have a perfect recipe for new practitioners of our medicine not being emotionally capable of charging and being paid what they could be and probably should be for their services.

In the case of the typical acupuncturist or other alternative health care practitioner, we must also acknowledge the common psychological stumbling block that some people encounter about charging people money when they are already sick or in pain. In this chapter, we'd like to try to help address some of these gut level issues that many people may have.

Money is such a fundamental and wholly integrated part of modern life that it touches every part of everything we do. In our culture, money can mean many things: survival, comfort, success, prestige, love, power, and access. Many books have been written on the subject and, if you believe that severe "money neuroses" are negatively affecting your personal or professional life, we encourage you to explore the resources listed in our bibliography. (See the Resources for Going Further section.)

> "Though mothers and fathers give us life, it is money alone which preserves it."
>
> —*Ihara Saikaku*

Within the scope of this book, however, we want to suggest several things with relationship to money. The first is that, as a businessperson, you need to understand your own money issues and figure out ways to work with them so that you don't sabotage yourself where making a living is concerned. We do have some suggestions with regard to this that we share in this chapter and others.

Second, with regard to "taking money" from sick people, we strongly suggest that you remember you are offering them services to help end or mitigate their suffering. If there is no appropriate exchange of energy for those services, it is commonly acknowledged among practitioners around the country that people are far less likely to actually get results from your treatments.

Third, and even more important and fundamental, we want to suggest to you that, *while greed or the love of money may be the root of all evil,* money itself is not. In fact, I'd [HW] like to suggest that very few, if any, good things come from poverty. If you truly consider all the worst ills in this world, many of them have a very direct relationship with poverty and its alter ego, greed. The desperation that leads people to become terrorists, to kill endangered species, to tear down the rainforests, or to murder or maim or sell others into slavery—these are most often due to poverty.

As you read this book, I encourage you to think about the good you can and will do with the prosperity that we hope to help you create. What would it be like if you could give away vast (or even modest) sums of money? Why do other types of health practitioners or other acupuncturists deserve more than you? Why can't you get to a place of financial comfort and prosperity similar to others? If you really don't like money and are uncomfortable with charging patients, can you come up with a practice that allows you to give it away for free and be supported in the world by some other method? However, if money and any discussion about it is *really that uncomfortable* for you, perhaps you need to find new ways to think about and relate to money in your life or get some help from a psychologist-money counselor. (Yes, these problems are common enough that such people do exist.)

Since we don't live in a fairy-tale world where no one needs to create a source of income, try for a moment to think of money in all its forms as a method of energy exchange, a form of qi, if you will. We all simply exchange our time and energy in lesser or greater amounts to get what we want or need to survive in the world. Our car requires so much energy per week to buy and maintain and no one expects to own a car and maintain it for nothing. Similarly, our house, food, utilities, and clothes all require some exchange of energy. No one should expect to get your services for free either. And, you should not feel that you are doing your patients a disservice by charging what you need to make a decent living. If you don't charge what you need and deserve, you will burn out and not be able to help anyone. Remember that 30-50% of acupuncture graduates are not in practice within five years of graduating, whether they have paid back their school loans or not! If you get your head and heart right with money, you are far less likely to be on the wrong side of these statistics.

> **Family messages**

Everyone "downloads" the family line (or lines) about money. Our deepest true beliefs about this mysterious stuff are probably pretty hardwired before we are five or six years old. So think back and look at what the cliches were that you heard in your household. Things like,

> "Money is the seed of money, and the first guinea is sometimes more difficult to acquire than the second million."
>
> —Jean Jacques Rousseau

"money doesn't grow on trees," "do you think I'm made of money?," "a penny saved is a penny earned," or "money is the root of all evil." (That is not, by the way, what it actually says in the Bible. It is the *love* of money that is the root of all evil according to the *Old Testament*.) In any case, we all got these messages, and, as young children, we mostly believed what we heard.

The problem with all this is that whatever we learned about this most fundamental part of life can have a way to come back and bite us if it does not mesh well with reality. For example, if we believe deep down that a camel has a better shot at getting through the eye of a needle than a rich man has of getting into heaven, this could make it difficult for us not to unconsciously sabotage our own efforts at financial success, even if practicing Chinese medicine is not really going to make us hugely rich. That is why it is important for us to really look at our personal money beliefs and become as conscious of them as we can. It is the "stuff" that is left unconscious that is most likely to stand in our way as people. When we know what our issues are, at least we can be more aware of and, hopefully, more in control of our responses.

Think about your parents and their money "styles."

- Was Mom a worrier and Dad a big spender?

- Was Mom always trying to get more money out of Dad, who tried to keep control of every last dime?

- Did you ever get into trouble as a child in relationship to money? What impact did these things have on your beliefs about money? What impact do you think this has or will have on your business life?

- What one thing in your relationship with money would you like to change?

- Can you give yourself a money assignment to become more conscious about how you work (or don't work) with money?

- What about keeping a journal about your responses to money: spending it, making it, accepting it, sharing it?

Almost everyone has some issues around money. It's pretty hard not to. However, if you think there are issues here that are beyond your ability to work with on your own, look for a counselor or psychologist to help you sort through this part of your life. For someone trying to operate a small business, it is more important than you might believe and can have an impact on your close relationships as well as your professional success.

One final note. If you have beliefs about money that are pretty negative and you don't want to change them for whatever reason but you still want to practice acupuncture, our suggestion is that you get a job. Find another practitioner, hospital, MD, or public clinic that will pay you a flat salary with no requirement for you to collect money, market your services to any extent, or have any money decision-making responsibilities. We have heard of such positions. Here's another possibility. You might try offering your services to an organization that will send you to somewhere in the Third World to do acupuncture in a free clinic. Such organizations do exist and can do wonderful work in the world. This allows you to leave the creation of money for your services and supplies completely to someone else. You will, in this case, probably not be paid at all, at least not in the form of money. But if you are not looking for money in exchange for your work, this style of practice is an option and not a bad one. However, even a life of voluntary simplicity that feeds your heart and not your pocketbook may take some work on your part to create. Either way, getting clear on your relationship to money and how you truly feel about it is fundamental to your success.

> ## PRACTITIONER POINTER
>
> "I believe that people decide where to go for health care based on where they believe they can get the best care and not based on who has the lowest prices."
>
> —Jonathan B. Ammen
> Boston, MA

255

POINTS TO PONDER FROM CHAPTER 1

- Do you have a healthy relationship with money?

- What if you could give away millions, or even just hundreds, every year?

- Patients who don't exchange anything for health services, often do not get well.

- What did you learn from your family about money and what is the impact of those messages on your business life? If the impact is negative, what could you do to change it?

- If you really have issues that are handicapping your life, get professional help.

- If you don't want money in exchange for your work, find a way to give it away that will allow you to live in harmony with your beliefs.

Methods of Payment for Your Patients | 2

As a health care practitioner, you are providing a service. As an acupuncturist, you are providing a very valuable service. In return, your patients are going to exchange some "green qi." There are at least nine different forms of payment that you may have to consider in your practice. It is wise to have at least thought about each of them and decided whether, when, and how to accept these methods of exchange.

When a patient comes into your clinic, some practice management gurus suggest that you should classify them by the way that they pay. Doing this not only keeps you abreast of how your clinic is getting its income, but it also helps you balance your payment spectrum. You may never want to have too many of one classification of payment type, except, of course, cash patients. It is best to keep things apportioned, sort of like a stock portfolio, so that your income has more than one stream. For example, if all you see is insurance patients for the one major company in town with 15,000 employees and they change their plan to no longer cover acupuncture, you are now out of luck for patients.

So, instead of keeping your entire set of patient eggs in one money-basket, try to spread things around a little bit. If you've got plenty of insurance and managed care patients, try to bring in some personal injury or cash patients. If you have plenty of cash patients, consider bartering to get some of the things you want and need without using cash at all. By maintaining a variety of patients based on their payment method, you will be better prepared to handle any economic challenge that may befall any one of those sectors.

"Not having a diversified cash base can have its drawbacks. The month that the U.S. went to war in Iraq (February 2003), the cash base in our clinic went from 75% to 45%. People everywhere were spending less money. Although our acute patients remained steady, the chronic ones were more likely to drop off treatment plans or space their treatments farther apart. Our solution? We spent time with each of our patients talking to them about their insurance coverage. Some of them were self-insured, while others had company policies that they could chose from. We gave all of them information on insurance companies that we bill for acupuncture with great success. Within 45 days, we had recovered our total patient base by increasing our insurance billing."

—*Eric Strand*
Canby, OR

➤ Cash

We all love cash. It is the green qi of instant gratification. Cash payments should and probably will make up the major portion of your patient payment pie-chart, especially in the early days of your clinical practice. Actually, cash payments come in three types: paper greenbacks, checks, and credit cards. These are all equal, which is one reason that you cannot offer patients a *cash* discount over insurance companies. The check the insurance company sends you *is* cash. While checks and actual greenbacks are nice, of course, you will find that many of your patients will use credit cards if they can. You will also find that patients and even visitors to your clinic buy more of the things you have on display for sale if they can use a credit card to make the purchase.

POWER POINT

On your clinic financial policies form that each patient must read and sign, you should state that while you are willing to bill for insurance payments if the patient's policy reimburses for acupuncture and the deductible has already been met, the patient is, at the end of the day, responsible for the payment of all fees. You may also say that payment is expected at the time services are rendered "unless other arrangements have been made in advance of treatment." If you are unsure of the patient's insurance status at the time they come in but the patient states that they want to bill insurance, you may tell them that until their insurance status can be checked you will give them a superbill in order that they can get reimbursement directly from their insurance company for all or any part of the fees they pay to you.

➤ Credit card machines

If you don't yet have a credit card machine, we highly encourage you to get one. There are a number of sources for getting equipment and processing. When you are interviewing banks to establish your business account, talk to them about their merchant services department and their charges for credit card processing fees and equipment. They are usually more than happy to send a representative to your office.

Costco is another good source for merchant services if you are a member and don't want to go the bank route. Some state and national acupuncture associations also have merchant services agreements for very low cost processing fees for group members. We caution you against using one of the companies that send out postcards offering low rate credit card machines and processing fees. Many times such companies go out of business quickly or stop providing customer service. Go with the larger companies that have been around for some time.

When you are shopping for credit card machines, there are a number of factors to take into account before signing up. First and foremost, there are usually at least three different charges that you must pay: 1) the lease or payment price of the machine, 2) the monthly fee for using the merchant services, and 3) a percentage fee taken from each transaction.

If you buy a machine outright, then your monthly charges will be less. However, your initial outlay of cash could be $250–900 depending on the speed and age of the equipment. Another purchase option is to make monthly payments, in which case you pay off the machine over a number of years with interest. This is a better route if you want to own a machine but don't have the cash up front to buy one. Be warned, however. Owning a credit card machine means that if it breaks or becomes outdated, you have to fix it or buy a new one all over again. You can also buy cheaply through E-bay. If you do that, however, check with your card services company to be sure the machine you want to bid on is still useable!

If you lease a machine, typically you sign up for some term of service, usually at least a year. If the machine breaks or becomes outdated, the company will fix or replace it at no charge. That's a nice feature. However, when you lease a machine, you never, ever pay it off. Instead of laying out money with an eventual end in sight, you are paying rent that does not stop. In my experience [HW], there is no right or wrong way to do this. I have both rented and purchased credit card machines. The equipment is usually reliable, rarely needs servicing, and will last several years before it is too outdated to use. If you can get used equipment for a good price, it's not bad to own it. We have two machines, one of which is a few years old and still works fine.

The percentage rates you pay on each transaction will vary depending on the company you go with and the volume of credit business you do per month. Also, if you only do on-site sales where the credit card is present, your rate will be better than if you are doing mail order sales. A good rate is anything less than 2.0%, especially if your company is in its infancy. Unfortunately, you may not get the best offers and the best rates until you've been taking credit cards for a year or more and the companies that offer these services can see that you are reliable. For this reason, we suggest finding the best rates you can with the shortest time requirements. After one year, start making phone calls to all of the local financial institutions. Tell them you are shopping for a new *merchant services provider.* Let them all bid their best prices to you and see what you get. You do not necessarily have to change the lease or buy out of your equipment in order to change service providers.

Time-of-service cash discounts

While you may wish to discuss any specific questions about this with the Office of the Insurance Commissioner in your specific state, in most states it is not illegal to offer a *payment-at-the-time-of-service discount.* According to an article by John Frostad, L.Ac., in the Winter, 2002 issue of *Extraordinary Points,* this type of discount is legally defensible because it saves you time and postage, reduces risk of nonpayment for services rendered, and means that you don't have to wait for payment. While there don't seem to be any guidelines on minimum or maximum discounts in this case, to be legally defensible the discount should be roughly the same as what the savings are to you for not having to bill for your services and wait for payment . . . say 5–10%. You do not have to offer such a discount to patients for whom you are billing their insurance, but you must offer the discount if they are paying you directly but billing their insurance themselves. You also do not need to offer this discount to a patient to whom you will be sending a bill after services are rendered.

> ## Fee for services insurance

Despite the obvious advantages of cash payments, if you take only cash patients you will shut out several other types of paying patients. Insurance patients are one of those types. The type we are discussing here is where you bill the insurance company every time you see the patient and they send you a check of some amount. The remaining balance, if any, is billed directly to the patient or to the patient's credit card that you have on file. This is likely to be the second largest group of patients that you will have.

Acupuncture coverage is, at present, the most common request of people who are buying new health insurance policies. It used to be that when an employee organization was asking for health coverage they wanted first major medical, then vision and dental. The number one request of employees today after major medical is acupuncture and alternative care. This means that more and more insurance companies are scrambling to add alternative care coverage so they don't lose their payers. When employees speak, employers listen and go shopping for the health plan that makes everyone the happiest.

People with insurance like to use their benefits. Usually they are paying some sort of monthly contribution to their insurance plan. So getting them to reschedule for more than one appointment is not that difficult. Therefore, insurance patients will typically follow through with any given course of treatment you suggest and often take more treatments than a cash patient, as long as your treatment plan shows that the care is *medically necessary.* That is a favorite phrase in the world of insurance companies. What it means in practical terms for you is that things like stress reduction and *zang-fu* balancing treatments are not usually covered under the plan and will be denied.

All insurance plans, however, recognize pain as a medically necessary treatment issue and will cover that if they cover acupuncture at all. All of the ICD-9/10 codes related specifically to pain are in the 7xx.xx series. For instance, low back pain is 724.2; shoulder pain is 719.41; and ankle pain is 719.47. Therefore, my suggestion with insurance companies (if you are *not* in the state of California and if the patient is *not* coming in with a diagnosis from an MD) is to bill for the pain. If the patient complains of RA or OA, then bill for the areas of the body where the pain is and you are far less likely to have difficulty getting your treatments covered. For more on the "ins and outs" of insurance billing, see Chapter 3 in this section.

P O W E R   P O I N T

A great idea to increase your insurance base is to canvas the area that you practice in. Find out what insurance programs the largest companies offer their employees and find out if your services are covered by the policy they use. By establishing some sort of relationship with the human resources (HR) director at this company you will be able to find out all of the answers you need. Once you find a local or regional company with coverage for acupuncture services, send the HR director some information on acupuncture and what it can do for people: treatment or prevention of colds and flu, quick pain management and resolution resulting in decreased downtime and increased productivity, or whatever you specialize in. Ask if you can send enough flyers to put something in each employee's pay envelope, or on the bulletin board in the employee break room, maybe a free lecture about acupuncture care as part of the company lecture series. Perhaps just letting those people know that acupuncture is a covered benefit is enough to spur an initial few patients. And, once the word gets around about the quality results you provide, you have yourself a nice patient population to draw from.

➤ Managed care

This is not usually the friendliest method of payment. However, it is one of the nine ways that patients will want to pay. Managed care is like insurance, only worse—for practitioners, that is. Managed care organizations function as the middleman between the practitioner and the insurance company. A managed care network is an organization that offers to collect a panel of certain providers for insurance companies for some set rate per insured each month. This does two things. First, it gives the insurance company a quick way to ensure that their clients are getting quality care from trained, licensed, and insured providers. Second, it limits the amount that the company pays for a type of medicine they know nothing about and haven't a real way of learning.

In order to participate with a managed care network, you have to be accepted to their panel. This is done by contacting the provider relations department of that network, getting and submitting an application, and sometimes paying an application fee. Once you've jumped through those hoops, the network will send you a copy of your signed contract and a fee schedule with acceptable billing codes. What this means is that you are limited not only in how much you can collect from the insurance company, but you are limited in what CPT codes you can bill for. Most importantly, being a provider for a managed care network means you cannot ever collect any other money from the patient other than a predetermined co-pay.

Think about this for a moment. If you typically bill $100 for an acupuncture visit but the managed care network only pays $50 (including the $10 co-pay you collect from the patient on the day of the visit), you have essentially cut your rates in half. The rest of that $100 bill is gone—poof. You cannot collect it from the patient, nor will you ever get it from the insurance company. So, is this necessarily a bad thing?

If you have done the budget exercises and have a clear idea of what your clinic needs to make per hour, it may be. If you only have the ability to see one patient per hour and your clinic needs to generate $65 per hour, then accepting this patient through this network means you are operating at a loss. You may as well give that patient $15 the moment they walk into your office. On the other hand, if you can see more than one patient per hour (by having more rooms or shortening the treatment to 30 minutes), then you are still operating in the profit zone.

Another way to think about managed care patients is not just on what the insurance company limits you to but to think of what that patient means to you over the course of a year or the potential life of that patient's need for your care, which could be several years. Chances are they can get X number of visits per year under the limitations of their policy. Say 12. Well, that means $600 to your bottom line. If you are not completely booked every day, wouldn't it be foolish to throw away $600 per year? You bet it would be. You may also want to consider the number of referrals that this patient can or will turn into who are *not* managed care patients. Also, you might consider only scheduling these patients on your least busy days when other, cash-paying patients are not wanting appointments.

Whether you decide to accept managed care patients or not will vary depending on your clinic's cost per hour, the number of patients you can successfully see in one hour, the overall income that patient means to your clinic, and what kind of referral base they may generate. In the long run, it is patient care that is important, but you need to determine why you will or will not accept managed care before doing so and have real numbers to back up your determination.

➤ Medicaid

This is a state insurance program for low-income individuals and children. The payment rate for these types of programs is typically extremely low. In California, the payment is only around $16–17 per visit, and they are only allowed two visits per month. This is by no means a decent payment for our services. However, it is ground-breaking. State-controlled insurance policies paying for acupuncture services is a governmental concession that acupuncture works.

Not all states cover acupuncture for their low-income people. Medi-Cal is the name of the insurance program in California, and it definitely pays—but not well. In other states, the program is called Medicaid, and the coverage of acupuncture varies from state to state. In Oregon, the Oregon Health Plan used to cover acupuncture but has been dropped in recent years due to budget woes. Your best course of action, if you are interested in working with low-income insurance, is to contact your state's Insurance Commission and find out if acupuncture is covered, at what rate it is reimbursed, and how many visits per month the patients are authorized. If such care is an option in your state, you believe in offering services to the economically disadvantaged, you have a clinic with multiple, semiprivate treatment spaces, and you can work on several patients at the same time with simple treatment protocols, you might be able to make this work at least a couple of days per week.

Everyone needs health care, even, and probably especially, the low-income and underserved of our nation. However, before you consider taking on this type of insurance, make sure you are still able to operate your clinic at a profit. The owner of your building will not take pity on you for lapsing on your lease payments because you are treating people out of the goodness of your heart. While your heart may be huge, you must balance out this type of work with treatments that net you more income. Again, the more you diversify, the more you are able to do things like treat people *pro bono* or for very small payments.

Medicare

As of this writing, acupuncture is still not a covered Medicare benefit. Medicare is federal health insurance for seniors and the disabled. The fact that we are not covered does not relieve us from needing to associate with this organization, however. Typically, many seniors will come to your office with dual coverage, possibly from a retirement plan or another supplemental insurance program. If this is the case, then Medicare is considered their primary insurance and, before you send a bill to the secondary insurance, you need to get it denied by the primary (insurance billing 101).

Here's the part of the system that works against us, but we will show you how to get around it. You see, everyone out there in the insurance world knows that Medicare does not cover acupuncture services. They know it, but the system is set so that you still have to get a denial of benefits. Ah, but there's a catch to getting that required letter of denial. When you send your CMS 1500 to Medicare to get your letter of denial, they will either take 2–3 months to return it to you or they will send it back with a letter telling you that since they don't cover acupuncture, they cannot even deny your claim. Ugh!

So here's what you can do. Instead of sending a new claim form to that great, big, red-tape organization each time you need a letter of denial, get one letter of denial that is generic and use that for all of your future billings. How do you get a generic "we do not cover acupuncture" letter? I'm glad you asked. If you look on the wonderful Website that comes with this book, there is a letter of denial in the insurance forms section which you can download and use. ● It will work in at least some cases. That being said, this type of patient should only comprise a *very* small proportion of your payment pie.

➤ Workers' Compensation

Workers' Compensation is another type of insurance program. It deals with employees that have been injured on the job. Not all states require the coverage of acupuncture by Workers' Comp. However, many do. Colorado is at the forefront when it comes to this type of insurance. The acupuncturists there are not considered primary care physicians and are not allowed to evaluate and diagnose Workers' Comp cases but they can be selected as the individual's choice of care once they've been seen by their primary care physician.

Workers' Compensation pays very well in some states. However, the plans and coverage vary widely from state to state and plan to plan. The best bet, if you are not in Colorado, is to call your state's Insurance Council and ask what the coverage policy for acupuncture is and what is the rate of reimbursement? Other questions you may want to ask:

> *Are there any special forms or reports?*
> *What CPT codes are acceptable and payable by Workers'*
> *Comp?*
> *How many treatments can a patient receive?*
> *And, most importantly, do you need a referral from an MD*
> *before treatments can be billed?*

Some practitioners have a very large proportion of this type of patient. If you have lots of medium to large manufacturing companies in your area, your clinic has multiple rooms, and you can stay focused enough to do a patient every 30 minutes for a few days per week, you may want to specialize in this type of patient. See Section 3, Chapter 5 for more specific information on working with Workers' Comp patients.

➤ Personal Injury

Auto-accident insurance pays for acupuncture in just about every state in the union at this point. This is another call and check issue. However, if you can bill auto insurance for personal injury (PI), then you should by all means do so. In the state of Oregon, personal injury payments include all *medically necessary* treatments or modalities up to $10,000. You don't have to be a rocket scientist to figure out that covers a whole lot of acupuncture.

The best things about billing PI is that, unless there is complex litigation going on with your patient's case, they pay what you bill (within reason), there is no co-pay, and there is no deductible. This means the patient can see you for relief and does not have to worry about amassing large medical bills that need to be paid out of pocket. See Section 3, Chapter 4 for more detail on dealing with PI cases.

P O W E R   P O I N T

A few words of caution on billing auto insurance companies:

- They have lawyers—lots of them. Make sure that the services you provide are indeed medically necessary and that you have very good, very clear chart notes. Do not try to string out a patient's treatment plan so you can make your overhead in the first week of the month.

- Make sure the patient signs in for each and every treatment. It is not unheard of that a patient will seek legal assistance when dealing with their insurance company. Your records could be subpoenaed regarding any case. If they didn't sign in on the date you say that they received acupuncture, the only proof is in your word

---

"Power Point" continues on the next page

and the patient's—and that may not be enough to hold up. Paying bills and taxes is hard enough. Don't be forced to send money back to the insurance company that you actually earned!

- Send in your CMS forms in a timely manner. If you save them up and the patient is getting other medical care at the same time, then the insurance company pays them in the order received. Obviously, we know that our services should be paid first as they are the most effective, but we are the *only* ones who know that.

➤ Trade or Barter

In the beginning stages of your clinic, this is a very good way to acquire services that you would otherwise have to pay for. Straight trades are just that. "I do this for you for free, and you do this for me for free." That's a trade. Bartering is, "I'll do this for you at no cost and you give me X number of dollars off of that" or the other way around. This is a fine system for any clinician to use some of the time. However, make sure the trade or barter terms are clear in advance.

If you are trading, then it is a trade across the board. For example, I [ES] do trades with a massage therapist. I get a nice massage once a month and she gets a great acupuncture/tui-na session once per month. Our services may be set at different rates, but we take the other's service as trade for our own. Another great trade that we do is for our CPA. She comes in for stress relief or headaches, and we get our books and taxes done *a gratis.* I have never used acupuncture to barter someone's cost of services down. However, I am looking for someone to restore my 1969 Mustang who is willing to trade or barter!

➤ Free

It doesn't sound like a very good method of payment, but this is an option for every practitioner. Friends, family, neighbors, or animals . . . at some point, we all give our services away. There are a variety of reasons for this and all of them sound good at the time. I [ES] don't charge my Mom when she is here visiting from Florida because I don't think she should have to pay. Would I bill her insurance if that was an option? Maybe.

P O W E R   P O I N T

Hardship Waiver Forms and Sliding Scales

It is not illegal to have a sliding scale or to discount your services based on the financial need of the patient. Many medical clinics, Planned Parenthood for example, have such discount programs, usually based on federal poverty guidelines. We have listed the most recently published federal numbers on the website along with a Financial Hardship form to have people fill out if they are requesting a discount based on financial need. ● You may wish to and probably should ask patients requesting a discount for some type of proof of their assertions. This can be three months of bank statements or last year's tax return.

You do not need to offer these discounts to patients for whom you are billing insurance. You also need not advertise that your clinic has discounted services but only provide information if they inquire about such a discount program or if you think it is appropriate for a specific patient. There are no minimum or maximum discount amounts mandated by law. In deciding what your discounts should be, remember that people will benefit more from your services if they exchange something fair for them in return.

Free patients are just that—free. Maybe you give someone a free treatment after they've come in for 10 paid sessions—kind of like a coffee shop. Or, perhaps you treat low-income people for free on the third Wednesday of each month as a sort of community service (and a great marketing idea if you've got the time and energy). The key with "free" is that it should not interfere with your clinic's potential to support itself and to support you. Also remember that, statistically, patients who don't pay anything for their treatment don't get well as fast as those who do pay something. So, whatever mix of payment methods you do accept in your clinic, it seems that there needs to be at least some kind of energy exchanged in order for patients to get the results they are coming to you for.

PRACTITIONER POINTER

"I pay myself first. Not the rent, the electricity, the herb company, or the phone company. I am the most important bill in my business. I have included my bill as part of the overhead and, as always, I 'goal' for the result and it always comes to fruition. When there are moments in the month that I think it might not happen, I think in my mind that I can cut back on my bill to myself. Then I call my mentor. She tells me that if I were electric or water, I would be turned off. So focus on your purpose and the practice will provide. Sounds like religion but, damn, it works month after month."

—*Susan Schiff*
Delray Beach, FL

➤ One final note about freebies and payments

We don't suggest that you give away "a first trial treatment" as a promotion. Oh, you will get calls and people coming in for those free treatments, but 90% of them are "tourists" who will not come back again when you discuss your fees for further care. They got it free the first time. So why should they consider paying you? These treatments do nothing for your long-term growth and even less for your self-esteem and sense of value. If you want to give away something, offer free 10-minute new patient consultations. This is a good idea and you can state this offer on your after hours phone message, on a little sign in your office, or on the back of your business card or your clinic brochure. When you do these, have a standard list of 5–6 questions that you ask (we give you a script you can tweak for this in Section 4, Chapter 3 under "script for working a health fair"). Then you give some fairly standard answers, which includes a closing statement something like:

"We have experience helping people in your situation, but we need to do a complete exam and intake to know everything about you and your specific case. I'd love to be able to help you with your health issues and I think Oriental medicine can be a wonderful resource for you. We take new patients on Mondays and Wednesdays. I'd be happy to have our front desk person schedule an appointment for you."

Hand the person some literature and your card. This is where your eye contact, tableside manner, and general demeanor sell you to that potential patient. But don't give away treatments except in rare situations or as demos at speeches and live events. Remember that in life, time is the one thing that you cannot ever get back.

POINTS TO PONDER FROM CHAPTER 2

- In order for your income to be balanced, it's a good idea for your clinic to accept more than one type of patient based on the various way patients can pay.

- Cash patients are great. However, you may find that insurance, PI, Workers' Comp, and managed care patients are more reliable sources of income for your clinic during tough economic times. So don't count them out.

- If you don't have a credit card machine, get one. You will find that patients are happier to pay you that way than to write a check. They may be more willing to take their herbs or buy other products you sell in your clinic if they can pay with a credit card. There are many companies who sell credit card machines and card services accounts. Shop around for a reliable, well-priced service.

- Regular health insurance, Workers' Compensation insurance, personal injury, and managed care patients can all be a part of your practice mix. If you have adequate clinic space, are well organized, and have a good front desk person, you can probably figure out a way to make each of these types of patients add to your bottom line.

- Trade or barter only for things you really want, not just to do someone a favor. You won't give them a good treatment if you don't really want what they are trading for in the first place.

- Be careful about free treatments. Patients who don't give back any kind of energy in exchange are less likely to get better than patients who do.

The Ins and Outs of Billing Insurance | 3

Insurance companies across the U.S. today are looking very carefully at acupuncturists and the services they offer. This is because acupuncture continues to grow in popularity and consumers want their insurance packages to include coverage for acupuncture. When you are deciding whether or not to accept insurance patients, remember that the insurance-billing process is both a blessing and a burden. While adding the ability to accept insurance can increase your income significantly, it also increases paperwork by the same percentage. And, you need to know that the amount of reimbursement for acupuncture services varies from company to company and from state to state. The purpose of this chapter is to help you decide whether or not to do insurance-billing, to explain how to work with insurance companies so that you have the smoothest possible relationship with them, to learn what forms you will need and how to complete them, and, ultimately, how to get paid promptly.

➤ The Gamble

The world of insurance-billing for anyone not trained in medical office administration can be, at first, rocky and stressful. However, once you conquer the insurance-billing learning curve, it can also open the door to a new patient population, leading to further financial growth. Furthermore, patients with insurance coverage are typically more willing to come in more frequently. You can see where this leads—straight to your bank account.

So why is it a gamble? Well, for starters, not all insurance companies pay the same rate for the same services. All companies will pay what they call a "usual, reasonable and customary" amount, of which you may only receive a percentage. While some insurance companies will pay whatever you bill (*e.g.,* personal injury insurance), at other times you may only get paid 50 cents on the dollar. The rules on whether you can retrieve the balance from the patient will be established by the type of insurance coverage as well as any contractual agreement you may or may not have with that company.

POWER POINT

Basics to Remember When Accepting Patients Who Want to Use Their Insurance Benefits

- Remember that the insurance policy you are billing for reimbursement is a contract between the patient and the insurance company. Fundamentally, it has little to do with the practitioner. The benefits are available to the patient, not to you specifically.

- The patient controls the monies paid out from the insurance policy. They can choose to pay or to stop payments to any and all providers.

- If benefits have been assigned to you, the treating practitioner, then your office procedure should without question have a system and procedure to verify the insurance benefits, *before you accept the assignment.*

- You must decide how much credit are you willing to extend to the patient before any payment is made. And how much time are you willing to extend that credit: 30, 60, 90 days or more.

- If you accept assignment of benefits, be sure the signature is on file for both:
  a. release of information form
  b. assignment of benefits form

"Power Point" continues on the next page

- Always follow the proper procedure for billing patients on a regular 30-day period. If the patient is not notified of the balance due to your office for any service you render, then the patient does not have to pay unless you have an agreement based on the time limit you are willing to extend credit. (See bullet point #4 above.) It is good business procedure to bill every 30 days for any unpaid balance, even if the insurance was supposed to reimburse for those treatments.

- Always remember that the insurance company will pay their percentage of what they deem is allowable under the benefit package of the patient. They may not pay the expected 80% of the total charges. They might pay only the amount that they (the insurance adjusters) deem "medically necessary." In most cases this is far less than the 80-100% you might be expecting.

Once you have read this chapter and understand all of the requirements for filling out the CMS-1500 form, you should have little problem billing insurance for your patients.

Types of Insurance

There are many types of insurance out there, and, in order to figure out whether and how they will pay for your services, it helps to understand how each type works with their clients.

Fee for service insurance:

This is insurance coverage that reimburses directly to the provider as long as they accept an assignment of benefits to the provider (in this case you) from the insured person. The amount of reimbursement is usually some percentage of what is called in the insurance world "usual, customary, and reasonable" charges. Each insurance company has what they call a *relative value schedule* (RVS) for all types of medical services, including acupuncture, by which they determine how much they should be required to reimburse for all the various services included in all their policies. Based upon the usual, customary, and reasonable RVS listing for acupuncture according to their company, they may pay for all, a portion, or none of your services. Based upon each patient's specific coverage, they may or may not be expected or required to pay you some additional portion of the total bill, which amount is called a *co-pay*. We will discuss below how you can find out if and how much they pay, and whether the patient is responsible for any co-pay.

Managed care:
Managed care companies are organizations that go to the insurance companies, offer to find and credential practitioners in each of the professional fields that they cover, and place them on a "panel." Patients using such managed care coverage have the option to select a practitioner only from among those on the credentialed panel. Services rendered by any practitioner on the panel are reimbursed by the insurance company at a predetermined rate. Some companies require a patient co-pay ($10-30 for example). Some companies require an application fee from the practitioner wishing to be included on a panel. Others take a piece of the amount being paid to the practitioner each time services are billed. This gives patients the financial incentive of lower out-of-pocket cost when they choose a practitioner who has been credentialed on their plan.

Medicaid:
This is a federal health care plan for low income Americans administered by state governments. The name of the plan varies from state to state. It pays, when available, similar to a fee for service insurance company. Reimbursement per service rendered is usually very low and usually no co-pays are allowed if you decide to offer your services to such patients.

Medicare:

This is a federal insurance plan for seniors and disabled persons administered under the Social Security Act. At the time of the printing of this book, there is no coverage for acupuncture under Medicare. There is, however, a bill before Congress, H.R. 1477, the Hinchey Bill, which would amend Title 18 of the Social Security Act and Title 5 of the U.S. Code so that qualified acupuncturist services will be reimbursable under Medicare Part B and also under the Federal Employees Health Benefits Program.

Workers' Compensation:

This subject is large enough that we have given it its own chapter below. Suffice it here to say that Workers' Compensation is industrial insurance required in all states to cover employees who may be injured on the job. Coverage for acupuncture varies from state to state but can be a good way to expand your income. The most important caveat for practitioners who want to bill this type of insurance is to learn the rules regarding billing and paperwork and follow them to the letter. See Chapter 5 below for complete details.

Personal Injury (PI):

This is insurance coverage for people involved in auto or other types of accidents. Such accidents could be the fault of the insured person or another party. Again, this type of insurance varies from company to company and may have state requirements as well. While some PI cases allow you to get paid as you go, it is important to note that, in PI cases where there is an unresolved lawsuit against the allegedly responsible party, you may have to wait some time to receive reimbursement. You also take the chance that the patient will lose their case and you may not get paid at all! If you choose to take on such lawsuit cases for the potential long-term payoff, it is important to have a good working relationship with the attorneys involved, maintain the proper paperwork to document what you are doing, and to be in touch with all parties involved regularly. (See the "skunk test" below to help you determine if an attorney is someone you do or do not want to work with.) It is also wise to have a clear assignment of benefits contract with the patient and possibly with the law firm working on their behalf. ● Most personal injury insurance billing requires regular accompanying chart notes and reports.

P O W E R   P O I N T

"Skunk Test" for Attorneys

1. Will the attorney sign your lien? Will the attorney return the lien to you?
2. Will the attorney send you a copy of the settlement statement?
3. Will the attorney provide complete insurance information?
4. Will the attorney give you all information on the defendant?
5. Will the attorney provide you with all of the information about the plaintiff's medical payment from the automobile insurance?
6. Will the attorney give you the information about the claims adjuster? This should include the address and telephone number as well as the claim number.
7. Will the attorney help you collect on the medical payment part of the auto insurance?
8. Who is the attorney's acupuncturist?
9. The attorney in PI cases often takes and sends the bills for professional medical services to the insurance company(s) involved. This means the attorney's office bills for all medical services and the checks are often being sent to the office of the attorney. Does the attorney deduct a fee (can be up to 30%!) of the checks before sending on the payment to the practitioner?

Finding out who pays what

When determining which insurance companies will reimburse for acupuncture services, you first need to determine the laws in your state regarding insurance payment for acupuncture. In some states, there is no requirement for insurance companies to reimburse for acupuncture at all. Other states, however, have mandated that insurance companies that pay for acupuncture by a medical doctor must also pay for acupuncture by a licensed acupuncturist.

There are a couple of ways to determine whether an insurance company will reimburse for acupuncture services. First, and most effective for building rapport in your area, call the human resources department of the major companies located within five miles of your clinic. You are trying to find out specifically what insurance carrier each company uses for its health care plans. Some companies give their employees a choice between two or more health plans, while others provide only one option. Ask if the company health plan(s) covers acupuncture and if they know the extent and type of that coverage. For instance, must it be administered by a medical doctor, is there a limit to the number of visits in a certain period of time or for a certain type of problem, and is there a co-pay? There is a form on the website to fill out with all the questions you need to ask.

> **PRACTITIONER POINTER**
>
> "It is wise to have a clear understanding with each patient that they are ultimately responsible for payment of all services rendered through your clinic."
>
> —*Anon.*

Gather this information into a file. When you have made all of the local phone calls, go to the Yellow Pages or online and look up the 800 number for each of the insurance companies mentioned. While it may take a bit of persistence to get a real customer service representative on the phone, there are several things you need to find out from them. Ask the representative:

1. For such-and-such patient with such-and-such policy number is there coverage for acupuncture treatment?
2. Is there a deductible on the policy and has it been met for this year?
3. Is there a yearly maximum for acupuncture benefits and has that been used?
4. Do they honor an assignment of benefits from the insured?
5. May acupuncture treatments be administered by licensed acupuncturists or only MDs?
6. Do they only cover certain CPT (Current Procedural Terminology) or RSV codes?
7. Do they require reports and at what intervals?
8. Do they require a medical referral from an MD?
9. Is there any other forms or paperwork specific to their company that they need to send you?
10. Do they prefer that you bill electronically? (Yes, this is coming and soon some companies may only accept electronic billing. There is more on this subject in Section 2, Chapter 1)

It is also possible with more and more companies that you can view specific policies and coverage at insurance companies websites. This may not answer all your questions, but can save time for those with a little Internet savvy.

POWER POINT

We have included a Phone Verification of Insurance Coverage form on the website that you may use when you call. You may also want to write down the phone number for provider services right on the patient's form. Once completed, this form should be kept in the patient's administrative file with all other financial records. FYI, it is now suggested that you keep two separate files for each patient. One includes all examination and treatment records, the other includes all financial, billing, insurance, HIPAA, and other administrative forms and records.

Some companies reimburse for acupuncture but at a different rate for "in-network" and "out-of-network" providers. If this is the case, you should try to get on the panel, also known as a PPO (preferred provider organization) or an IPA (independent physicians association). Ask to be transferred to the provider services department. The staff in the provider services section can tell you if they are looking for acupuncturists in your area, if the panel is accepting applications, or if the panel is closed (meaning they have enough practitioners in the area). Regardless of the panel status reported to you on the phone, request an application. When you get the application, fill it out and mail it back. You never know when their situation may change or who will be accepted next.

A second path to discovering which insurance companies cover and pay for acupuncture services is to wait until prospective patients call you to ask if you accept a specific company's insurance. Politely let the patient know that insurance plans vary and that if they would mail or fax you a copy of their insurance card and give you their name and birthday, you would be happy to contact the insurance company to find out if coverage is available. (They can also give you the number of the policy and company contact numbers on their card if they are unable to get you a copy of the card immediately.) Alternatively, they may already have insurance paperwork that they will ask you to help complete, but you'd be wasting your time if no coverage is available.

While it would be less time-consuming to have a potential patient call their company and fill out forms, you cannot always be sure that they will understand the questions they are asking or the answers they are given, nor can you assume that they will be completely honest with you! Thus it's better to do these calls yourself, and, after you've done a few, you will know red flags or potential problems when you hear them.

P O W E R   P O I N T

Forms that You Will Need to Use if You Are Going to Accept Insurance Patients ●

1. Assignment of Benefits form
2. Power of Attorney to cash checks written-to-the-patient-but-sent-to-your-office form
3. Superbill forms
4. CMS-1500 forms
5. Claim forms provided by the patient
6. Insurance tracer letter/form
7. Insurance company basic information form
8. Patient Confidential Information form
9. Notice of Doctor's Lien for PI cases
   See the website for samples of all these forms.

As of 2007, you also need a National Provider Identifier (NPI#) to bill insurance. See Appendix A for how to apply.

When you are given a prospective patient's insurance card, make a copy of both sides for their administrative file. Somewhere you should find a 1-800 number directing you to the office that gives eligibility information. Call the number and tell the customer service person that you are calling to *verify eligibility for benefits.* The representative will ask you a number of questions regarding the patient and the type of benefits requested. You may also be asked to provide your social security number (or Tax ID number), clinic name and telephone number. Be sure to write down all information you receive or use the form on this book's website.

Once you have either the confirmation or denial of coverage, you can provisionally add that company to your list of those that do or do not cover acupuncture. Be careful, however, as each company may have many plans with different coverage.

Blue Cross/Blue Shield, for example, has many health plans available in our area. While we were happy to learn that one local business using Blue Cross/Blue Shield offered acupuncture and alternative medical benefits to their employees, the policy used by a slightly larger company next door to them also using Blue Cross/Blue Shield did not cover acupuncture.

POWER POINT

When you are starting out on your quest to work with insurance companies, tell the representative on the phone just that. Inform the person on the other end of the phone that you are new to the world of insurance-billing. They will usually help you. Insurance companies want you to succeed and want you to communicate with them effectively. The more successful you are as a practitioner, the more people want to sign up for their coverage of your good work. Before you call, always have a pen in hand, call the person by name (Miss Jones, Mr. Smith) and thank them sincerely for their patience and help. If you can make a friend at every insurance company you bill, there may be someone to help you if things don't go smoothly later on.

Getting on a Panel

When dealing with a *managed care organization* or a *health management organization,* you will most likely be asked to join a panel. Panels are groups of practitioners assembled and certified by a management organization so that it is easier for insurance companies' clients to use your services. Since many insurers don't really know much about acupuncture and Chinese medicine (who you are, what you do, the nature of your training, or how to find you), the certifying agency functions as a go-between to ensure that the insurance company's clients are only allowed to frequent practitioners who have the appropriate training and credentialing, an accessible and professional clinic that affords patient privacy, and who carry adequate malpractice insurance.

Getting on a panel can be as easy as calling the desired company and asking if they are accepting applicants for their acupuncture or other health service panel. The company will send out an application and certification packet, a contract for you to sign, and may require an application fee (which is usually non-refundable). This packet is used to gather all information regarding the practitioner's education, license status, malpractice insurance, previous claims and/or settlements, practice setup, including patient privacy and ADA accessibility, and possibly other information as well, such as *curriculum vitae* (see Section 4, Chapter 5), and/or professional references.

Once you receive the application, read through all of the instructions prior to filling it out. A poorly completed application will not inspire confidence in the certifying agent or committee. Make sure that all information is filled out neatly in *black* ink. If your handwriting skills are not very tidy, ask for some help from a friend or find an old typewriter. If you have to do it by hand, make a copy of the form beforehand so that you can start again if you flub the first one. You may also ask if the application can be filled out online.

Also included with the application will be a contract for you to read through and sign on various pages. *Make sure to read the contract thoroughly.* It will tell you how much and for which services/codes you can bill. It will also contain instructions for conduct, filing grievances, how disputes will be handled, and whether you may bill patients for any difference in the billed and paid amounts.

Once the company has received your application, they will follow up on and investigate all educational and licensing claims, call references, and verify your malpractice and general liability insurance if required. At this point, the company may send an inspector to your clinic. Their job is to ensure that many conditions are indeed met, some of which relate to patient privacy and safety. Others are centered on acupuncture practices and disposal of hazardous medical waste. These inspections do not always take place, nor may they even be required. As an individual practitioner, I [ES] am now on at least 11 panels. Of those, there was only one company that required on-site inspection. However, since they are located in another state, they sent me a camera and a list of things to photograph!

After the background work has been done, the completed application and all results of investigation and inspection will be forwarded to a panel of people who vote on your candidacy. Once the vote takes place and you are accepted to the panel, you will receive notice from the company as well as a list of acceptable billing codes and fees and a copy of the contract that you signed which now contains a signature from a representative of the company.

There is no limit to the number of panels in which you may participate. Once you are on a panel, your name and clinic information will be added to the list of available practitioners for selection by the members of that insurance group. Getting placed on a panel can be considered another form of marketing and, in the first years of practice, may help to establish immediate cash-flow. While some managed care panels are controversial within the profession because low reimbursement amounts are not a great precedent to set within the insurance industry as a whole, they may be a way for you to expand your business and offer service to a larger slice of the public.

➤ Know the Code

There are two sets of codes that you must become familiar with in order to effectively bill insurance and *get paid.* While not as esoteric as the behavioral code of a Samurai warrior or the secret handshake of the Knights Templar, they can seem complex at first! These are standardized codes for billing that tell the insurance company what diagnosis the patient has and what procedure you are performing to treat the patient. These codes are known as CPT (Current Procedural Terminology) codes, and ICD-9 or 10 (International Classification of Diseases, 9th or 10th edition) codes. There are books available that list these codes in lengthy detail. These codes are important to you because, without both a thorough exam and history and a specific diagnosis for each patient who wants to use their insurance to reimburse you for services, you cannot establish *medical necessity.* Without adequate proof of medical necessity, an insurance adjuster is likely to deny coverage for your services.

Current Procedural Terminology (CPT) codes are five digit numbers used to bill for the procedures you administer. These procedures include, but are not limited to, intake and examination, follow-up evaluation, acupuncture and electro-acupuncture, moxibustion, cupping, and tuina or other bodywork and manipulation (if allowed in your state). Listed below are typical CPT codes, their associated procedure, and when you are allowed to use them. Remember, however, that the types of codes required or accepted may vary by company. So make sure to ask.

CPT codes are written in block 24D of the CMS-1500. (Never fear. There's more on CMS forms later in this chapter.)

➤ New Patient Codes
(Evaluation and Management [E&M] Codes)

These may only be used for the first time you see a patient, or if you are seeing a patient whom you have not seen for three years or more. In California and some other states' Workers' Compensation law, you may use these codes for any new injury even if you have seen the patient within three years prior. Typically, the new patient exam code is separate from any acupuncture or other service you provide and, as such, is billed separately from your treatments. The codes are followed by the number of minutes typically spent face to face with the patient or patient's family and the severity of the chief complaint.

99201 – 10 minutes; presenting problems are minor
99202 – 20 minutes; presenting problems are low to moderate
99203 – 30 minutes; presenting problems are moderate
99204 – 40–50 minutes; presenting problems are moderate to high severity
99205 – 50–60 minutes; presenting problems are high severity
97041 – Colorado and some other states' Workers' Comp New Patient E&M code (no matter the number of minutes)

All the above codes have three requirements for use. These are:

1. You must take a medical history, the scope and comprehensiveness of which increases from: a focused history regarding the problem (99201), an expanded history regarding the problem (99202), a detailed patient history (99203), or a comprehensive patient history (99204-99205)

2. You must perform an examination, the scope and comprehensiveness increasing from: focused on the problem (99201), an expanded examination regarding the problem (99202), a detailed patient examination (99203), or a comprehensive patient examination (99204-99205)

3. You must also make a medical decision of increasing complexity from: straightforward (99201-99202), low-complexity (99203), moderate complexity (99204), and high complexity (99205) These last two codes will require an accompanying report proving necessity in most cases.

At the time of this writing, it is not clear if insurance companies are going to continue to pay for E&M codes billed by acupuncturists. There have been reports that some insurance companies have stopped paying for these codes if not billed by an MD office. Other practitioners say no, they get these codes reimbursed all the time. We will continue to monitor this situation and post any information we receive on the Blue Poppy website.[HW]

➤ Established Patient Re-evaluation and Management Codes

These are used for a follow-up examination, re-evaluation, and for an established patient who presents with a new condition. In order to bill this code, you must again take a history of the problem, perform another examination, and make a medical

---

POWER POINT

Using Evaluation & Management Codes (E&M)

These codes are used instead of office visit codes. E & M codes include various components and the provider is paid one fee for all of these parts:

1. Medical history
2. Physical examination
3. Medical Decision Making (MDM includes diagnosis and creation of a treatment plan)
4. Counseling of the patient
5. Level of severity of the problem
6. Co-ordination of benefits (time for phone calls, report writing, etc.)
7. Time. This is the most important for oriental medicine practitioners because the acupuncturist/herbalist spends more time with a patient than most other types of medical providers.

Find out what each insurance company will pay for specific codes. You can contact the benefits department of any insurance company directly to get this information.

---

decision. As stated above, these codes are separate from any acupuncture or other service you provide and, as such, are billed in conjunction with the service. The codes below are followed by the number of minutes typically spent face to face with the patient or patient's family and the severity of the chief complaint.

99211 – 05 minutes; presenting problems are minimal

99212 – 10 minutes; presenting problems are minor

99213 – 15 minutes; presenting problems are low to moderate

99214 – 25 minutes; presenting problems are moderate to high severity

99215 – 40 minutes; presenting problems are moderate to high severity

97044 – Colorado and some other states' Workers' Comp Re-evaluation code (flat fee no matter how many minutes are spent.

Acupuncture-specific CPT codes

These codes are used to bill for acupuncture services and they changed significantly at the beginning of 2005. These changes have been accompanied by great confusion and worry by practitioners wanting to continue to get their insurance billings paid promptly and to stay out of trouble. Below we will try to illuminate the dark corners of the CPT code dilemma as well as we can. We think it is important to understand from the beginning that there can be just as much confusion with how to use these codes with insurance adjusters as there are with practitioners. That being said, we encourage you to keep sending in your bills and keep working with all the companies that you can to clarify what they will and will not cover. Here goes:

97810 – This is the basic acupuncture treatment code. It is a "time-based" code and is used to bill for the application of one or more needles and active one-on-one patient contact for 15 minutes. That means the time spent palpating and preparing points for treatment, positioning the patient, washing your hands, disinfecting points, inserting and manipulating needles, checking on the patient in the middle of the treatment, and taking needles out. It can include up to three minutes of what is called "pre-service" or "post-service" activities such as charting time. Neither this nor any other 15-minute increment includes the time the patient spends lying on the table quietly.

97811 – This is the code for a second (or third) increment of time (a minimum of 7.5 minutes up to 15 minutes) working one-on-one with patients. It usually has to do with the insertion of a second group of needles. Not the same needles, however. The first set of needles should be disposed of according to this billing model. This code is used for each subsequent application of needles (without electronic stimulation) regardless of whether you reposition the patient. This code may be used whether 97810 or 97813 was used for the first 15-minute increment; in other words, you could have used electricity for the first increment and not for the second increment. You bill this in 15-minute increments of time or any portion thereof.

97813 – This is the primary electro-acupuncture code. It is used the same as 97810 except that, in this case, there was the application of one or more needles with electro-stimulation. This code should not be used with 97810 or 97811. For a second time increment of electro-acupuncture, bill using the following code,

97814 – This is the second 15-minute increment code for electro-acupuncture. To use this code, you must have first used 97813 or 97810. The time requirements for this code are the same as 97811. Please also note that, in some cases, electro-acupuncture will be reimbursed at a slightly higher rate than regular acupuncture, perhaps $1-2 per increment.

97782 – Cupping. This code; may not be billed concomitantly with either acupuncture code with some insurance companies. This code is not accepted for Workers Comp billing in every

writing there have been huge changes in worker's comp in California and it is still very much in flux. See Chapter 5 in this section for more details). Whether acupuncturists will be included at all in the California worker's comp system in the future is not known and in the current economy not as likely.

97783 – Moxibustion; may not be billed concomitantly with either acupuncture code with some insurance companies and is not accepted for workers comp billing in many states.

97803 – California worker's comp code for moxibustion

97124 – Massage/tui-na; billed in 15 minute increments. Time blocks are billed after 7.5 minutes up to 15 minutes. For example, 15 minutes of tui-na is billed as one unit of 97124, while 22.5 to 30 minutes of tui-na is billed as two units of 97124. This code is listed once on the CMS-1500 and then modified in the unit block for each 15- minute period. (Use same code for each 15 minute increment. Some companies will not reimburse when billed with acupuncture codes.)

97250 – Myofascial release

97140 – Workers comp code for manual therapies in some states; *i.e.*, trigger point therapy. This code may not be reimbursed by some companies as it is considered to be a part of acupuncture.

Remember that, if you provide services through managed care or PPO plans where you are a paneled member, your level of reimbursement for any and all of these codes will be specified in advance. If they are not, (or if you've lost the paperwork!) call and find out from the provider services department any limitations or specifics they can give you about which codes will be reimbursed at what level and which ones may be used on the same billing form.

OK, how do you put this together so it works for you as well as for your fee-for-service insurance patients? Here's my suggestion [ES].

First, remember that there has been just as much confusion within the insurance companies as there has been in your offices with regard to the use of these codes. They were comfortable with the old system as well. To make things simple, however, what many of them have done is to split up their old rate of reimbursement between one unit of 97810 and one unit of 97811. For example, a payer who used to reimburse $48 for 97780 will now pay $33 for 97810 and $15 for 97811. The unfortunate reality of this is that, if you want to make the same income accepting insurance, then you have to do twice the needling (sort of).

Now, I never advocate anyone lying, nor to cheat or steal; but you do deserve to be paid for your time. So, I will tell you what we are doing in my office that is working. I also encourage others to email either Honora or myself and let us know where you are coming up against pitfalls or having great success.

As always, when we see the new patient, we bill one of the new patient EM codes (such as 99203, etc.). Once the interview is complete, I ask the patient to lie supine on the table (gowned for further treatment depending upon the patient's needs) and I start to insert my first group of needles. My initial repertoire usually consists of Liv 3 and LI 4 contra-laterally or bilaterally, and then a hand/ankle pair for one of the extraordinary vessels that may play a part in the patient's main complaint. I may also insert a needle at Yintang, GV20 and/or GV24 as seems appropriate. At this point I leave the room, giving the patient instructions to rest and I will return in a few minutes to begin the treatment.

After about five to ten minutes, I re-enter the room, remove the face/scalp points and start my treatment. This would be acupuncture session number two for those of you who are counting and will be billed as 97811. After those needles are inserted I will leave the patient for 15-20 minutes. Depending on the amount of time remaining and the severity of their condition, I may then have them change positions for a third session of needles on the back or simply remove a few needles and insert any others that may be called for. In this way, I can bill for one 97810 and one or two 97811 codes. Remember that each 97811 code requires *at least* 7.5 minutes of hands on time in addition to the 15 minutes of hands on time for 97810. These sessions may include point location, sterilization, or other required preparation of points as we have described above under each code.

This is just one recommendation about how to make the new system work for you *and* for the insurance company while giving your patients the best possible care for their insurance dollars. It is working well in my clinic so far. The key is to bill only one unit of 97810 or 97813, and then add any number of units of 97811 or 97814 depending upon the number of extra sessions you perform.

Remember to document everything that you do. Under the **plan** section of your SOAP notes, be sure to delineate between each insertion/re-insertion sessions. For instance, note them as "Acu1, Acu2, Acu3" or "Acupuncture: 1st; 2nd; 3rd." As always, accurate chart notes are required by law and can be reviewed by the insurance company at any time. Do not bill for that which you do not do. But, by all means, bill for each acupuncture session that you *do* do during each appointment!

▶ International Classification of Disease (ICD-9) Codes

These are diagnosis codes that are universally accepted by the insurance industry. ICD-9 codes consist of a three digit number followed by a decimal and may be followed by one or two more digits called modifiers. These numbers are written in block 21 on lines 1–4 of CMS-1500 in order of severity. The diagnosis codes are chosen based on the chief complaint(s) the patient presents. However, you will want to be careful with what codes you choose as many insurance companies are restrictive with the selection of diagnoses acceptable for acupuncture treatment. Many companies will tell you what types of disorders are covered under the patient's plan when you call to verify eligibility. Others will not. So it is best to be conservative when choosing them. For example it may be easier to get paid for treating shoulder pain than to get paid for fibromyalgia.

Although we are providing you with some of the more common ICD-9 codes in use for acupuncture, we recommend you purchase a book of codes. These are available at most book stores or online. If you purchase medical patient management software, such as Gingko or AcuBase or TCM Pro, there are some pre-loaded codes. It is a good idea to check for code changes once in a while as these codes are updated occasionally.

▶ Tips for getting your codes reimbursed

Many insurance companies have a limited number of disorders that are allowed for acupuncture reimbursement. Therefore, it is best to ask if the diagnosis is covered when you call the insurance company. They may be willing to tell you, especially if you have already made a friend at the company. Also, it is never wrong to scale the diagnosis down to a symptomatic ICD-9 code that is a part of the overall diagnosis. For instance, some companies only pay for the treatment of pain. Should a patient present with a diagnosis of **847.2 Lumbar strain/sprain** for treatment, this may not be a covered disorder. However, if a patient has a lumbar strain/sprain, then they most definitely are suffering from **724.2 Back Pain, Low.** The person at the insurance company has a list of codes that are acceptable. If your code is not on that list, it will be sent back posthaste with a statement of noncoverage. So, if you cannot get specific information about acceptable billing codes from the insurance company you are billing, use the most

P O W E R   P O I N T

Sample of Frequently Used ICD-9 Codes

Headaches:

784.0	Headache
951.9	Cranial nerve(s) injury
307.81	Tension headache
625.4	Premenstrual headache
627.2	Menopausal headache
346.1	Migraine, common
346.2	Migraine, variants of
346.8	Migraine, other forms of
346.9	Migraine, unspecified

Musculoskeletal pain:

789.0	Abdominal pain
781.2	Abnormality of gait
756.10	Abnormalities of m.s. system, unspecified
724.6	Arthritis, gouty
714.30	Arthritis, rheumatoid, juvenile
733.22	Bone cyst
848.42	Chrondosternal sprain or strain
737.4	Curvature of spine, unspecified
737.41	Curvature of spine, kyphosis
737.42	Curvature of spine, lordosis
737.43	Curvature of spine, scoliosis
719.7	Difficulty walking
839.61	Dislocation of sternum
737.1	Kyphosis, acquired, postural
905.6	Late effect of dislocation
907.9	Late effect of injury, unspecified nerve
905.7	Late effect of sprain/strain
905.8	Late effect of tendon injury
908.9	Late effect of unspecified injury
737.2	Lordosis, postural
354.8	Neuralgia, intercostal
729.2	Neuritis, neuralgia, radiculitis, unspecified

"Power Point" continues on the next page

297

715.9	Osteoarthritis, unspecified
712.0	Osteoarthritis of spine
268.2	Osteomalacia
306.0	Osteomyelitis, unspecified
733.02	Osteoporosis, idiopathic
733.01	Osteoporosis, senile
733.00	Osteoporosis, unspecified, wedging of vertebra
733.99	Other bone disorder
782.0	Paresthesia
720.0	Rheumatoid arthritis
848.3	Sprain/strain, rib
845.1	Sprain/strain, ankle, unspecified
719.59	Stiffness in joint, multiple sites

Please note that ICD-9/10 codes can change every year. You may need to replace your ICD-9/10 book every few years to stay up to date. You may also want to get a copy of the *AccuCodes Book* from the H.J. Ross & Co. by calling 1-800-562-3335. This book is easy to use, well organized and covers all the major pain codes that acupuncturists commonly use.

generic codes possible when you fill out your CMS form for that patient.

▶ Filling out the CMS-1500

Insurance companies like paying us for our services as long as we play the game by their rules. In fact, they want you to succeed enough that they have made it easy to bill for services if you understand how to use their standard form, the CMS-1500. CMS stands for Center for Medicare/Medicaid Services. Of course, before you can send the insurance company your bill, you need to understand what goes where and what is required on a CMS-1500.

You can also purchase these from several organizations online or by phone. ● However, for now, let's just go through the CMS, block by block. (It really is not difficult after you have done two or three of them!)

Starting at the very top of the CMS, there is a large margin with "PLEASE DO NOT STAPLE IN THIS AREA" in large letters in the left hand corner. This space is for the name and address of the insurance company. This information should be placed directly above and to the left of the bold face words on the form "HEALTH INSURANCE CLAIM FORM" which is written towards the upper right corner.

The numbers below correspond to the numbered items that must be filled out on the CMS form.

1. Make an "x" in the appropriate box related to the type of insurance policy you are billing. For patients with insurance through their employer, the Group Health Plan box is appropriate. For Workers' Comp or PI cases, use the box that says "other." For private health plans that are not purchased through an employer, you may also use the Group Health Plan box. Champus is a type of U.S. military coverage but is mostly not applicable to acupuncturists.

1a. Insert the insured's identification number. It is on their insurance card. It may or may not be their Soc. Sec. number. Some insurance companies assign their own number.

2. Insert the patient's last name (ALL CAPS), first name, middle initial.

3. Insert the patient's date of birth using eight digits. (You must use four digits for the year.) Check box male or female.

4. Insert the insured's last name, first name. (This is not always the patient's name.)

5. Insert the patient's street address.

6. Insert the patient's relationship to the insured.

7. Insert the insured's address.

8. Insert patient's marital and employment or student status.

9. Leave blank.

10. Insert appropriate type of case (*e.g.,* Workers' Comp, PI.)

11. Insert insured's group number if there is one on their insurance card, date of birth and sex (a), and employer (b).

1500	Name and Address of the Insurance Company goes here.	CARRIER

HEALTH INSURANCE CLAIM FORM
APPROVED BY NATIONAL UNIFORM CLAIM COMMITTEE 08/05

PICA — PICA

1. MEDICARE (Medicare #) ☐ MEDICAID (Medicaid #) ☐ TRICARE CHAMPUS (Sponsor's SSN) ☐ CHAMPVA (Member ID#) ☐ GROUP HEALTH PLAN (SSN or ID) ☒ FECA BLK LUNG (SSN) ☐ OTHER (ID) ☐ 1a. INSURED'S I.D. NUMBER (For Program in Item 1) **123-45-6789**

2. PATIENT'S NAME (Last Name, First Name, Middle Initial) **Doe, John A.**
3. PATIENT'S BIRTH DATE MM **11** DD **08** YY **51** SEX M ☒ F ☐
4. INSURED'S NAME (Last Name, First Name, Middle Initial) **Doe, Sally M.**

5. PATIENT'S ADDRESS (No., Street) **1234 Main Street**
6. PATIENT RELATIONSHIP TO INSURED Self ☐ Spouse ☒ Child ☐ Other ☐
7. INSURED'S ADDRESS (No., Street) **1234 Main St.**

CITY **Anywhere** STATE **NY**
8. PATIENT STATUS Single ☐ Married ☒ Other ☐
CITY **Anywhere** STATE **NY**

ZIP CODE **11234** TELEPHONE (Include Area Code) **(315) 222-3333**
Employed ☒ Full-Time Student ☐ Part-Time Student ☐
ZIP CODE **11234** TELEPHONE (Include Area Code) **(315) 222-3333**

9. OTHER INSURED'S NAME (Last Name, First Name, Middle Initial)
10. IS PATIENT'S CONDITION RELATED TO:
11. INSURED'S POLICY GROUP OR FECA NUMBER **H8374521 X**

a. OTHER INSURED'S POLICY OR GROUP NUMBER
a. EMPLOYMENT? (Current or Previous) YES ☐ NO ☐
a. INSURED'S DATE OF BIRTH MM **05** DD **10** YY **53** SEX M ☐ F ☒

b. OTHER INSURED'S DATE OF BIRTH MM DD YY SEX M ☐ F ☐
b. AUTO ACCIDENT? YES ☐ NO ☐ PLACE (State)
b. EMPLOYER'S NAME OR SCHOOL NAME **ANYWHERE DAILY NEWS**

c. EMPLOYER'S NAME OR SCHOOL NAME
c. OTHER ACCIDENT? YES ☒ NO ☐
c. INSURANCE PLAN NAME OR PROGRAM NAME

d. INSURANCE PLAN NAME OR PROGRAM NAME
10d. RESERVED FOR LOCAL USE
d. IS THERE ANOTHER HEALTH BENEFIT PLAN? YES ☐ NO ☒ If yes, return to and complete item 9 a-d.

READ BACK OF FORM BEFORE COMPLETING & SIGNING THIS FORM.
12. PATIENT'S OR AUTHORIZED PERSON'S SIGNATURE I authorize the release of any medical or other information necessary to process this claim. I also request payment of government benefits either to myself or to the party who accepts assignment below.
SIGNED **SIGNATURE ON FILE** DATE **9/1/2006**

13. INSURED'S OR AUTHORIZED PERSON'S SIGNATURE I authorize payment of medical benefits to the undersigned physician or supplier for services described below.
SIGNED **SIGNATURE ON FILE**

14. DATE OF CURRENT: ILLNESS (First symptom) OR INJURY (Accident) OR PREGNANCY(LMP) MM **09** DD **01** YY **06**
15. IF PATIENT HAS HAD SAME OR SIMILAR ILLNESS. GIVE FIRST DATE MM DD YY
16. DATES PATIENT UNABLE TO WORK IN CURRENT OCCUPATION FROM MM DD YY TO MM DD YY

17. NAME OF REFERRING PROVIDER OR OTHER SOURCE **Dr. Mark Smith**
17a.
17b. NPI **Dr. M. Smith NPI#**
18. HOSPITALIZATION DATES RELATED TO CURRENT SERVICES FROM MM DD YY TO MM DD YY

19. RESERVED FOR LOCAL USE
20. OUTSIDE LAB? YES ☐ NO ☐ $ CHARGES

21. DIAGNOSIS OR NATURE OF ILLNESS OR INJURY (Relate Items 1, 2, 3 or 4 to Item 24E by Line)
1. **848.3** 3. **719.59**
2. **354.9** 4.
22. MEDICAID RESUBMISSION CODE ORIGINAL REF. NO.
23. PRIOR AUTHORIZATION NUMBER

24. A. DATE(S) OF SERVICE From MM DD YY	To MM DD YY	B. PLACE OF SERVICE	C. EMG	D. PROCEDURES, SERVICES, OR SUPPLIES (Explain Unusual Circumstances) CPT/HCPCS	MODIFIER	E. DIAGNOSIS POINTER	F. $ CHARGES	G. DAYS OR UNITS	H. EPSDT Family Plan	I. ID. QUAL	J. RENDERING PROVIDER ID. #
1 09 05 06	09 05 06	11		99202		1-3	75 00	1		NPI	YOUR NPI GOES HERE
2 09 05 06	09 05 06	11		97810		1-3	45 00	1		NPI	NPI #
3 09 05 06	09 05 06	11		97811		1-3	45 00	1		NPI	NPI #
4 09 05 06	09 05 06	11		97124		1-3	25 00	1		NPI	NPI #
5										NPI	
6										NPI	

25. FEDERAL TAX I.D. NUMBER **84-1234567** SSN ☐ EIN ☒
26. PATIENT'S ACCOUNT NO.
27. ACCEPT ASSIGNMENT? (For govt. claims, see back) YES ☒ NO ☐
28. TOTAL CHARGE $ **190 00**
29. AMOUNT PAID $ **Ø**
30. BALANCE DUE $ **190 00**

31. SIGNATURE OF PHYSICIAN OR SUPPLIER INCLUDING DEGREES OR CREDENTIALS (I certify that the statements on the reverse apply to this bill and are made a part thereof.)
SIGNED **Sally Jones, L.AC** DATE **9/5/06**
32. SERVICE FACILITY LOCATION INFORMATION **ABC Acupuncture Clinic 1111 Broadway ANYWHERE NY 11235**
33. BILLING PROVIDER INFO & PH # **(315) 211-1222** **SALLY JONES, L.AC. 1111 Broadway ANYWHERE NY 11235**

a. b. **Your NPI# GOES HERE**

NUCC Instruction Manual available at: www.nucc.org
OMB APPROVAL PENDING

If you want to get some of this paperwork off your plate, consider hiring Office Ally (www.officeally.com) to do your billing electronically.

12. Insert "Signature on file" and date. (You must actually have a form on file signed by the patient, at least on the patient confidential information form in order to fill in #12 this way.)

13. Insert "Signature on file." (Same as #12 in parenthesis.)

14. Insert date of current illness or injury or the first day you saw the patient.

15. Leave blank.

16. Complete only if you took the patient off work.

17. Complete only if referred by an MD and this type of insurance only covers services referred by an MD.

17b. The referring physician's NPI# goes here.

18–20. Leave blank.

21. Insert appropriate ICD-9 diagnosis code. You may use up to four of these. If there is more than one, put them in order of severity, the most severe first. You may also want to list the codes in order of the level of specificity, the most specific diagnosis first. For instance, 737.4 is the code for a general curvature of the spine, whereas 737.43 is the code for scoliosis specifically. So 737.43 would be listed first since both are applicable.

22. Only complete for Medicaid.

23. Only complete for MediCal in California.

24a. Insert date of service.

24b. Insert place of service. The number 11 means at an office. The number 12 means at the patient's home.

24c. Leave blank.

24d. Insert appropriate CPT code.

24e. Insert "1-3" if you've used three diagnostic codes, 1-4 if four

24f. Insert fee for specific service.

24g–i. Leave blank.

24j. Your National Provider Identifier (NPI) number must go here and must go on each line where a CPT code is listed.

25. Insert your Tax ID # or Social Security #.

26. Insert patient's account number.

27. If marked "Yes," check will be sent to the practitioner.

28. Insert total charges for the claim.

29. Always "zero."

30. Insert total charges for the claim.

31. Insert signature of practitioner and date.

32. List the address where the services were performed.

32a. Insert your clinic NPI number here. If your clinic NPI is the same NPI as your personal one, list your personal one.

33. If you are doing the billing from the same location as your clinic, list *your name* with the same address as in 32. This is where the check will be sent and how it will be made out.

33a. List your personal NPI# here again.

Send the original to the insurance company. Keep a copy for your records.

One more piece of information about the CMS form. Recent word on the street is that HIPAA regulations may require everyone who does any type of insurance-billing to use the CMS form, even replacing the super-bill when the patient has paid for services and is being reimbursed directly. This is still rumor at the time this book is going to press.

> ## What to do if you don't receive timely payment

Of course you may call the company. If you have created any friends at the company, contact them first and see if they can help you find out what happened to your bill. If you have no "insider" to contact directly, send the company a copy of the CMS form with an *insurance tracer letter.* Insurance companies are required to respond to tracer letters in writing with an explanation within 10 days of receipt. What usually happens when you send an insurance tracer is that, instead of a letter response from them, you will simply get the delinquent payment.

POINTS TO PONDER FROM CHAPTER 3

1. If you're willing to do the paperwork to play the insurance game successfully, you can increase your income significantly by taking insurance reimbursement.

2. There are several types of insurance you could agree to accept. These include basic fee-for-service private or group plan insurance, Workers' Compensation (see Chapter 5), personal injury, managed care, or Medicaid.

3. Before agreeing to take an insurance patient, you must find out if their policy covers acupuncture, under what circumstances, for up to how many treatments, with what type of required reports, and with or without a co-pay.

4. It is usually easy to get on managed care insurance panels by calling for a copy of their application, but find out how much they reimburse and for which codes before you decide if you can afford this use of your time.

5. You must know how to use CPT codes and ICD-9 codes in order to prove medical necessity and get reimbursed for care.

6. Workers' Compensation CPT codes may be different from other insurance codes.

7. All insurance companies require the use of the CMS-1500 form. Instructions for filling out a CMS-1500 are listed in detail above.

8. If you don't get paid in a timely manner, file an insurance tracer letter and they must respond to you in writing within 10 days.

9. See Appendix A on applying for your National Provider Identification number.

Personal Injury Patients: Yes or No? | 4

Personal injury [PI] patients are people who have sustained some type of injury or injuries from an accident. The most frequent type of accident is "auto versus auto," the common car accident. With the growing number of cars, trucks, and motorcycles on the road, the number of accidents is growing every year, as is the number of potential PI cases that could end up in your clinic. Other incidents that may become PI cases include auto/pedestrian accidents, bicycle accidents, or a fall in a grocery store, restaurant, or the parking lots adjacent to any business establishment.

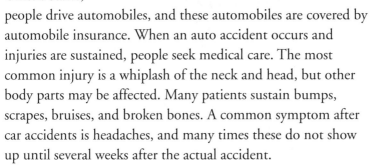

In every state within the United States, people drive automobiles, and these automobiles are covered by automobile insurance. When an auto accident occurs and injuries are sustained, people seek medical care. The most common injury is a whiplash of the neck and head, but other body parts may be affected. Many patients sustain bumps, scrapes, bruises, and broken bones. A common symptom after car accidents is headaches, and many times these do not show up until several weeks after the actual accident.

If you decide that you are going to treat such accident victims, there are many things you will need to know and consider. First, we suggest that you find out if your state auto insurance system is *no fault* or *tort liability* in nature. If your state is no fault, it means that an injured person's auto insurance will usually reimburse for the medical treatment rendered to the patient. This situation is often easier, since any litigation over who was at fault in the accident will probably not affect the reimbursement for medical services in most cases. If your state has a tort liability system, then medical treatment coverage responsibility will depend upon whether the patient was the party at fault in the accident or if the other driver was at fault.

If the injured party was at fault, usually they will be using their regular health insurance or paying out-of-pocket. If the injured party was not at fault, they may be covered by the insurance of the at fault party or under the injured patient's own auto insurance in the bodily injury coverage and/or the uninsured motorist coverage. If they don't have such coverage as part of their policy, they may, again, be forced to use their regular health insurance. In such cases, the health insurance company may sue the party at fault or their insurance company. This is called *subrogation.* If the issue of who is at fault is unclear, such cases may result in litigation or complex insurance company mediation that can take many months. Whether medical bills will be paid in advance of the completion of these legal proceedings is something you must find out on a patient-by-patient basis.

One place to start doing research is with your own auto insurance carrier. Your personal auto insurance agent will, at the very least, be able to explain the fault/no fault situation in your state. You may also be able to find out a great deal about how they handle PI cases, the extent of uninsured motorist coverage for injuries on your own policy and their most standard policies, and whether acupuncture care is a reimbursable service. If it is, under what circumstances, does the patient need an MD prescription for your care, what types of progress reports are required, and how are the funds disbursed? If you have a good relationship with your insurance agent, you may be able to get all sorts of information about the best way for you to involve yourself in PI cases, if at all.

If you do make the decision to treat auto accident or other accident-related injury patients, there will be more paperwork, your chart notes must be written with detail, and supporting objective exams to justify the treatment will likely be required. This is because all the paperwork will be part of a medical-legal file in most cases. There must be comparative exams to document progress throughout the course of treatment, the possibility of the need for future medical treatment related to the injury, and the possibility of residual problems in spite of whatever treatment is given.

In states where you are not considered a primary care provider, your patient may also need a referral or prescription for acupuncture from a medical doctor. In such cases, you may have to prove medical necessity for more than a specified number of treatments with reports that show specific progress such as increases in range of motion or mobility, lower levels of pain, improved functioning of specific bodily systems, etc.

When any new patient calls your office to make an appointment, it is important to determine if they are seeking care because they were involved in a car or other type of accident. If it is not something that you discuss in your initial phone conversation, then the patient confidential information form you use should have questions about the method of payment for the expected treatment as well as other demographic information that will reveal if any type of accident has played a part in their major complaint and if they expect their own (or any other person's) auto insurance to cover their fees. If so, you will need to contact the insurance company(ies) involved to find out if your services can and will be reimbursed and in what amount of time, if there are specific paperwork or reporting requirements, if you will be reimbursed for the time required to create these reports, and if there are any limitations on your regular fees or procedures for care. If you need to contact the patient's or the at-fault party's legal counsel, you need to find that out as well before you begin caring for this patient.

Upon determining that a patient is a PI case and what the expected payment method and time frame is, there are other special forms that need to be completed by the patient with regard to the accident and the injuries sustained. Additional paperwork necessary for payment may include the following:

- **Auto Accident Information Form** ●
  This form provides demographic information about the patient, the attorney, insurance coverage and other information about the accident.

- **Phone verification for Acupuncture Benefits** ●
  This is a form that can be completed by anyone in your office to learn the information regarding a patient's insurance. This will include insurance information about the medical payment benefits on their auto insurance. Health insurance benefits should be verified.

- **Assignment of Benefits to you or your clinic** ●
  This form is to be completed and signed by the patient and then is sent to an insurance company to guarantee that the check will be sent to the acupuncturist.

- **Rescission of Attorney Assignment of Benefits** ●
  There are some attorney's that want to bill for all medical services through their offices. In such a case, when the insurance company pays for the medical services the check is sent to the office of the attorney. Some attorney's then take up to 30% of the insurance reimbursement for medical services and send the remainder of the money to the acupuncturist or other health care practitioner. This is a scheme that allows the attorney to take extra money for the case. It is illegal and not fair to the provider of medical services for an attorney to take part of the medical payments.

If this happens to you, then send the Rescission of Attorney Assignment of Benefits to the insurance carrier.

- **Power of Attorney** (limited to endorsement of checks) ●
  The patient signs this form so that if a check comes to your office made out to the patient you can endorse the check and deposit it directly into your checking account.

- **Medical Lien** (agreement between medical provider and attorney) ●
  In a PI case, the practitioner has paperwork completed and signed by the patient and the attorney has paperwork completed and signed by the patient. The medical lien is a legal agreement between the acupuncturist and the attorney that allows your office to get paid.

- **Copy of Accident Report** (this usually is obtained by the patient from the local law enforcement authorities)

- **Personal Injury Questionnaire** ●
  This form can be used in lieu of the auto accident information form listed above. It is completed by the patient and provides demographic information about the patient, the attorney, insurance coverage and other information about the accident.

Most of this paperwork is completed by the patient and it should supply information to you without involving additional time on your part, but these forms do need to be in your files even if you don't need all of them right away. If you are lucky, there will be several of these forms that you never have to use.

Another key factor in most PI cases is the attorney or attorneys involved. They can either make your involvement easy or very difficult. Listed below are questions that should be asked and answered if there is legal representation and especially if you will be dependent upon their office in order to be paid.

- Who is the attorney?
- What is the address and telephone number?
- Who is the paralegal if there is one involved?
- Who is the secretary in the attorney's office that you will usually deal with?
- Will the lawyer sign the lien if there is one?
- Will the lawyer return said lien to your office promptly?
- Will the lawyer send you a copy of the settlement statement?
- Will the lawyer provide complete insurance information?
- Will the lawyer give you all information on the defendant?
- Will the lawyer provide you with all of the information about the plaintiff's medical payment from the automobile insurance?
- Will the lawyer give you the information about the claims adjuster? This should include the address and telephone number as well as the claim number.
- Will the lawyer help you collect on the medical payment part of the automobile insurance?
- Who is the lawyer's acupuncturist if he or she has one?
- Does the lawyer's office ask your office to send the medical bills for professional medical services to their office as intermediary to the insurance company? (This usually means that the lawyer's office will bill the insurance company for your medical services. The insurance payment is then sent to the office of the lawyer who will take up to 30% of the check before sending it to the medical provider's office. This practice is illegal in most states.)

If the answer is "no" to any or all of the above questions or "yes" to the very last one, there is the possibility that you, the practitioner, may not get paid, the attorney may ask you to cut your bill, or that the money will only be paid in the distant future. In any PI case, what you want and need is a PI attorney that will help both your patient to get the care they need and you to get the payment you deserve. If you have any suspicions about the lawyer, do some digging to check out their reputation. Make sure the patient knows about your concerns. And remember, if this all seems like too much work and too many problems, you do not have to accept the patient for care.

Many times within the process of a PI lawsuit, an insurance company will ask for an "independent" medical examination of the injured patient. This is a normal proceeding within a lawsuit or under the policy conditions of the insurance policy. As a caregiver, you may apprise the patient of their rights which should include the following:

- You, the acupuncture patient, have the right not to be verbally abused.

- You, the acupuncture patient, have the right not to have to wait an unreasonable time for the scheduled examination.

- You, the acupuncture patient, should not be submitted to disrespect regarding your choice of medical providers for your injuries.

The insurance company's doctor may ask questions concerning the injuries your patient received as a result of the accident in question. They may ask how your patient sustained the injuries. The insurance company's doctor may not ask the following questions:

- Questions about the patient's personal life.
- Questions about how the accident took place.
- Questions about the patient's medical condition before the accident.
- Require the patient to take an X-ray examination.
- Questions about the patient's lawsuit.
- Questions about other medical problems the patient may have but are not connected with this lawsuit.

Your patient may be examined but not cross-examined. As an acupuncturist, you may put the above "Bill of Rights" on your own personal letterhead and hand it to the patient and have them take it with them when meeting with the insurance company doctor and keep it for personal reference.

Sometimes a PI lawsuit will go to trial. If you have been treating a patient whose case does go to trial, you may be asked to testify or at least to give a deposition. You may testify as an expert witness or a percipient witness. You may be reimbursed for your time in either case, but the amounts paid will differ. Regardless of whether you have been designated as an expert witness or as a treating medical provider, you need to know if you will be testifying about some or all of the following issues:

- History and examination of the patient
- Subjective complaints verses the objective findings
- Diagnosis and treatment plan
- Mechanics of the accident and the biomechanical issues
- Whether your treatment was necessary
- Whether your treatment was reasonable
- Opinions made by other doctors
- The possibility of long-term disability
- Prognosis and the cost of future care
- Whether your billing was reasonable and in line with the community.

➤ How to dress for a court appearance

As a professional health care provider, you need to dress and groom yourself in the same professional manner as anyone going to a trial. Anything less than professional attire will give the jury a sense that you and your profession are not credible or reliable. On the other hand, it is important that you do not give the appearance of being too flashy. Avoid gold chains, big rings, and gaudy jewelry. A business suit, conservative dark shoes, and a tie are mandatory for men. Women practitioners should wear a business suit, plain stockings, and conservative shoes, no sandals. Remember, the judge and jury will probably only see you once, and a first impression will be the only impression. Make sure to dress appropriately and conduct yourself as a medical professional.

If asked to testify in the court proceedings or in a deposition, the following is a list of potential qualification questions:

1. Could you please state your name?
2. What is the address at which you practice acupuncture?
3. You are a doctor of what specialty?
4. What professional schools have you graduated from?
5. What colleges did you attend prior to your professional acupuncture-Oriental medicine school?
6. When did you first enroll in undergraduate college?
7. What courses did you take at undergraduate schools?
8. How many years were you in attendance at your undergraduate school?
9. What year did you enroll in your specialty college?
10. What year did you graduate?
11. How many years of acupuncture-Oriental medicine college or how many semesters of acupuncture-Oriental medicine college are required to be completed before you graduate?
12. Did you attend acupuncture-Oriental medicine college for three or more years?
13. What degree did you receive upon graduation?
14. Can you tell us, please, some of the courses that you study in a professional acupuncture-Oriental medicine college?
15. Are the books used in acupuncture-Oriental medicine school accepted in other medical or health healing professions?
16. Do acupuncturists have an internship?
17. Are you licensed to practice in this state?

18. What type of license is that?

19. When were you first licensed in this state?

20. Have you been involved in the acupuncture profession as a practicing health care provider since the inception of your license?

21. Are you required to take relicensure classes or do you take postgraduate classes each year?

22. How many cases have your treated involving the spinal column?

23. Approximately how many cervical or neck problems or conditions did you treat in the past year?

24. How many years have you been practicing?

25. During the period of time that you have been in practice from your start until now, approximately how many patients have you treated?

26. What percentage of those patients would you say have cervical or neck injuries?

27. Do you have hospital privileges?

28. So, if you do have a patient that requires surgery, are you able to refer or recommend them for surgery?

29. Have you written or published any articles within the acupuncture-Oriental medicine profession?

30. Has this patient reached the maximum improvement under your care?

31. Have you done all that you can do for this patient?

32. Do you feel that treatment will need to continue or extend beyond this courtroom proceeding?

As the treating medical professional in a PI matter, you may be required to write a *medical-legal report*, especially if there is a court case or insurance mediation. The following is an outline for such a report:

- Written on personal-office letterhead stationary
- The inside address of the attorney
- Identifying demographic information:
    Patient's name
    Date of the accident-injury
    Employer
    Insurance company
    Social Security number
- Inside greeting
- History of the Accident: how did the accident occur and the mechanics of the injury
- Occupational History, Job Description: what does the patient do at his or her employment?
- Initial Complaints at the Scene of the Accident
- Presenting Complaints: the original subjective complaints, the patient's view of the problem created by the accident
- Past Medical History
- Physical Examination Report
    Vitals
    Orthopedic tests
    Muscle strength
    Range of motion
    Palpation findings
    Acupuncture-Oriental medicine findings/diagnosis
    X-Rays taken, date, views, and report
- Treatment Plan Administered
- Review of Records
    Emergency room
    Other doctors
- Diagnosis using ICD-9 terminology and criteria as related to Oriental medicine
- Disability—if any
- Lifestyle
- Prognosis, the discussion, summary and conclusion

- Attachments
    Accident photographs
    SOAP notes
    Police report
    Laboratory findings and report
    Hospital report
    Orthopedic report
    Psychological report
    X-ray report
- Closing
- Signature

As you can see, there is, potentially, a great deal involved in caring for PI patients. That being said, if you can create a good relationship with one or more reputable PI attorneys, if you can find ways to streamline the paperwork involved, and if you are not uncomfortable with the fact that your reports will be legal documents, you may get many referrals for this type of work.

One word about PI patients—similar to Workers' Comp patients—there may be some malingerers who will choose not to get well no matter what treatment they are given. If there is a lawsuit with potentially a great deal of money involved, it may be difficult to know when or if they are or are not really suffering from the complaints they report. It can be a sticky business to be involved with such patients. On the bright side, PI patients usually come in for many, many treatments over a reasonably long period of time. And, as acupuncture and Oriental medicine become more and more a part of the medical mainstream, more practitioners will undoubtedly participate in such patients' cases. Depending upon your situation and personal connections in your town, this type of patient could become one part of your income mix and should not be completely discounted without some investigation.

POINTS TO PONDER FROM CHAPTER 4

- Personal injury (PI) patients are people who have been injured in some type of accident, most commonly auto accidents.

- PI cases require a great deal of paperwork, reporting, and careful chart notes which may become part of a medical-legal record.

- If you consider taking PI cases, do some research about the fault/no fault auto insurance situation in your state. No fault insurance states may be easier to navigate as a PI care provider. Contact your own auto insurance agent and ask questions.

- Know what forms you will need to have on file for PI patients. ● Most of these will be filled out by the patient, but they need to be completed and in your file.

- If lawyers will be involved in a patient's case, find out the answers to the questions for lawyers listed in this chapter before you decide to treat the patient!

- You may be required to testify in court or be deposed by either the plaintiff or defendant's legal counsel. Find out if you will be paid for your time. If you are asked to appear in court, dress professionally.

- We have included here a list of the things that may be included in required progress reports in PI cases. This list may also be downloaded from the website for you to craft your own reports. ●

- If you have personal acquaintances who are PI attorneys or can become a part of their referral circle, PI patients often require many treatments and it can be a financially rewarding part of your practice mix.

Working with Workers' Compensation | 5

▶ Workers' Compensation and You

Worker's Compensation, also sometimes called Industrial Medicine or Occupational Medicine is the type of insurance that pays for medical services for employees who get injured on the job. Each state has different laws regulating Worker's Compensation insurance and what types of care must be paid for at what rates.

Once you have decided in what state you will practice, a call to the state Department of Insurance to ask for information regarding Worker's Compensation is a good place to begin. The reason to start here is that in most states there are several private companies that sell worker's comp insurance to businesses or all sizes and these companies are strictly regulated by each state's specific policies and guidelines. If this call does not yield adequate information, follow up by another call to the regulatory body that oversees Industrial Medicine in each state. You can get these phone numbers for every state by visiting the website www.comp.state.nc.us/ncic/pages/all50.htm or linking to their various websites directly from our website. ● Once you have determined that acupuncture services can be covered in your state, ask if they offer seminars to help you learn all the rules for managing Worker's Comp patients properly. If the reimbursement levels are good, it's worth the money to go to one of these seminars and really learn the rules and regulations.

> **PRACTITIONER POINTER**
>
> "The most important thing with Workers' Comp patients is that you have to find out all the rules for what and how you can bill in your state, and follow them to the letter."
>
> —*Neal Stuart Miller*
> *Sherman Oaks, CA*

P O W E R   P O I N T

How to Get Worker's Comp Patients

Once you have established that Worker's Comp in your state will pay for acupuncture treatment and under what circumstances, then you might consider developing a marketing program to meet and work with varying referral sources. There are three general groups of people that you need to network with in this case.

*   First, we suggest sending information about why acupuncture is a cost-effective resource to the Human Resources directors of any and every company in your area that has 25 or more employees. You want to emphasize the idea that you can save their company money by getting workers back on the job more quickly than any other type of medicine.

*   Second, this same information needs to be sent to every insurance company that sells Worker's Comp policies to large and small companies. It is wise to call these companies first and find out who would be the best person in the company to communicate with. If you can find an ally inside one or two companies that carry lots of policies in your state, it will give you someone to call when and if your claims are not reimbursed quickly or to help you know how to navigate the maze the insurance company creates to slow down payments to folks like us.

*   Third, if you can find out the names of any attorneys who specialize in Worker's Compensation or *employment law*, you might also send them information about your services since they often have some influence over their clients' choices.

Acupuncture services and procedures are covered and will be reimbursed with minimal difficulty in a number of states including Alaska, Florida, New Mexico, Nevada, Arizona, Colorado, New York, and others, as long as you find out and follow the guidelines for billing in your state and as long as you can create reports that support what you are doing *in Western medical terms.* More on what I mean by that in a minute. In most states, acupuncture services are only paid for if there is a referral from a doctor, dentist, or chiropractor. Some states do not require a referral but do require acupuncture treatments to be pre-authorized by the insurance company. This may mean filing a report showing medical necessity and will at the very least mean a phone call to the claims adjuster for the company where the patient works. In some states, injured workers may request a specialist of their own choosing after 30 days of being treated by the employers' or insurance companies' specialists. However, even after 30 days, most acupuncturists will still be required to get pre-authorization for their treatments. Also, most states have a limit to the number of treatments that may be given or a limit that may be given before reports are required. Usually there are only certain CPT codes for which you may bill and specific amounts at which these codes will be reimbursed. There will also be varying requirements for documentation, which you must ascertain from the specific insurance carrier or HR department where the patient works.

In terms of required documentation for treatment, these reports must be written in the same language that orthopedists, chiropractors, and other Western medical providers use. In other words, it won't help your case for getting authorization for six more treatments by saying "the patient feels better" or "the flow of qi and blood is greatly improved." The reports must state specific improvements in function such as "patient's range of

POWER POINT

The situation in California

At the time of this edition, the Worker's Comp situation in California is not good. The reimbursement rules have been changed so that all cases require pre-authorization which is now based on the American College of Occupational and Environmental Medicine Guidelines and the AMA Impairment Rating Guidelines. Since these guidelines do not include research suggesting that acupuncture is a useful therapy for most common on-the-job injuries, authorization is being denied even with MD or HR department referrals to acupuncturists who once treated hundreds of Worker's Comp patients. Some acupuncture groups are trying to document research supporting the use of acupuncture for work-related complaints, but the long term status of Worker's Comp in California is very much in question. Budget shortfalls in that state have not helped the situation either. Also, how this situation may impact practitioners in other states remains to be seen.

motion in shoulder abduction has increased by 30 degrees after two treatments on the following acupoints…" or "after three treatments on the acupoints listed above to increase general stamina, the patient can now work three hours more per day," or "after three treatments to increase blood flow to the lower back on the following acupoints, patient can stand up without leg and back pain for more than four hours."

On your Patient Private Information form, there should be a line to fill in when a prospective patient has been injured on the job. When you get a Worker's Comp case, you need to contact the company that covers the patient similarly to how you contact any other insurance carrier and fill out your insurance information form. In this case, you may already know that they will cover the patient's claim but you need to find out:

- Do they require pre-authorization for the treatments?
- Are there a certain number of treatments that you may do before any authorization is required?
- Are patients allowed to choose their own providers in your state? If not, how can an acupuncturist get chosen for doing treatment? Does the patient require a referral or prescription for acupuncture treatment?
- Is there a limit to the number of treatments allowed?
- What types of reports do they require and how often?
- Do you need to send them an assignment of benefits form in order to get paid?
- Do they have any standard forms they need to send you?
- How long does reimbursement usually take once your forms are filed?
- What is your scope of practice limited to according to the Work Comp system in your state? Do they only allow reimbursement for specific ICD-9 codes? If so, where can you get the list of acceptable codes?
- Do they expect you to use regular CMS forms or do they require some other form for billing?

This is where having a friend or two inside an insurance company can come in very handy. You may be able to get all these questions and more answered if you have already made a friend on the inside of the company you are billing. But we suggest you do as much homework as you can with the Worker's Compensation or Industrial Medicine department in your state. We cannot give you specific answers to the above questions because the answers in each state are different.

If reimbursement levels are low in your state, you may have to consider doing shorter sessions with this type of patient or scheduling more than one patient at a time. If you have more than one treatment room and an assistant, you could possibly treat two patients per hour and still do a good treatment for each one. Can you schedule such cases on your quietest day of the week so they don't interfere with higher paying patients? Go back to your figures of how much your clinic needs to generate per hour to thrive and see how you can make this work. Also, consider that if you do a good job for these patients, others in their company are likely to hear about it. You may get some non-Worker's Comp patients as referrals and the patient may come back to you for a non-work related complaint at a later date. Remember, as we suggest in Section 3, Chapter 2, it is wise to have patients from more than one category of payment and many practitioners make a very good living caring for people who have been injured on the job.

POINTS TO PONDER FROM CHAPTER 5

- Workers' Compensation or Industrial Medicine is the name for insurance that covers people who are injured on the job.

- Many states' policies reimburse for acupuncture. To find out if yours does, go to the website www.comp.state.nc.us/ncic/pages/all50.htm and call the numbers given.

- Call some insurance carriers that cover Workers' Comp policies for the industries and large companies in your state. See if you can make a friend or two with claims adjusters inside these companies. Get as much information as you can in advance of taking your first Worker's Comp case.

- Consider creating a brochure that discusses the

"Points to Ponder" continues on the next page

benefits of acupuncture for getting people back on the job fast to send to Human Resources directors at large companies and to adjusters at all the insurance companies that carry policies in your state.

- When you do get a Workers' Comp case, take a look at our list of questions to ask the insurance company before you take the case.

- If reimbursement levels are low, be creative in how you manage these cases. Can you do shorter treatments, schedule appointments during slower hours, or treat more than one patient at a time in order to accommodate these patients' needs?

- Before you dismiss them, consider other ways that these patients will help you grow your practice if you give them good care.

- Workers' Comp patients can be a very nice slice of your income pie and a great source of referrals! But in order to get paid easily for Workers' Comp, the most important thing is that you have to find out and then followed all the rules.

Selling Products from Your Clinic | 6

Most of the really successful practitioners we know make a significant percentage of their income through product sales. While the most common product lines sold in acupuncture clinics are Chinese herbal medicinals, there are many other groups of products that practitioners might want to consider offering to their patients. We encourage you to consider several possibilities for your clinic depending upon your physical space limitations and the kind of products and information that you would like to offer to patients.

Some practitioners do not like the idea of "selling" anything or they feel it is a conflict of interest, like having an MD sell Western pharmaceuticals out of their medical office. To these people we offer the following thoughts.

1. As we discuss in the marketing chapters, think about the fact that, by offering products for people to purchase from you, especially the herbal medicine, you are providing a one-stop shopping opportunity for your patients. This is a convenience to everyone in our busy world.

2. In most cities and towns across America, Chinese herbal medicine is not widely available in regular stores or pharmacies, if at all. If you do not provide these products for your patients, they will simply not be available.

3. Even if you live across the street from Chinatown in New York City, people may not want to schlep somewhere else to have to purchase their herbal formulas. This may be changing with the Internet and its convenience for purchasing almost anything, but that option may not where herbal formulas are concerned and it also takes more time. Furthermore, at the

present time, few herb companies are willing to sell their products directly to the general public because of insurance liability issues and athe FDA.

4. Studies show that compliance is much better and understanding of how to use products more accurate with patients who receive herbal formulas directly from the practitioner. Thus, patients are likely to get better faster because you were there to educate them about the products you offer.

It is also useful to consider that your pharmacy or other product lines are a profit center that continues to generate income even when you are on vacation or whether you are seeing patients or not. As we say in our live courses, we'd like you to think of your income as a chair with at least three legs, because a chair typically needs at least that many legs to stand up effectively. Your treatments are, of course, the main leg of the chair. Classes that you teach might be another. Rental of space to other practitioners might be a third, but these two are likely to be relatively small income streams compared to the fees for services that you collect. However, product sales can and should be a steady and profitable source of income if managed properly.

➤ Possible product lines to sell

In our chapter on setting up your pharmacy, we suggest that you carry at least one or two good lines of prepared or "patent" medicines as well as either a powder "singles" line or a bulk pharmacy line to create your own formulas.

In addition, there are several other types of products that you might consider:

- A vitamin/mineral line if you are allowed to sell these within your scope of practice.

- If you practice either dermatology or acupuncture cosmetology, consider carrying a line of skin care products.

Many people love to use a special product line that was
personally recommended for them.

- If you do largely Worker's Comp or PI cases, a line of
orthopedic supports and supplies can often be billed to
insurance and will sell well in that practice environment.

- In the interest of providing your patients with information
about Chinese medicine, it can be effective to sell a small line
of books that are easy for patients to read and understand.

- Aromatherapy products and/or essential oils are a nice
adjunct to any practice that treats mostly women. This may
include candles, soaps, oils, or creams. Some practitioners do
extremely well with products such as these.

- If you participate in any type of multilevel marketing group
which sells any type of health-related product, you have a
better chance of success given the constant stream of people
through your office who will be likely to see your product(s)
displayed.

▶ Soft and easy selling strategies

Once you decide what types of products you'd like to sell, how
do you go about getting patients to buy them without a great
deal of brain damage and without the products sitting around
for weeks and months eating up space and cash flow?

While some products are more likely to "sell themselves" than
others, it will also depend upon the type of specialty you have
and, therefore, the type of patients as well as the physical layout
of your space. If you have a nice counter space where people
check in and out at your clinic, use this space judiciously to help
you sell things. You can find nice plexiglass stand-up frames in
varying sizes at office supply stores in which you can put
friendly signs about a specific product or group of products that
you like. On the next page is a sample of what we mean by this.

Unfortunately ours is in black and white, but if you have a color printer and colored paper, yours can be more visually appealing. These signs can be as simple as, "Ask About Our Aroma Therapy Products. They Make Great Gifts," or "Ask Us To Create Your Personalized Essential Oil Formula. Only $6.95 for a one-oz. bottle."

Allergies Got You Down?

Ask Your Practitioner About Our Favorite Herbal Allergy Formulas!

10% Discount During August
(Good for up to four bottles per person)

If you are carrying a good product line, the company may provide you with a sales brochure to give to patients or leave out next to your product display. If not, you might want to create a simple brochure or flyer about your favorite products and their various uses. Keep this simple and conversational. Just make sure it is proofread well and easy to read.

> "Anyone can make soap. It takes a wise person to sell soap."
>
> —*Anon.*

If you want to sell books, you can purchase all types of nice display materials either on-line or through companies like Siegel Display Company (1-800-626-0322). If you plan to have only one or two books, you can buy small, single books stands at many office supply stores. A sign next to your book display might say something like, "Easy to Understand Information on Chinese Medicine. Get One for a Friend Today." You can get small stickers that are easy to remove and mark the prices on the front so that people can make a price decision without having to ask anyone, although most books will also have the price on the back cover. We suggest you choose books that are not too large or too complicated. If you are willing to buy in reasonable amounts, say 6–10 copies, many companies will give you a discount as long as you have a resale Tax ID number (TIN), which you can get from the state government and from the federal government (www.irs-ein-application.com). You will have to have these numbers if you become a corporation or an LLC.

If you have a product line that is beautifully packaged or the products themselves are lovely or they smell good, such as candles or soaps, you want to make sure they are out where people can see them without being in a location that makes them tempting to carry away without paying. A small wall display shelf right next to the reception desk can be quite effective in these cases. If you have a line of nice scented candles, you might keep one or more lit in your treatment rooms or in your waiting area. If you have creams or lotions, an open sample with a sign saying "Try Me" can be all the marketing effort you need to make. Also, be sure to find out from the companies you work with for these types of products whether they have special lines for the holiday season and special display materials or brochures to help you sell the products. Consider changing your product lines or at least the product displays every several months to give things a fresh look.

If you have a great nutraceutical line, you might create a quote such as, "I take such-and-such vitamins and they have doubled my energy level in the last six months. Ask me for more information." Put your name at the bottom and frame the quote to put up in your bathroom.

And, last but not least, your various lines of herbal products will sell because you prescribe them for your patients' patterns. If you choose your product lines well, your patients will feel better and be happy to buy them when they need them with not much prompting from you. Finally, remember that there are new products coming on the market all the time. Once in a while, we urge you to consider another professional product line than the ones you've been using or the ones you were introduced to in school. You might find better technologies, better crafted medicinals, or something new that works better for you and your patients than what you've tried so far.

➤ What should your markup be?

With the exception of grocery chains and car dealerships, most stores with whom we all do business every day have to mark up their products at least 50% in order to make a profit because of inventory tax, storage and space usage, shipping costs, and because a certain amount of cash flow is always tied up in the product line. Your situation is really no different. You cannot afford to sell products at cost! No retailer can afford to do that. If an 80–100% mark-up feels like too much, find an amount over 50% that you can live with for most products. A markup lower than 40% will work only if your turnover is really excellent or they are very specialized products and you simply don't feel you can sell them for a higher price. For example, if a product is sold to you for $10 and the shipping per unit is between $.50 and $1, you cannot really afford to stock it for more than a few weeks without getting $15.95 or better when you sell it—and $17.95 is better. Many product lines will give you the suggested retail price. You can, of course, choose to charge either more or less than that depending upon your situation, shipping costs, amount of shelf space, type of market, or other factors.

If you have a real problem with markups or if even having this discussion makes you squirm, I ask you to consider the situation of other retailers from whom you buy. Would you expect them to operate at a loss or in a manner that forces them out of business? Of course you don't. Most of us are more interested in value for our money than we are interested in something being cheap. This is true for the products you sell as well as the services you offer. Price is not the only criteria people have for choosing what to buy. If it were, we'd all be driving around in a Ford Focus or a Yugo, which is clearly not the case. It does not serve you to price your products or your services too low. It only creates financial stress in your life and a perception of less value to your patients.

Our suggestion is that your markup for herbal products and nutraceuticals should be between 50% and 80%. External herbal products, such as liniments and ointments, usually have a smaller markup . . . say 25–30%. In the world of books, the standard markup for retailers is 20–40%. Be sure to ask publishers how many copies you need to order in order to get a discount of 30–40%. Skin care product lines and aromatherapy products may have different suggested markups. Of course, on any kind of product line you sell, you will be able to get better pricing on larger orders, which will increase your profits. While pricing varies, you need to make sure that you are consistently making some profit on everything that is purchased in your clinic. In most cases, you need not use a "hard sell" approach, and we don't even suggest that as an appropriate sales method. Good products displayed well will sell without too much effort and can make a real difference in your income as well as the ambience of your clinic. Remember, if you have someone to fill patients' herb orders or deal with other sales, you can be making money on your products even when you are on vacation! If you have a product line that you·have done very well with, we hope you'll drop us an email about it so we can share your success story with others.

POINTS TO PONDER FROM CHAPTER 6

- There are many types of products you can sell in your clinic to create another "leg" on your income chair. In addition to herbal medicine, consider skin care products, books, aromatherapy products, and nutraceutical products.

- Some people may consider sales in their clinic to be a conflict of interest, but there are few other options for patients in the world of Chinese medicine than to buy their products from a professional clinic.

- Other advantages are that people prefer one-stop shopping and are always more compliant with products that their practitioner recommends.

- Use small friendly signs and displays to sell products. No hard sell approaches are necessary.

- Make sure you mark up your products enough to make them profitable without gouging. People expect good value but not give-away prices.

- As long as there is someone in your office to fill people's orders for herbs or other products, you can be making money even when you are on vacation.

Buying or Selling an Acupuncture Practice | 7

➤ **Here's what you need to know**

In the last year or two, I [HW] have received calls or emails from people asking me advice about buying someone else's acupuncture practice. This was not a common event in the world of acupuncture until recently, but as our profession grows, it will become more and more common. Since it has come up several times in recent weeks, I decided it was time to do some research and find out what people really should know no matter whether they are on the buying or selling side of the equation.

First of all, let me say that there are many web resources available on this subject, although all the ones I could find specifically discuss the sale of either a medical (MD) practice or a chiropractic (DC) practice. So the information I am presenting here is as generic as I could make it for acupuncture practices based upon the resources currently available.

Second, because the information available on this subject is not acupuncture specific, there may be some wiggle room on the numbers I present here, although it's my gut feeling that they transfer pretty well to any medical profession and may be used as a safe rule of thumb for buyers or sellers.

Third, if you have bought or sold a practice, either successfully or unsuccessfully, I'd love to hear from you with your experiences and what you learned from the experience. If we all shared information about business experience with each other, we would all do better as business people. At the end of the day, the more of us who are successful, the better it is for the profession as a whole.

With those things in mind, I have tried to divide the information below into concerns for buyers and considerations or advice for sellers.

➤ Buying a practice

There are many things to consider when purchasing someone's practice. The most important considerations are as follows:

1. What would be the difference in cost between starting and successfully growing your own practice down the block as opposed to buying the practice that is for sale? Be as honest as possible with yourself about start-up and growth costs for a practice.

2. What are you really buying? Are there hard assets such as equipment, furniture, or real estate involved in this transaction? If not, are you buying the accounts receivable or the bank account balances?

3. If there are no cash or hard assets, you are then buying what is called "goodwill." In that case, a medical or chiropractic practice is considered to be worth no more than 30% of the annual gross receipts of the clinic. If there are any hard assets, those are added on to the value of the "goodwill."

➤ Practice assessment for a potential buyer

1. There are a few ways to determine or prove the value of gross receipts. Most sources suggest that you require access to two years of tax returns and financial records. If a practitioner selling a clinic cannot provide these records, it is questionable whether they will have kept their patient records in any more organized a fashion! At that point I say, "Buyer beware." If they refuse to give you access to this information, then you certainly don't want to do business with them.

2. Intangible assets may include:

a. The clinic market position (monthly patient visits, positive cash flow, take home pay of the practitioner[s], number of total patient records, income and expense projections, base overhead expenses per month).

b. Regulatory history (are there any suits or legal problems)

c. Operational systems in place and quality of patient record keeping

d. Quality of the facilities and capacity for growth staying in those facilities

e. Soundness of the balance sheet and up-to-date financial record keeping

f. Size and current status of the mailing list

g. Reputation of the clinic in the community

h. Staffing situation (will the current staff stick with you)

i. Visibility of the location

3. Other considerations you need to research:

a. How flexible is the financing and payment structure for this purchase?

b. How many months or years is the current practitioner willing to stay in the clinic and work with you? The longer this transition process, the better to introduce you to the client base and the more valuable the practice is to you.

c. What does an analysis of the local demographics reveal? Is the area gaining or losing population? What is the average age of the population and what was the average age a decade ago? Are there many third party payers serving this community that require you to be paneled in order to serve the largest

PRACTITIONER POINTER

"My advice is don't be afraid to buy a practice. I sold my first practice in 1985 for a very reasonable price. It had supported me well enough, but the new owners expanded it to support two practitioners very quickly. Then they sold it again after a decade or so and now it supports three practitioners. The practice is still there and still growing 20 years later.

For the sale of my second practice, I consulted with a professional business valuation expert to help me come up with a fair price. Again, it is a growing practice with great potential for a good, young, ambitious practitioner.

Remember, if you are buying a practice, that has created goodwill, is obviously growing, and the price is fair, it can be so much easier than starting your own from scratch. Get the practitioner to introduce you to as many of the patients as you can and get out into the community and meet people. Tell them you are the person who is taking over so-and-so's practice and you'd love to see them at the clinic. You still have to do your marketing and introduce yourself to the community, but at least you have a potential patient list to start with."

—Don Beans, L.Ac., Ph.D.
Whitefish, MT

segment of the population and what do those panels pay?

d. What does an analysis of the clinical appointment book for the last year reveal? Are there many repeat patients? What is the average number of appointments per patient? What type of hours and workload is the practitioner maintaining and does that work for you?

e. Will the seller send out a letter informing the entire patient base of their upcoming departure and supporting you as their practitioner of choice for referral? Will they pay for that mailing?

f. If you only keep 40-50% of the patients who have come to this clinic, would that be enough to support you while you build the patient base and would the price still be worth it?

g. What is the status of the current lease? Are there opportunities for expansion? Are there any legal or zoning problems with the building that could affect you?

h. What is the seller's definition of an active patient? Is it the same as yours?

i. Who is assuming responsibility for the inactive records and what will it cost you if you must store them?

j. Who owns the clinic name and logo if it is not the person's name? For example, John Smith Acupuncture Clinic is not a name you want to buy as part of the purchase, but you might want to keep the name Whole Woman Health Clinic if it is well established in the community.

If all this seems like too much and you are really serious about wanting to do this purchase, you might consider hiring an independent valuation expert. This is usually a shared expense between buyer and seller whether you end up buying the practice or not.

Finally, buyers, don't ever think that buying a practice absolves you of marketing efforts in the community. Remember that most people who become your patients are buying "*You*" and you will still need to embed yourself in the community in a positive way.

➤ Selling your practice successfully

The first and most important word for sellers is "transparency," If you try to keep secrets from potential buyers or are tempted not to tell the truth about this or that, they will be immediately suspicious and shy away from the purchase pretty fast. If they dig a bit, they will most likely find out what you don't want them to know anyway. So it pays you to be up front about everything, especially anything that is less than the perfect image you wish to project.

That being said, what can you do to help yourself sell the practice smoothly and for the best possible price?

Assess your market position

Before you even think about placing an ad or putting it out in the ethers that you want to sell your practice, you'll be better off if you carefully assess all of the following.

1. How much competition is in the area, and how have you managed that competition successfully?

2. What is your payer mix of cash, fee-for-service insurance, insurance panels, worker's comp, PIP, trades, and pro-bono? If you have accounts receivable, what is their average age?

3. Know the local and regional demographic trends (age, income, employment, stability) in advance and make this part of your seller's information package. Cite or footnote your sources with dates.

4. Are there any other practices for sale in your region of the country? If so, can you compare and contrast your practice in a favorable light? If yes, this is a great marketing point.

5. Are there any recent or potential changes in the regulatory climate in your state?

6. Take a close look at your overhead and all expenses and decide if you could be more efficient in your use of resources. Is there anywhere that you could cut costs without losing quality or efficiency? Do you have the best phone service deal (bank service, draft capture service, laundry service, etc.)? If you can do better, you can make your net profit better and your profit/loss statements and balance sheet more attractive.

7. How is cash flow managed in your business? Could you improve internal controls to keep costs even lower, improve the terms on money you owe to vendors, get a better float or a lower interest rate on company credit cards?

8. What are your fixed and variable expenses? Can any of those numbers be improved? If so, do it now.

9. Consider various ways to advertise this sale and write your ad copy carefully. Consider state and national publications, online services, word-of-mouth, through your state association meetings and publications, and in school newsletters and on school bulletin boards.

10. Consider carefully your exit strategy. The longer you are willing to stay in the practice and introduce the new practitioner, the more valuable the practice will be and the better the selling price. Also, if you plan to stick around for a while, you can give a potential buyer longer to pay for the practice using their work as part of the pay-off. (They do the work, you get some or most of the income for that work.) Having three years to actually pay off the entire practice price is optimal and may, again, increase the value of your practice. The better the terms and the longer your exit strategy, the more you can charge for the business.

11. When creating a realistic exit strategy, define carefully the patient distribution and work load and how that might/will change over the months of your exiting. Who is responsible for what types and amounts of work by what dates? Be very clear about your final departure date and stick to it.

12. Be clear as to how and how much money needs to change hands and by what specific dates.

13. The more you do to let your patient base know about this

transition (letters, postcards, phone calls, open houses, personal introductions), the more valuable the practice is.

14. Give yourself adequate time. If you are planning to retire altogether in, say, five years, start looking for a partner or younger associate now. By bringing someone into your practice, you can avoid selling off your accounts receivable and your equipment for nothing more than their depreciated value.

If this is all too complicated, then you probably are not ready to sell your practice. Even hiring a professional valuator will not exempt you from the work that you must do to assess the value of your practice, because they will require you to provide much of the information that we have listed above in any case.

As I stated at the beginning of this chapter, there are many books and websites that give you information about how medical practices are bought and sold. Whether you are buying or selling, the more you have read on the subject and the more research you have done, the fairer a deal you will be able to create.

POINTS TO PONDER FROM CHAPTER 7

- Buying and selling of practices in our profession is increasing in recent years.

- Buyers need to know that 90% of what they are buying is goodwill and carefully assess the value of that good will. In medical practices, goodwill is usually valued at 30% of the last year's gross receipts.

- Before entering into contract negotiations, buyers must carefully assess the following:

  - the clinic market position
  - regulatory history
  - quality of patient record keeping
  - quality of the facilities and capacity for growth
  - soundness of the balance sheet and up-to-date financial record keeping
  - size and current-status of the mailing list
  - reputation of the clinic in the community
  - staffing situation, visibility of the location, status of the current lease agreement

- Sellers can sweeten any deal by lengthening their transfer/exit strategy.

- Sellers will gain the trust of potential buyers by total transparency and by having done some serious homework to assess and improve the real value of their clinic prior to putting it on the market.

- Honesty and fair play are the most important qualities to bring to any contract.

SECTION FOUR

Marketing Your Practice

What's in this section:

- First Things First for the New Graduate
- Marketing Inside Out
- Be a Community Team Player
- A Good Mailing List: How to Build One; How to Use One
- Creating and Using a Presentation Folder
- Writing a Successful Press Release
- Marketing Your Practice on the Internet
- Marketing Odds and Ends

The difficulty of writing about marketing is that you could write an entire book just on marketing, even just on marketing for a private practice in Oriental medicine! If you go to a library or bookstore, you will find scores of books on marketing. And, we encourage you to read books on marketing once or twice a year just to keep your head in the marketing mind-set. At the end of this book, in the section called "Going Further," you will find a list of books that we especially recommend.

Just to keep things tidy, we have divided this voluminous information into several chapters and done our best not to be redundant. In trying to decide what and how much to include in this section, we've focused on the things that we believe to be the most effective for acupuncturists. These fall loosely into three categories: 1) marketing from within your clinic, 2) marketing outside your clinic, and 3) things that don't really fall into either of those categories. For any excessive cheerleading or mentioning the same idea in a different context more than once, we apologize in advance.

Also, if you have read other chapters of this book, you have probably noticed that marketing is sprinkled throughout it. That is just the nature of marketing. It easily creeps into everything else you do and how you think as a businessperson. Which is another way of saying that marketing is not just a bunch of stuff you do. Marketing is an attitude, a way of thinking about your business to make it as visible as possible and as attractive as possible to the people who might benefit from your services.

Good marketing is not dishonest or slippery. Good marketing does not invite or produce buyer's remorse. Good marketing, fundamentally, is merely having a good thing to say (and the chops to back up your words), saying it well enough for anyone to notice, and saying it often to those who may be interested in listening. Marketing can be as complex as creating a fund-raising event with a cast of thousands or as simple as having a cup of coffee in the same café every morning for six months. So, here we go.

Marketing From Day One: First Things First | 1

hat things do you need to consider right away upon graduation with regard to marketing? Hopefully, you have given some thought (and action) to this question well before you receive your diploma. (See Section 1, Chapter 3.) The information below picks up where that chapter leaves off.

➤ **Whether you think you can or think you can't, you're right.**

You have just finished a 3–4 year process to digest a body of clinical knowledge that will allow you to help people be healthier and happier. You deserve to feel good about that accomplishment. Now you need to focus on staying upbeat and positive about sharing your skill and knowledge with whatever community of people you desire to serve. While you cannot usually expect to have a full practice from day one, you can expect success over time, and you can expect people to respond to you and what you are offering in a positive manner. The more you are able to maintain and project this positive attitude, the faster you will find the success you desire. Even on the days when there are few patients or none at all, stay as upbeat as you can. Look at the temporary breaks and slow times in your schedule as opportunities to find more ways to connect with your community, improve the look and feel of your clinic space, write articles or schedule speeches, and to take care of yourself. If you start each day asking the universe for what you want and intend to happen and then follow through on your marketing strategy, you will get where you want to go.

As Mark Victor Hansen says in *The One Minute Millionaire,* think, work and plan "from your dreams, not toward them." That means starting your days visualizing and believing in what you are trying to create. As discussed in the chapter on goal-setting, we further suggest that you write down what you want your practice to look like, what you want your clinic to look, feel and smell like, draw sketches in your notebook or journal, make a collage, write a poem, or do whatever helps you stay focused on creating what you want in a practice in as much detail as possible. If you can actually keep this discipline of keeping your goals and dreams in your mind, the ways and means of creating it will come if you are paying attention.

Strategic planning

No matter what group of people you plan to serve or whether you will be in a small town or a large city, one of your first tasks as a new graduate is to create a well-organized plan for building your practice or revise the one you (hopefully) created in school or in doing your business plan. This means writing it down and deciding how much work to do on your plan each day and each week. Of course, if it all works really well and your practice grows really fast, your plan must be flexible. You could have a lot worse problems than this! What might this look like? Well, here's what it would look like for us if we were graduating tomorrow.

> "Test all things; hold fast what is good."
>
> —*1 Thessalonians 5:21*

Start by creating a list of the possible ways you might build your practice. These could include but are not limited to the following:

1. If you already have a location for your practice, call everyone you already know who lives or works within a 10–15 mile radius of your clinic and tell them you are open for business and may you please send them a few business cards to give to friends, family, and coworkers.

2. Send an announcement to the business editors of the local newspapers and let them know you are opening a clinic (or are now working at XYZ clinic that is already in business).

You might also invite those editors as well as the health editors for all local papers in for a free consultation and/or treatment.

3. Walk around the neighborhood of your clinic . . . four or five blocks in every direction. See who is there and what sorts of businesses are in the neighborhood. How could you serve them? How could you partner with them? Would they let you put your cards up on the employee "break-room" bulletin board? Could you do any trades with them for products or services?

4. If you have family in the area, will they take cards and give them out to everyone they know that you don't know? Do they have any influential friends to whom they could introduce you, such as media moguls, hospital administrators, MDs, wealthy socialites, or famous sports figures?

5. If you have any well-known friends such as sports, music, literary, film, or media personalities, organize a practice opening bash with them as the featured speaker or performer, autograph signer, or schmoozer. Send announcements about your party to everyone you can think of. Be as adventurous as you can with this event. The more unusual you can make it in terms of theme, invitation design, food choices, or live entertainment, the more people will come. If you want to create a practice for a certain niche market, make the theme somehow relevant and exciting for those people in particular.

6. If you have created a presentation folder, create a list of MDs, DCs, TV and radio personalities, or anyone else you need to send these to in your area. That part is easy, but here is the hard part: Create a follow-up calling schedule and stick to it. We suggest you get these calls out of the way early in the day so the dread of them does not hang over your head. When you get the front desk gatekeeper, talk to him/her about who

you are and what you do. If he or she sounds at all interested, offer to provide an in-service lunch for their entire office so that you can go and tell them about what you have to offer their patients and what conditions you will help them to treat more efficiently. (See Chapter five about presentation folders below for more on this strategy.)

7. If you are planning to specialize in one area of practice, call every other practitioner in the area where you will practice and ask them for referrals *for only this type of patient.* You also might consider putting a classified ad in the state newsletter about your specialization. Let the other practitioners know that you will refer in turn to other specialties.

8. If you are planning to specialize in a discipline that you think MDs would find helpful, see if you can find books, brochures and research (or create your own literature) about your specialty emphasizing how and why your services will help them treat their patients more successfully for less money and time. Send this information to every MD in that field of expertise. Offer to speak to them in person to discuss ways that you can help them treat their patients. Emphasize how you would work together with them.

9. Start collecting a mailing list. This can be used for a wide variety of strategies that we discuss below. A mailing list of interested people is one of your most valuable tools.

OK, there are nine ideas that you could use as is or expand upon. We hope they give you a dozen other ideas. What you have to do is take only *a few* of these and write them down as an organized plan with a schedule that you can follow through on day by day. At first, this type of work may take up most of your week. As you get patients, it will take up less and less of your week. However, it is our experience that if you create a plan *and follow through on your plan in a systematic manner,* you will build a practice unless you are simply wrong for this work. Some things will work better than others. So revisions and adaptations to your plan will happen as you go along. You may find that teaching classes at the local community college works better than free talks at the library or that one part of your plan morphs into something completely different. That's great. Be flexible, but be regular and systematic as well. Sometimes this will all be scary and there are always days when everything you try leads down a blind alley. Do your best not to let worry or fear drown you. Remember that failure is always "the path of least persistence" and keep working your plan.

We *do* suggest that you keep track of your activities other than seeing patients. At the end of each week, make a practice management/practice building "to do" list for the next week. This helps you avoid chaos, manage your stress, and stay on top of your plan. And, it feels great to check things off your list as the week goes by. See a sample below.

Week Beginning Monday June 21

To Do List:
1. Write and send letters to all local OB/GYNs
2. Create text for new brochure/call designers to create barter
3. Speak to local community college class co-ordinator, write and send follow-up course description
4. Call herb distributors for new catalogs
5. Create copy for website FAQ
6. Place classified ad for front desk helper/place ad at local acupuncture school
7. Follow-up meeting at All Women's Health Clinic
8. Research case from last Thursday before his next visit

Monday
8AM   Review charts for today's patients

---

9 AM   Call to follow up with Dr. Jones and Dr. Boswell, offer a lunch meeting; write blog article
10 AM   Patient appointment. Nancy Sinclair (get signed form to her MD requesting records)
11 AM   Patient appointment. John Rafferty
1 PM Find research articles to post at website
2 PM   Appointment at All Women's Health Clinic to talk to practitioners
3 PM Patient appt. Joan Stanley . . . talk to her about insurance deductible issue
4 PM Reminder Calls for tomorrow's patients
5 PM Yoga class at YMCA

This is a pretty sane schedule for the first month out there. Staying organized with ongoing marketing efforts and tracking them each day, this practitioner will have four patients per day next month, and five per day the month after that.

▶ Being remarkable

> "Trust your crazy ideas."
>
> —Dan Zodra

In your graduating class and all the ones before you and after you, people mostly take/took the same courses from the same instructors and came/come out with the same skill set. A few people are "naturals" in both their intelligence and aptitude, but most practitioners have approximately the same skill set and are selling the same thing in the marketplace that you are selling. That being the case, unless you are in a small town or rural area or otherwise the only game in town, you need to come up with other ways to be remarkable. What does that mean and how can you do this?

POWER POINT

We have talked to many people about how they got their first patients. While there are variations, of course, the most successful practitioners tell a similar story: networking, networking, and more networking, which usually started before they graduated.

- One new graduate started by treating the guys on her husband's construction crew for various sore body parts. They came in after work to her small rented clinic space. They told their buddies and wives, and she was off and running.

- Another woman lives in the same city as her family and she had all of them giving out her business cards to their friends and coworkers. She had five patients waiting to see her before the paint was dry at her clinic.

- Another new practitioner went to see a local chiropractor and gave him a series of free treatments in exchange for using his clinic on his day off "on a trial basis." The DC is now referring his patients to her for care and has put her name on his signage. More important, he is including an announcement of her services in his next newsletter to his 700+ clients. She is expanding to using his clinic on Saturday as well.

- One new graduate has moved back to his hometown of 15,000 folks in upstate New York. Because he knows almost everyone in town, coaches Little League, and has joined the PTO at his children's school, it took him less than a year to have a full practice.

Remarkable means exactly what it implies: being someone and something worth remarking about . . . someone that someone will tell others about. One place to start is to visit all kinds of professional offices, stores, cafes, museums, restaurants, and retail experiences that you can find and take notes. Which ones really light your fire? Why? When you go into a place that really makes you want to spend your money there, try to analyze what it is about that experience that is so attractive. Could you take that idea (the feel, smell and sound) and "cross-pollinate" it somehow into how people experience your clinic and your services? How can you take the best parts of the limitless possibilities that living in the developed world affords you and make your clinic medically credible and yet so beautiful, interesting, unusual, exciting, soothing, stimulating, singular, or magnetic that everyone who goes there will want to tell all their friends? That's your goal.

There are many possible ways to be remarkable. Could you create the best customer service, the coolest peripheral product options, the best lending library, always-available on-line research access, the best playroom for kids, the most authentic and beautiful replica of an 18th century Chinese pharmacy, free reflexology for all customers one day per week (choose a day that does not fill up as easily as others), available spa services, walk-in availability, crystal chandeliers, house-calls one day per week, an over-the-counter Chinese herb vending machine (for safe products like Curing Pills, Cold Quell, etc.), the most beautiful clinic rooms, an evenings-only practice with a video-game room for the kids, an annual organized fund-raiser for the local women's shelter, an ATM machine in your office, or... ? What would your ideas cost in money, administration, and personal bandwidth? What

> "A ship in a safe harbor is safe, but that is not what a ship was built for."
>
> —William Shedd

would be your potential return on investment? Then, try to assess your personal risk tolerance financially, socially, and aesthetically? Once you have done that, pick a marketing "limb" go out as far on it as your risk tolerance can handle. That's where the fruit is. By this we mean think and dream of the most remarkable, outrageous ideas you can for your clinic. Don't be a clone.

POINTS TO PONDER FROM CHAPTER 1

- A marketing plan is one of the first things to create upon graduation unless you have already created one. It should be flexible but put into effect immediately and carried through day-by-day, every day.

- There are literally as many marketing plans as there are practitioners; consistency and follow-through are what matter most.

- Be flexible with your plan as your patient base grows.

- In a sea of practitioners offering the same services and products, research creative ways to make your clinic remarkable. Assess your risk comfort, and then go for it.

Marketing Inside Out | 2

At the most generic level, disease causes in Chinese medicine fall into three categories, internal, external, and neither internal nor external. Marketing is similar, *i.e.,* there are things you do inside your clinic, things you do outside your clinic, and then things that don't fall neatly into either category. In this chapter, we discuss internal marketing—the things you do inside your clinic—to attract and keep new patients.

First, it is important to always keep in mind that you, your clinic, and your services *are* the primary marketing for you, your clinic, and your services. Everything from the cleanliness of the bathrooms, friendliness of the front desk "staff," prompt and efficient phone service, and your caring, effective treatments are part of your marketing effort. And those are simply the things that people expect. Beyond that, there are whatever special touches you can create as discussed above. Then there needs to be at least a few of the following:

➤ Information

Remember that informed patients usually make better patients and better "sales reps" for your clinic services. When people can understand what you are doing and why, they tend to respond better to treatment and they are more likely to talk to people about what they have learned. So, for the first 3–5 treatments, we suggest that you never send your patient out the door without a book, brochure, research report, flyer, clipping, or some other reading assignment. There are a number of ways to display this information or otherwise let your patients know that they have access to information on Oriental medicine.

1. **The fun scrapbook**

   Create an information scrapbook in your waiting area. This is exactly what it says it is: a scrapbook with all kinds of interesting and fun information in it. This may include articles you see in the media, research or articles that you download from the Internet or other sources, articles that you have written, letters from satisfied patients, photos of you on your recent study trip to China—whatever information to which you would like your patients to have access. Put each piece in a clear sleeve in the notebook. Make sure that it says on the fun and creatively designed cover that patients may ask for up to three or four or however many pages you feel you can afford to be copied for free. Then get a rubber stamp with your clinic address, phone, email, and website and make sure you stamp each page on the top or bottom or the back. That way, when your patients ask for copies, your clinic contact information is clearly visible. You never know into whose hands these pieces will fall.

2. **The always-available on-line database**

   This requires a digital cable hook-up in your office and possibly the help of an IT consultant, but it is a cool idea given what is available on the Internet. You connect your internet to 3–4 websites that have voluminous information about Oriental medicine (like Blue Poppy's website, for example) and put a sign next to the computer saying that patients may look up research on their condition at these "favorite" sites. You may also want to say something like, "Please inquire at the front desk to print out articles." Have the computer connected to a behind-the-counter printer. You may charge a nickel per printed page or give the information away. Make sure that after each page is printed out, it is stamped with your company rubber stamp as described in #1.

3. Visible brochure displays

There are many types of brochure-holders on the market. These can be attached to the wall or sit on a table or counter. Again, you need to make sure that your card or contact information is on each brochure. We suggest that you either create or purchase several different brochures, at least four or five, on various specific health conditions that you like to treat as well as more general brochures, such as "What Is Acupuncture," "About Chinese Medical Diagnosis," or "How Chinese Herbal Medicine Works." Rotate which rooms these brochures are in for patients to pick up or take charge of the situation and hand the appropriate brochure to the patient, actively requesting that they read it and write down questions before their next visit.

4. Book sale displays

You can educate your patients and create a separate income stream with this idea. A small book-rack for a few favorite health books on your counter and a small sign is all you need for this one. The sign says in one sentence that these informative books are available for sale or that they will help the patient understand more about Oriental medicine. If you buy books several at a time, you can often get a nice discount from the publisher or distributor and then make the price of the books one dollar less than the retail.

Another idea is to charge enough on your initial visit to simply give each patient a book and ask them to read it before their second appointment. Patients are impressed with this, you can be sure. Don't mar the books by stamping them, but do put a card in as a bookmark. You don't know where the book or the card may end up.

5. Monthly or quarterly newsletters

This can be a hugely successful way to keep yourself in your patients' minds. It does not have to be long. Indeed, people don't want it to be long. One or two pages are enough. You can offer a free healthy recipe for the season, an article about in-the-news health care issues, an interesting bit of research on Oriental medicine, articles about Oriental medical politics in your state (if the issue will affect your patients' lives), special upcoming classes or events you are offering, seasonal preventive health suggestions, or information about specific herbs or formulas. These need to be very short articles, by the way. Bullet pointed articles usually get read . . . things such as, "Five Tips for Preventing Seasonal Allergies." Put a newsletter sign-up form in with other new-patient forms that people have to fill out. Most will want the information as long as you agree not to rent or sell your mailing list. Also take newsletter sign-up forms if you do public lectures or classes and mention how to sign up for your newsletter with your author info at the end of any articles you get published.

Of course the cheapest and easiest way to do this is by email, and there are lots of software options for creating a nice email (or print) newsletter if you have a little computer savvy. Or you can use very simple text-formatting if it is in email form. If you do it by regular postal mail, it costs quite a bit more money and brain damage, but, if your list is not large, this may not be a problem and will help bring in customers. You can shift to an e-newsletter later on as your list grows.

Remember, in every newsletter, to tell your patients how much you appreciate their referrals. It is the best way for them to thank you for your services. It is okay to actually ask them for this assistance. If you do an email newsletter, you can put this message into a small "box" in a different color than the rest of the text. If you are doing this on paper, make your request stand out at least a little bit.

6. Clipping/research file

Put up a small sign in your clinic waiting area stating that you have a research file and that patients may ask to see the list of articles currently available. You might even want to simply post a list of these articles and state that people may request copies at five cents per page. Again, make sure your stamp is on at least one page of each article that goes out the door. This does require you to keep adding to your research articles on a regular basis so that the information remains fresh. One clinic I know combines this idea with the scrapbook idea and has over 100 research articles in clear sleeves in a notebook with a notice on the front saying that patients may buy copies at 25 cents per article.

7. Signage or framed clippings on specific diseases

This is especially good if you only want to treat a certain range or type of conditions. Take short articles about Oriental medicine and specific conditions and frame them as information "art" in your treatment rooms, bathroom, and next to your front desk. Keep extra copies in a file if anyone requests one for a friend.

> **Artistic touches**

- Think about what is the image you want to project with your clinic: medical efficiency, warm and homey, ancient esoteric China, sleek Euro chic, or what? Every piece of furniture, the art on the walls, the picture frame style, and the colors down to the toilet paper, can and should project the same image throughout.

- Buy or add artistic pieces selectively. Spare is often better than cluttered. Usually, you want people to notice a few beautiful things rather than be overwhelmed by visual excess. Also, if you have signage or other marketing messages around your office, clutter can keep people from noticing what you

> "If you give people what they want, you will get what you want."
>
> —Zig Ziglar

have to say. (Unless, of course, you go for the cluttered, 19th century antique Chinese pharmacy look with lots of fun and esoteric visual stimulation. There is always a reason to break almost any rule.)

- Whatever look you choose for your clinic, make sure it communicates a healing message. You want your clinic to be a haven, a place that, by its very nature, supplements and nourishes yin, warms but calms yang, and rectifies stagnant qi.

- One way to connect with the community and use an element of artistic surprise in your clinic is to offer a local artist(s) a place to exhibit their work. Displays could change quarterly or semiannually. While there is a small hassle factor with this idea, you get some potentially nice art in your clinic while becoming known as a team player in your community. You might even work with a group of local artists and go together to organize an open house. Everybody gets some free publicity and there is more than one person to help publicize the event.

One-stop shopping

I have heard some practitioners say that they don't want to have the hassle of selling things in their clinic or managing inventory. Or they believe it is a conflict of interest to prescribe and then sell herbal medicinals in their clinic. To these practitioners we have this idea for them to consider. Until and unless Chinese herbal medicines are available by prescription in drugstores across America (and Canada), your patients have nowhere to go to acquire Chinese medicine other than your office. You are providing a service and helping your patients sort from among dozens of products at the health food store that may or may not be right for their pattern(s) of disharmony.

Furthermore, people are busier and busier these days. By offering quick and easy access to these products, you are saving your patients something that is not replaceable and that is everyone's most precious commodity, time. Even for those of you who live in large cities with a bustling Chinatown, do you think your patients really want to schlep off to another store to pick up their prescription or wait for you to have it drop-shipped?

So, beyond the obvious Chinese herbal products, think about what other health-related products that you personally love. Whether it be books, aromatherapy products, other nutraceuticals, special soaps, or a line of wonderful skin care products, people love to have special products from a personal referral. It saves them time and decision-making energy. You have become a buying advocate or advisor, which, if you think about your own buying habits, most of us really need and appreciate.

➤ An effective phone system

In the same way that an acupuncture channel connects the outside world to the inside of the body, your phone is your company's lifeline from the outside world to your checkbook, the "spleen-stomach" of your practice. The presence or absence of prompt and effective phone access can make or break your clinic. It does not matter how well you do the rest of your marketing or how good a clinician you are if no one can reach you by phone promptly or if the phone part of patient management is handled poorly. While we freely admit that the lack of availability and effective phone communications within the acupuncture practitioner community is a pet peeve of ours, it is, truly, a vital element in your success or lack of it!

What can a skilled phone-answerer-office-manager do for your clinic?

We cannot stress enough what we hear from practitioners who have hired a staff person to help them manage their business. You are trained to treat patients and the power of your treatments is based on being able to focus. This is also where you can make the best income. Think about how much better work you could do if there were someone to answer your phone, manage product inventory, keep the office clean, help with outbound patient contact, help with insurance forms and other business correspondence, proofread anything you write before it goes out the door, greet your patients, handle patient payments, and make copies of charts, articles, and promotional materials. A really good office assistant can do all these things, allowing you to practice the skills you worked so hard to learn. Most seasoned practitioners tell us that they pay their office help as much as they possibly can because that help is so valuable. The $25–50K this person costs you per year could earn you twice that much. Really. If you don't have any office help, make a short-term goal of hiring someone to help you as soon as possible.

There are several elements to an effective phone system.

- **Availability**

  If you are not available by phone easily and reliably, you will lose business to those who are. Period. If you believe that you cannot afford office help for answering phones, confirming appointments, marketing assistance, and product ordering, get an answering service, a call-forwarding service that vibrates the cell phone which never leaves your body, or some other method of being able to get back in touch with callers within 10–15 minutes at the longest. That being said, we have heard the same story from practitioners ad infinitum that, "After I hired someone to manage my office and answer the phone, my practice doubled in a month." Think about it.

- **Courtesy**

  If you have never studied acting, sales, or patient management specifically, we suggest that you consider taping yourself or your office staff and listening to how you sound or even taking some audio courses in medical patient management. Learning how to script your calls with potential new patients, angry patients, persistent telemarketers, and missed appointments, all while remaining absolutely courteous on your busiest days, is an acquired skill. Letting each caller know that you care about their needs and issues without being a pushover to everyone who calls requesting that you come in early, stay late, give a discount, buy their product, or otherwise make a special case for them is not something most of us are trained to do. However, we can tell you from personal experience that courtesy to every person who calls, every time, and effective patient management on the phone will go a long way toward helping you build your business, no matter what sort of business it is. Just think about the last time you ordered a product from a catalog and the person on the other end of the line was tired, short, or monotone-voiced. Then think of the times when you spoke to someone on the phone who was helpful, knowledgeable, and you felt like they were in the room with you. It's obvious which company you are more likely to order from again.

- **Adequate numbers of lines**

  If you have a fax and a modem in addition to your regular phone, get at least two phone lines. Three is better. That way, if you are on the phone with one patient, have an in-coming fax or email, and another patient calling in all at the same

When you or anyone on your office staff answers the phone, it's nice to say something like "Thank you for calling White Crane Clinic. This is Sarah. How may I help you?" Or "Good afternoon. White Crane Clinic. Sarah speaking." Also, speak clearly and not too rapidly so people can understand what you said the first time. When your phone answerer (you or a staff person) speaks too fast, without good enunciation, or with a strong foreign accent, people may think they have reached a wrong number and hang up!

time, the phone will at least ring and you can keep your fax available all the time and/or be on-line all the time. If you are an on-line all the time sort of person, it is possible to get fax software so that your computer becomes your fax. The important thing is that patients have as easy a time as possible getting in touch with you.

- **Using your phone to market directly**
  If you have a hold function on your phone, it is great to record a hold message to be played while someone is waiting. In many businesses, this is merely music, but you could also tell patients about an upcoming class or event, a new herbal product you are selling that will help allergy or cold sufferers, or why they should schedule a treatment at the spring and fall equinox. Some of this same information could also be a part of your answer recording for after-hours.

- **Calling your patients**
  Outbound calls are an effective way to keep you and your services in your patients' minds. There are several legitimate reasons why you might want to call them, and most will be flattered by the attention because it is not something they are used to from a health professional.

- Courtesy calls within 24 hours after a first treatment just to see how they responded to the treatment and if they have any questions.

- A call after they have been using herbs for 3–5 days to see how they are doing or if they are responding as you feel they should. During this time you may make dosage adjustment suggestions and/or schedule a short follow-up appointment.

- A call after someone has not been in for six or more months to tell them about a new procedure that you think could help their condition, just to check up on them and say hello, or tell them about a lecture you will be giving, or a class you are going to teach that they might find interesting.

On the companion website you will find the names of several companies who offer business telephone-marketing tips, classes, and related services. One of the best is www.teldoc.com.

P O W E R   P O I N T

Make sure your patients know that you want and need their referrals and that referrals are as important as the checks they write! You can put up a sign in your waiting area or give out cards to satisfied patients and ask them to refer their friends and colleagues. Then find a way to reward your best referrers. (Dinner coupons, movie certificates, free herbs or free foot massage with their next appointment, a free book on Chinese medicine . . . Be creative.)

▶ Other internal marketing tips

• This one we got from a very successful, award-winning realtor. Whenever she sends out anything to a client, she closes the envelope with a colorful small sticker that says, "I always appreciate your referrals." Notice this is active, not passive voice, *i.e.*, it is personal from her to her client. It is visible but not aggressive. Or, you could make stickers that say something like, "Cold season is here! Ask about my favorite cold remedy." These little messages help keep you in your patient's mind in a pleasant way.

• Small stand-up plexiglass signs in various places in your office that tell your patients about an upcoming class, a lecture you are giving, an open house you are giving, a local fundraising event you are participating in, a product that you think helps many people, or about why they should come in for a fall checkup can be quite useful. The bathroom sink is a particularly good marketing location.

• Books and toys for children can make a mother's visit easier. Many of us have had the experience of the young child who wants to be on Mommy's lap and is inconsolable that she is on a table with pins sticking out of her. A good toy corner can be very helpful in such cases.

• Good signage is really important for people to find your clinic easily. It is always unfortunate when someone is twice as stressed as normal when they arrive five minutes late for their first appointment because there were no signs outside, in the lobby, on the door, or anywhere that helped them find you easily. We've all been through this type of experience, and we can and should do whatever we can to make a good clinic experience start before they ever even get out of the car and into your building.

• If you keep in prompt contact with patients by using a cell phone, keep it on vibrate and keep in on your body. That way you can leave the treatment room at the first convenient moment without disturbing your current patient's experience.

• A spotless, shiny bathroom is not optional. Someone needs to give it a quick once-over every day and a serious cleaning at least once per week.

• Keep your reception area as tidy, artistic, and uncluttered as possible. That way people are more likely to experience your clinic as a haven that is calming and healing from start to finish.

• Remember that the way a patient is spoken to on the phone, as they enter or if they have to wait, and, most importantly, when they are paying and leaving is most effective if it is at least somewhat "scripted." This topic is discussed in detail in the patient management chapter (Section 2, Chapter 11).

• Make sure the last thing each patient hears when departing from your clinic is, "Thank you for your business," or, "Thank you for coming in." Remember that they don't have to be your patient. People like to know that their business is appreciated.

You are your marketing

As we are fond of saying, "Every minute is a marketing minute." This is especially true when you are working in your clinic. Your services, your skill, your demeanor, and the way your clinic feels, smells, looks, and acts are the most important part of any marketing effort you can create. You cannot afford to be a lazy practitioner with regard to any of these points. Take classes and continue to improve your skills. Make sure your patients feel that coming to your office is like entering a safe and healing space. If your clinic is humane and yet run as an efficient, clean, well-oiled machine with just a touch of magic, you are way ahead of the game as a marketer. That is why I [HW] always tell graduating students that running a private practice requires the passion of a Romeo, the patience of Saint Francis, and the intellectual curiosity of a Socrates.

POINTS TO PONDER FROM CHAPTER 2

- You and your clinic itself are the most important aspect of your marketing. Don't skimp on how your clinic feels, looks, or operates.

- There are lots of other ways that you market from inside your clinic: lots of available information and education for your patients, excellent and prompt telephone customer service, engaging artistry and aesthetics in your clinic, one-stop shopping convenience, good signage, spotless bathrooms, and toys for kids.

- Your telephone is your lifeline. Make sure you are easily available, your phone patient management skills are honed, you have adequate incoming lines, and that your hold message or after-hours recording includes simple marketing messages.

- A successful clinic is both humane and run like a well-oiled machine, but with just a touch of magic.

Community Team Builders and Marketing | 3

This chapter is about outside marketing. Outside marketing means everything from pounding the pavement in your neighborhood handing out cards, volunteering for community projects, using the same service people and companies in your town over and over and getting to know them well, to writing articles for the local media or giving free speeches to every possible organization who will let you in the door. While we truly believe that inside marketing (Chapter 2 above) is fundamentally the most important in your overall marketing efforts, few new practitioners can grow a full practice without ever doing any outside marketing. No matter how great your clinic or your skills, you have to do some things to let people know about you in the initial few years of your professional life.

PRACTITIONER POINTER

"My experience has shown me that networking is very important. I tend to be shy, but I've forced myself to be as social as possible, and every event I attend helps my practice to grow. I took an acupuncturist out to dinner when I first arrived here, which was a big investment for me at the time. That relationship has grown since and now her office regularly refers patients to me. And she provides moral support and encouragement!"

—Elizabeth Liddell
Philadelphia, PA

Below we have included as many ideas as we can think of or have heard about that can be effective for practitioners of Chinese medicine and acupuncture. Not every idea will work for everyone, but there are some very effective marketing ideas here. Unless you are really not meant for this work, some of these ideas will appeal to you and bring patients in your door.

➤ Effective pavement-pounding methods

Above we said that one good strategy is to walk concentric circles around your clinic in a five block radius and see what is there. Take a notebook and pen with you. There are all types of marketing possibilities here. You could:

- At every business location find out if you can post a flyer on the staff break-room bulletin board.

- Is there a service or product from a business down the street that you can help promote? See if you can create a you-scratch-my-back-I'll scratch-yours relationship. Where you can sell their products in your clinic or give out their cards and vice versa.

- At every company that has more than 25 employees there is likely to be a Human Resources (HR) person who is in charge of medical insurance, Worker's Comp referrals, payroll Cafeteria Plans, and other personnel services. It's a great idea to meet these people, offer them a free treatment, provide them with educational materials, brochures, or bring them a complete presentation folder about your clinic services.

- If you are specializing in any specific niche market, note every business that has any relationship to your specialty. For example, if you do acu-facelifts or dermatology, you want to make sure that any and all day spas, beauty salons, or beauty supply retail outlets have your cards and brochures. Perhaps you could do a trade with the owner… treatments in trade for putting your cards out next to their cash register? Perhaps you could do a free in-service lecture for their entire staff on how your services compliment theirs?

- Introduce yourself to the wait staff at every restaurant and coffee shop that you can. Give them cards and tell them you'd love their referrals. Then pick one or two that you frequent as often as you can. Get to know everyone there on a first name basis. Go early in the morning when it is the least busy and start conversations with them. That is to say, become their friend. One practitioner we know gets over 50 referrals per year from one coffee shop near his clinic.

- If you are in a large office building, make sure every receptionist at every office in the building has your card and that you take the time to learn about all his or her aches and pains and other assorted health problems. If there are MDs or DCs in your building, are there ways that you could enhance their services to their patients without being a threat? Find out if the office staff would be interested in a lunch time in-service about Chinese medicine. You provide the sandwiches and drinks and let them convince the MDs in their clinic to let you educate them about your services.

- If you are in a residential neighborhood, write a short letter of introduction about your clinic and leave them in every screen door. Offer them a "good neighbor" discount on their first treatment or a free consultation. Put a smiling photo of yourself on this letter or brochure. Or, even better for more courageous souls, knock on every door, introduce yourself and offer them a brochure and a free consultation at the new clinic in the neighborhood.

➤ Corporate marketing strategies

If you are in an area with a few large companies (100+ employees), it is really useful to find ways to connect with them. Again, the HR department is a good place to start.

- Find out the name of the head of the HR department and send or bring in a presentation folder to them. Try to get an appointment to find out what ways you might serve the company's employees. Find out what insurance company they use and whether their policy reimburses for acupuncture. What Worker's Comp insurance carrier do they use? Will they share their insurance rep's name with you?

- Do they have a company newsletter and would they like some free, short articles on relevant topics?

- Do they have any in-service lectures on health for their employees? Could you give one of these on stress management, repetitive strain injuries, managing low back pain, graceful aging, preventing the common cold and flu, etc.?

P O W E R   P O I N T

Tips for Writing for Corporate Newsletters
- Keep your article to a half-page unless the editor asks for something longer.
- Use bullet points for things like, "Five Tips for a Healthy Holiday Season."
- Don't use jargon, Chinese words, or difficult to read words and sentences.
- Don't write in long sentences with lots of commas, clauses, phrases, etc.
- Keep articles friendly and think about the "what's in it for the reader" message.
- All you want in return is your name and contact info at the bottom of the article.
- If they don't ask you for a follow up article for next quarter, take the initiative and call the editor to see if there has been any feedback and if they want another article. Better yet, bring them three or four short articles all at one time.
- Find out what digital formats they prefer and send them both a disk and a hard copy for proofing.

➤ Community participation

Almost every city and town in the U.S. has a myriad of opportunities for community involvement. You can get yourself on all sorts of committees for fundraising, riverfront cleanup, hospital auxiliary, homeless shelter, school music program, AIDS relief, battered women, humane society . . . the list goes on and on. The idea here is that the more you can participate in the community, the better known your name will become. People instinctively like to buy products and services from people they know and trust. While you can create trust by running a really great clinic with effective services humanely and efficiently delivered, in your early years of practice you will also need to find ways to weave yourself firmly into the warp and weft of your chosen community. And who knows, you may make some wonderful friends while you are building your practice. Here are just a few ideas.

➤ Health fairs or community fairs

These are tricky, but they can be effective if you really work them and don't just stand around behind your table under your pop-up tent smiling. If you live in a small town or city, these are probably more effective than a large city. Here are a couple of ideas that have appeal.

One woman gets her patients to come and be treated for free. She actually sets up appointments for them as if it were a regular day, each one 45 minutes apart. She gives simple pro-forma treatments, nothing complicated and she does not do an interview with them, just a treatment. But there's lots of rubbernecking as people stop to talk to her and to her patients while they are on the table with needles sticking out. She then gets the benefit of on-the-spot referrals from her patients telling passersby how great she is as well as the fascination with needles curiosity factor working in her favor. She has people to talk with all day, gives out lots of cards and brochures, and definitely gets patients from these events.

Also consider bringing a fish bowl and put a sign on it saying that people may put in their business cards for a prize drawing. You should give away something really good, not just one free treatment. A great piece of Chinese art work that you brought back from China could be attractive, a package of wonderful general health-promoting herbs that you normally sell in your clinic, or a set of Chinese medical self-care products. Your prize should be worth at least $100. You might also have some second or third place prizes that you display on the table, such as an interesting book on Chinese medicine for the general reader or two bottles of AllerEase for hay fever sufferers if it happens to be either spring or fall. This is all just to create traffic at your booth. What you will find is that if you have two or three people hanging out at your booth, more folks are likely to stop to see what the other people stopped for. After you pick your prize-winners at the end of the weekend, you can use the rest of the business cards as contact information for later. After the fair, send a postcard to each person who stopped by your booth and left a card or signed up for the newsletter. Thank them for stopping and let them know that they did not win the prize but that, if they have any more questions about Oriental medicine or acupuncture, you'd be most happy to hear from them on the phone during regular business hours. If you want to be really aggressive, you can tell them that the card is good for their first bottle of herbs free when they come in for an initial examination and treatment.

These events are easier (and cheaper for the booth rental!) if you share the booth with three or four other practitioners working in two-by-two shifts of a few hours each. Here are some more ideas for creating traffic and conversation.

- Stand in front of your booth, not behind it. Wear an easy-to-read name-tag. Keep your cards handy or a basket of giveaway goodies (pens, herb samples, magnets, etc.). Smile and start as many conversations as you can.

- Bring an acupuncture doll and different sizes of needles in a case or laminated onto something. A display of various bulk Chinese herbs can be a visual attraction.

- If you have a newsletter, make sure to have a sign-up sheet on your table for anyone interested. Put up an easy-to-read little plexiglass sign that says, "Sign Up Here for a Free Health Tips Newsletter."

- Give out ginger snaps and licorice ropes, explaining that they have Chinese herbs in them or have a large dish of Chinese "trail mix" with lycium berries and black date pieces and walnuts.

- Invest in some brochures on different conditions that you treat well. Don't just leave them on the table but actively hand them to people. (Make sure your contact info is on each one!)

- If your fair is near Thanksgiving or Christmas, you might give away little tubes of Curing Pills and put up a sign explaining how to use them after consuming a large meal to avoid indigestion.

- If there are several practitioners sharing a booth, you can do pro-forma treatments on each other because people like to see the needles. They will inevitably ask, "Doesn't it hurt?" to the person on the table.

- Consider giving free pulse diagnosis sessions for 10 minutes each, explaining just one simple thing to each person about their health.

- If you put up a large sign above the booth, don't make the sign say "Ace Acupuncture Clinic." The sign should have a what's-in-it-for-me-the-passerby message like "Acupuncture Works! Any Questions?" or simply "Improve Your Health Today!"

- Make sure all your current patients and friends know that you are doing the fair. Ask them to stop by with their friends and family.

P O W E R   P O I N T

Script for a Health Fair

"Hello, I'm Honora. I'm an acupuncturist licensed by the state of Colorado. I see you're looking at the low back pain brochure. (Hand them the brochure.) Do you have a health condition that you have some concern about?

Then you let the person talk for as long as they need to and don't interrupt. When they have finished, ask several questions:

1. How long have you had this?
2. How frequently do you get the pain (or other symptoms)?
3. When did the problem start?
4. On a scale of 1–10, what is the intensity of your pain?
5. What do you think is causing this problem?
6. What other doctors have you seen about this condition?
7. Did their treatment help you?
8. What else have you tried?
9. What will you do if this gets worse?
10. Is it bad enough that you want to solve the problem if you could?

Then, if it is a condition that you feel capable of or have experience treating, tell them that you think you may be able to give them some relief. Give them your card and a brochure or take their name and phone in order to follow up with a phone call if they are not willing or able to schedule an appointment right then and there.

The key here, no matter how you set up your booth or how you staff it, is that you have to really "work" the event. If you do this right, you will be tired after a few hours, but you will get lots of people stopping by, signing up for your mailing list, asking questions, taking cards, and, hopefully, becoming your patients. One final word, don't do this type of event if you are shy.

➤ Playing the media card

There are lots of ways to interact effectively with the media. Get the names of every health editor, feature editor, city editor, or Sunday magazine editor at every newspaper in your

NEWS FLASH
Acupuncture Works!

area you can find. Send them a presentation folder with a cover letter offering your services as an authority on Oriental medicine and acupuncture. Tell them you are always happy to hear from them or write an article or column for their section of the paper. If you have had any articles published elsewhere (like those corporate newsletters we mentioned above), send them copies. Offer to have them come to your clinic for a tour or a treatment.

If you always had a fantasy about your own TV or radio show, it is not really very hard to get on cable TV or public radio. With an effective presentation and a short how-to class, you could have a talk show on the radio about health-related issues. If someone in your town already has such a show, you can at least get booked in as an expert once or twice a year. The same is true of cable TV. Call several TV stations, especially the local public TV stations, and talk to the manager about what the possibilities are and what hoops you'd need to jump through to do this. Even if you get taped for a show that airs at 2 AM, you could do "Health Tips for Insomniacs" as your theme! If you want to get on a local or even a nationally syndicated talk show as a guest, do some digging on the internet and send out information to every producer you can find. Of course it helps if you are a published author or have some special expertise about a relevant in-the-news topic, but it could be worth it to fish in this pond. Somebody has to be the "expert" the next time Oprah wants to talk about Oriental medicine, so why not you?

When contacting the media, use odd times of the day. These people often work weird schedules, but the gatekeepers who work for them work regular 9–5 schedules. Thus, if you call at 7:30 AM or PM, who knows who will answer and what access you may have?

If you have something really exciting to share and the chops to do it well, you can contact every syndicated columnist in the U.S. (almost). *Editor and Publisher* magazine has a list they sell very inexpensively (888-612-7095). Just make sure whatever you send them is professionally done. You can also go to www.radio-locator.com for a list of radio stations and then contact producers with your great idea.

If you want to be an expert on a specific subject (improved sports performance, preventing anorexia, treating fibromyalgia, whatever is currently the hot health topic), go to your local/regional paper and TV station websites and find the names of relevant editors (health, special features, modern living, etc.) and send them a short, powerful e-mail message. Keep it to three paragraphs max and use powerful words and sentences to get across your message. If possible, it's even better to reference or tie to a previous story that this journalist has written or covered. So do some homework first . . . and never use attachments. Give them the guts of what you have to say in a sound bite. Deliver it in a way that makes their job easier and, who knows, you might become their main contact for alternative health for years to come.

> **POWER POINT**
>
> Be paranoid in reverse. Assume that people are plotting to make you happy and help you to fulfill your dreams. What you believe matters!

➤ **What other skills do you have that may help you market yourself?**

Can you teach t'ai chi, yoga, qi gong, cooking, calligraphy, or anything at all related to health and Oriental medicine? If so, find a way to teach it in your community. This could be through the local community college, the YMCA, the city recreation department, or a lifelong learning clearing house or a local related business. If you are good and you do this regularly, at least some if not most of your students will become patients at some point.

Are you a great organizer? If so, consider organizing an event (golf tournament, walk-a-thon, food drive) for your favorite charity. Involve other local acupuncturists or even your state association. This is a great way to get media coverage! If you cannot find the juice to create an event yourself, participate in as many such events as you have time for. All the people you work with, march with, call on the phone, and raise money from are prospective patients. People want to do business with others who are active in promoting good things in their community.

After any committee or event that you work on, follow up on those connections. After you've worked on the breast cancer walk-a-thon committee (or whatever), send follow-up notes to everyone you worked with that say something like:

> *Dear Sally,*
> *Just a note to tell you how much I enjoyed working with you in the last month on the walk-a-thon. I feel great about what we were able to accomplish together. If I can ever be of service to you or your family when it comes to your health,*
> *or if you ever have questions about my acupuncture services, please don't hesitate to call. I'd be happy to speak with you. Thanks again for your great energy working on the walk-a-thon committee.*
> *Yours sincerely,*

Don't forget to include your business card with the picture of you on it.

Remember, everybody will be somebody's patient someday. Why shouldn't they be yours?

POINTS TO PONDER FROM CHAPTER 3

- At least when you are starting out, you will need to do some proactive outside marketing. This may include but is not limited to events, committees, health fairs, volunteering of any kind, writing articles, teaching classes, becoming a media darling, giving lectures, and following up on those contacts.

- Search out and make contact with the Human Resources departments of any and all companies with more than 100 employees. Can you write for their newsletter, give free classes or talks to their employees, post your business cards on the break-room bulletin board? Find out what type of insurance they have and if it reimburses for acupuncture. Can you become a regular recipient of Worker's Comp referrals with these companies?

- People like to do business with people they know and like.

- Media folks are always looking for a new story and a new angle. If you find ways to help them write the story or gain access to something of interest, you will get in the news and could become a regular 'source' for articles on complementary and alternative medicine.

- Do you like to write, teach, organize events, or give public lectures? Consider your talents carefully and how you can give your best back to your community. That's how new patients will find you.

- Never go anywhere without your business cards, don't be shy, and remember that everyone is someone's patient someday.

Building & Using a Mailing List | 4

Whether you are a tiny one-person show or a large, multi-practice clinic, a good mailing list is an important asset to your business. This, of course, means both an e-mail and regular mailing list. You can and should start on this very early . . . even while you are still in school. Your goal should be a minimum of 200 names if you use a postal mailing list and as many names as you can get your hands on if you use an e-mail list. In either case, more is always better.

➤ **Where to start**

There are several ways you can collect mailing list names and addresses.

- Ask your friends or family in the area where you are going to practice for likely referrals. Ask your patients for referrals of friends who would be happy to receive information about your newsletter, classes, lectures, etc.

- When you give a free lecture, do a health fair, or attend any other public event where it is possible, put out a mailing list sign up sheet. Be sure to put on the top of the sheet what kinds of things you will be sending. Also put a statement saying that you never rent or sell your mailing list to other companies or organizations.

- When you teach a class for a community college, pass around the same type of sign-up sheet as described above.

- Your intake forms packet should include one giving you permission to send cards, newsletters, or other general information from your clinic and HIPAA requires this now anyway. Explain on the form the kinds of things you will be sending and that you don't sell or rent your list out to any other company. If a patient signs this form, you have been given permission to include them on your list.

- Are there local businesses that serve the same niche of people that you serve? If so, include these businesses on your mailing list. The same is true of local MDs or other health providers. While you might not send them every single piece that you publish, there will be occasions when you want to include them in a mailing.

- Look for the names of local/regional newspaper editors, TV and radio producers, or other media folks who should be on your list. Keeping in regular touch with these type of people can lead to all sorts of unforeseen marketing opportunities.

- Mailing lists grow faster than you might think. Keep a paper file for cards and signup sheets but put them in a digital file as soon as you can and always keep a backup!

- If you write articles for a local paper, parenting newsletter, corporate newsletter, chronic fatigue support group website, or wherever, your contact information and the fact that you publish a newsletter, recipe-of-the-month, health tips articles, etc. should be at the end of every article. Say something like, "Honora Wolfe is a licensed acupuncturist in Boulder, CO. You can sign up for her free Health-Tip-of-The-Month newsletter by sending your contact info to honora@ bluepoppy.com or calling 303-447-8372."

So, the point here is that there are lots and lots of ways to build a mailing list. Now let's discuss what to do with those names and addresses.

Using your mailing list
This makes me think of the statement, "Vote early and often." The greatest mailing list in the world won't do you any good if you don't use it. On the other hand, you need to consider

P O W E R   P O I N T

Even when people sign up for something, they may change their mind or not even remember that they signed up. If it feels like spam or they decide they are not interested, you are required by web etiquette to give them a way out. When you do e-mail newsletters, always include a "Click Here if you wish to opt out of this newsletter" link at the bottom of your letter, article, or announcement. Make sure you or your staff takes care of these requests promptly... the same for your postal mailing list.

timing your use of any mailing list both in terms of costs and the kinds of things that people like to receive.

• Divide your list into categories. You may do a mailing to MDs or DCs that does not go to patients. Or you may want to do a media-only mailing of a *press release* or offer yourself for interviews or a corporate mailing to offer a series of free lectures. You may want to divide your list as to whether people are or are not already patients.

• Speaking of dividing your mailing list into specific groups, if you use Microsoft Access or Excel or another major database or mailing list program, there are many ways to subdivide or segment any list. You can create various categories when you set up your digital file. Then, when you want to print labels or envelopes or merge a letter, you can choose from those specific categories whom to include in the mailing.

• Remember that e-mailings are cheaper by far than postal mailings. Make sure all your sign-up sheets and forms have a line for e-mail addresses. Most on-line interface software such as Firefox, Explorer, and Outlook, provide a way to create large e-mail groups. However, remember that most people don't want everybody and their brother to have their email address. So whatever software you use has to be able to send to each person as if they were the only one, while all the other people in the group are like "blind" copies. There are, of course, other more sophisticated software options that you might use to create e-newsletters or announcements.

- Start using your mailing list right away. One of the most important principles of marketing is to have a good message, say it well, and say it *often*. Not all the plums on any tree ripen at the same rate. But shame on you if you are not there when each one does ripen. The only way to "be there" is to stay in touch regularly with anyone and everyone who has given you permission to do so or who is a public entity and does not have to give you permission. Ideally, that means you send out a postcard, e-mail, newsletter, course announcement, or other missive every 8–12 weeks to some segment of your mailing list.

- Keep your cards, e-mails, press releases, and newsletter articles short and sweet, at least most of the time. People don't have time to read a lot. And, very important, always try to craft a headline that explains what's in it for them if they do read the whole thing. Say something as funny, compelling, dynamic, poignant, or outrageous, as you can. Then you can explain (quickly and to the point) the message you really want to get across.

- Here's a fun e-mail newsletter idea for good cooks or nutrition aficionados (we mentioned this idea in Chapter 2 above). Create a Recipe-of-the-Season newsletter or a Nutrition News newsletter. The entire newsletter is simply a recipe with an introduction on why you like this recipe, its nutritional or Chinese medicinal qualities, etc. Or you can write about a specific herb or formula (in easy-to-understand layman's terms) and why you like it for the current season.

This type of message allows you to send out something fun and useful while simply staying in the patient's (or potential patient's) mind. As we said before, everybody becomes someone's patient someday.

- Mail out an autumn card about preventing the common cold and winter flu. Something like, "Why Does Everyone Need Three Bottles of XYZ Chinese Cold Remedy?" or "What Chinese Medicine Makes a Great Stocking Stuffer?" This is followed by something like, "You can stop a cold or flu before it starts if you have one bottle at work, one in the medicine chest, and one in your car's glove box. Buy three bottles and get 10% off. This offer is good through 12/15/0X." This could also be a reminder to come in for an autumn constitutional strengthening/flu prevention treatment or treatment series.

- You can do the same thing for spring or fall allergies, post-Halloween sugar blues, or post-holiday digestive tune-ups. Or you can tie your reminder to Breast Cancer Prevention Month or Diabetes Month. The possibilities are endless.

As you can see, the point here is to find reasons to stay in touch with your patients, your possible future patients, people with businesses related to the niche market you want to serve (bicycle clubs, women's groups, skin care spas, etc.), the media, possible referrers such as MDs, DCs, DOs, PTs, CMTs, and RNs, and make your messages something they will be happy to receive because of useful content, humor, or because they already love you. A mailing list is a very powerful and important part of your marketing tool-kit!

POINTS TO PONDER FROM CHAPTER 4

- A good mailing list is one of your best communication tools to potential patients or referrers.

- There are lots of ways to build up a mailing list. We've listed eight possibilities.

- A mailing list does you no good unless you use it often. We list lots of ideas and you could easily come up with a dozen more.

- The chapter is only five pages long; we suggest you read the whole thing.

Creating Your Presentation Folder | 5

A *presentation folder* (PF) is a public relations tool with many uses. It describes, formally, beautifully, and in organized detail, everything you want any specific group or person to know about you and your clinic services. There are several things that should always be included in a presentation folder and many optional pieces. They can be formal and slick, like a corporate media kit, or done more simply on your office computer and inkjet printer. Either way, we encourage you to create one and update it regularly as your professional situation changes. You will find many uses for this tool.

➤ What goes in a presentation folder?

Your folder should include at least the following pieces:

- A cover letter explaining why you are sending them this information and how you hope they will respond to it.
- A curriculum vitae (CV)
- Prescription pad
- Information flyer or brochure about your clinic and the services available, hours of operation, and prices.
- Your business card
- A map with directions to your facility.
- Letters of reference from a patient or another practitioner (MD, DC, PT, DO, JD, other professional).

Optional pieces for your presentation folder:

- A short, nontechnical book on Oriental medicine
- Articles from magazines or newspapers about acupuncture or Oriental medicine.
- Articles or research papers you have written on any subject related to Oriental or alternative medicine.
- Your clinic mission statement

- Articles or brochures about specific conditions (*e.g.,* sports medicine if you are sending the PF to an orthopedist).
- Printed research supporting the ability of acupuncture and/or Oriental medicine to treat a specific condition effectively.
- Any other relevant or interesting information about you, published articles about your clinic from the newspaper
- Copies of any letter received from a satisfied patient regarding how much your services helped their condition.
- A small notepad with your name and phone number.
- A magnet with your clinic name and phone number or a business card magnet.
- Evidence of malpractice insurance for your practice.

Remember, most of these pieces can also be used for a website!

Okay, let's go back and talk about each one of these elements separately.

⟩ Writing an effective cover letter

A cover letter should be short and to the point. A good cover letter can mean the difference between someone actually reading through your PF or not bothering to look further. Below is a sample cover letter. This same letter and others specific to different audiences are on this book's website and can be downloaded and tinkered with to your heart's content. ⦿

What you will notice about this and other letters on the website is that these are one page, to the point, specific, and friendly. They tell the reader exactly how you hope they will respond, *i.e.,* they give the reader a next step to take that is low risk: look through the PF and call for more information. Other options in this type of letter are to offer a free luncheon in-service, times that you are available by phone, or references upon request. Letters to the media, other acupuncturists, or corporate HR managers would, of course, be completely different in content. ⦿ Consider creating different cover letters for different uses.

VITAL HEALTH ACUPUNCTURE CLINIC
SARAH SMITH, L.AC.
1234 FOREST STREET
DES MOINES, IA 60000
515-123-4567

August 14, 200X

Des Moines Health & Orthopedics
Attention Dr. John Doe
4444 Main St.
Des Moines, IA, 60000

Dear Dr. Doe,

My name is Sarah Smith and I am a Licensed Acupuncturist in the state of
Iowa, certified by the Iowa Board of Medical Examiners.

I have recently relocated my clinic to the above address and would be happy
to accept referrals from your office for patients whose conditions may not be
responding well to traditional health care options. I offer safe, competent, and
effective care with acupuncture, Chinese herbal medicine, and nutritional
counseling to help people with problems in the following areas:
- pre- and post-surgical care
- pain management
- migraines and chronic headaches
- chronic insomnia
- environmental sensitivities and food allergies
- fibromyalgia and chronic fatigue immune deficiency syndrome

Enclosed is a packet of information about the benefits of acupuncture and
Chinese medicine. I would love to offer my services to your patients and to
work with you to improve their chances at full recovery from the conditions
listed above. My clinic is also able to provide documented research on a variety
of other health care concerns and proof of malpractice insurance upon request.

I believe that the integration of our two medicines is the future of modern
health care and I look forward to being of service to you and your patients.
Please feel free to contact me at any time with questions or requests for
further information.

Yours sincerely,

Sarah Smith, L.Ac.

➤ The curriculum vitae or CV

A *curriculum vitae* means, basically, what you have done with or the "curriculum" of your life. It is short, preferably one page long, and mentions only the most important aspects of your professional history. There is a sample CV on the website that you can print out or download and imitate. ⊙ There are also web sites and books that can help you do a really good CV. Basically, you need to include the following:

1. Your name and contact information at the top.

2. Educational history. This includes your BA or BS undergraduate degree, any advanced degrees, your acupuncture school certification, and other professional training certifications that are relevant. Do not put dates, but do put them in chronological order.

3. Licenses and credentials. Here you will list your NCCAOM certification, your state license, Red Cross First Aid training, certification in Clean Needle Technique, and any other licenses (nursing, massage, midwifery, psychotherapy) that you have.

4. Professional experience. If you are a brand new graduate, you may list the college clinic as one listing. Again, list no dates. If you have other professional experience in another field put that down. If you are young and were waiting tables or tending bar, we suggest putting down something like, "Consultant to the Food Industry." If you were cleaning hotel rooms, put "Consultant to the Hotel Industry." You may need to be a little creative if you don't have a lot of professional experience at anything.

5. Societies and memberships. Are you a member of Rotary, Kiwanis, Big Brother, or the Chamber of Commerce in your town? If so, by all means include that information here. Have you joined your state professional association or a national professional association? It looks very good to be a member of a few associations; so consider joining. Many associations get discounts from various professional product suppliers, which could easily pay for the membership each year.

6. Publications. At least list a couple of papers you wrote in school. If you have written for your state professional association newsletter, a corporate newsletter, a local newspaper, or any other publication, list it here.

That's it. Be concise, spell out acronyms such as NCCAOM because no one outside the profession knows what they mean, and leave out dates. Proofread to make sure it is spelled correctly. If you are a lousy speller, get someone else to proof it for you. Actually that advice goes for every piece you create for your PF!

➤ What is the definition of a good business card?

We get asked to critique a lot of practitioners' business cards, and we have created a list of what's helpful and what's not as helpful from a marketing point of view on a business card. There is still lots of room for interpretation here, but these are the basics.

1. Your business card is your calling card and should be easy to read. Don't make people work to find the information they want. That means using an easy to read typeface. We suggest that you stay away from *Flowery*, **Chinesey**, or 𝔥𝔦𝔤𝔥𝔩𝔶 𝔰𝔱𝔶𝔩𝔦𝔷𝔢𝔡 typefaces. Pick fonts that allow people to find and read the information immediately. Don't use more than two different typefaces on one card.

2. Your name is the most important piece of information.

3. Your phone number is the second most important piece of information. Don't make it smaller than 11 point type and make its placement on the card prominent enough to find in an instant.

4. Fax number, email address, and regular and website address if you have one, are the next most important pieces of information on your card.

5. If you have a logo, a color scheme, or a USP (see Section 2, Chapter 1) for your clinic, these help identify your clinic, especially if they are repeated on your signage, brochures, or other written promotional pieces.

6. On the back of the card, you might include a map to your clinic, hours of operation, or a "Your Next Appointment Is" section.

7. If you don't have a logo, it's really nice to do a photo of yourself on your card. When people meet you at a public fund-raising event or health fair and find your card two months later, your photo helps them remember the conversation they had with you.

8. In terms of papers, use a nice textured card stock or high gloss stock for your card. If you put your photo on the card, always use high gloss stock.

9. We don't suggest plastic cards. They're cute but people cannot write on them.

Creating a prescription pad

Most of us have had the experience of being in a doctor's office and the doctor wanting to refer us to a specialist. Behind their appointment counter, the office staff person checking you out looked through a pile of prescription pads and tore off one saying, "Here is the name of the specialist Dr. Smith wants you to see." They may even have made the appointment for you right while you were there.

In the world of medicine, practitioners refer patients to each other all the time. It is simply standard operating procedure. If a

389

referring office has a prescription pad from your office, you are more likely to be able to participate in this network.

What should be on a prescription pad?

These are pretty simple. We have included one sample below and a couple other samples on the website. ● Basically you want "Acupuncture Prescription" at the top, your name and contact information next, then the patient's name, date of the referral, diagnosis, space for any specific requests from the referring practitioner, and the name and contact phone for the referring practitioner. It should not be larger than one-half page, but one-quarter page can also be fine.

Once you have created a digital file for a prescription pad, take the disk or email the file to your chosen printer and have them print 100 pads, 20–25 sheets to a pad. Like your business cards, give these out liberally to any other practitioner who will refer to you, even if you have not sent them or don't need to send them a PF.

Your name and address here
Acupuncture Prescription

Patient Name: _____ Phone: ( ) _____ Date: ___ / ___ / ___

Primary Diagnosis: _____

Secondary Diagnosis: _____

Instructions/Precautions: _____

Frequency of Treatment: _____ /wk   Duration of Treatment:: _____ wks   Re-check with Doctor: _____ wks

Treatment Plan   Evaluate and Treat as Necessary ☐

Modalities ☐	Procedures ☐	Exercises ☐	Functional Rehab Prog ☐
☐ Heat	☐ Myofascial Release	☐ Flexibility	☐ Knee
☐ Ice	☐ Massage	☐ Strength	☐ Cervical
☐ Electrical Stimulation	☐ Traction (Mechan/Manual)	☐ Endurance/Cardio	☐ Shoulder
	☐ Cerv ☐ Lumb ☐ Spinal	☐ Trunk Stabilization	☐ Lumbar
☐ TENS Trial	☐ Acupuncture	☐ Posture/Body Mech	☐ Hand
☐ Interferential Trial	☐ Pilates	☐ Home Program	☐ Other:
		☐ Gait Training	
		☐ Therapeutic Exercise	Evaluations ☐

Referring Physician: _____

➤ **Clinic brochures. The byword is keep it simple!**
Your clinic brochure needs to grab the reader's attention within
a two-second perusal. That really is all the time you have.
Following a few simple rules will make it more likely that
anyone will actually read what you spent so much time to write.

1. Your headline must be a what's in it for me statement that
   grabs attention because it responds to a need or problem.
   That means, don't put the name of your clinic or a picture of
   your clinic on the front. Or, if you must put your name on
   the front, put it at the bottom of the front panel. A headline
   like, "Post-op Patients Return to Work in 50% Less Time
   with Regular Acupuncture," "Chinese Medicine Treats
   Insomnia No Side Effects," or, "Modern Research Shows
   Relief for Menopausal Patients with Chinese Medicine," is
   likely to get the health care practitioners you are trying to
   reach to actually read the rest of your words. Of course you
   will need to quote some research to support your statements,
   but such research is available on a wide variety of subjects.

2. On your general clinic brochure, put your photo on the
   inside or the back cover. If you don't have enough for a three
   panel fold brochure, a two panel fold can be just as effective.

3. Use a serifed typeface for the body copy of your brochure
   (such as Times Roman, **Century Schoolbook**, Garamond,
   or Goudy) and a sans serifed typeface for the headlines
   (**Futura**, Ariel, **Univers**). Serifed faces are easier to read for
   lengthy body copy, sans serifed faces pop out if used sparingly
   for headlines and subheadlines.

4. It is usually easier to read text lines that are less than two
   inches across and not more than four inches across and at
   least 11 points tall. Also, the longer the line, the larger the
   text and the more space between lines, called leading, you
   will need. It is also easier to read text that is flushed left or
   right, not justified on both sides (see below).

391

Notice that the headline below is bold, large, and sans serifed. The body text in the first paragraph below is flush left, ragged right, and 12 points tall. It is easy on the eye.

What is Chinese Medicine & How Does It Work?

Chinese medicine is the oldest, professional, continually practiced, literate medicine in the world. This medical system's written literature stretches back almost 2,500 years. And currently 1/4 of the world's population makes use of it. One can say that modern Western and traditional Chinese medicines are the two dominant medical systems in the world today.

Notice that the paragraph below is justified on both sides, causing "rivers" of uneven white spacing between the words, as often seen in the newspaper. It is harder to read than the paragraph above.

Isn't Chinese Medicine Just a System of Folk Healing?

No. This system has been created by some of the best educated and brightest scholars in Chinese history. These scholars have recorded their theories and clinical experiences from generation to generation in literally thousands of books…

The message here is, as much as you can, design your brochure to make it easy to read.

5. Bullet points get read first. Short paragraphs are more likely to get read than long ones.

6. Don't use too much Oriental medical jargon. On the other hand, don't write as though you were speaking to a first-grader.

7. Proofread by reading forward for context errors, then backward for spelling errors, because the eye tends to see the spelling of words the way it thinks they should be.

8. It is useful to have one brochure about your clinic and others about specific subjects or disease conditions.

9. If you cannot do your own clinic brochure, see if you can trade for treatments with a graphic designer, copywriter, and proofreader. For brochures on specific diseases or other topics, Blue Poppy as well as other companies now have many from which you may choose for use in presentation folders and at public events.

Letters of reference from patients

If you don't get any of these spontaneously, ask your best patients if they would be willing to write one for you to use in your presentation folder. Tell them exactly to whom the folders will be sent. Many, if not most, will be happy to do so if they have seen good results from coming to you. Tell them you are trying to get more referrals from MDs, DCs, or whatever and would they mind you using their letter of referral to send to their family doctor (or specialist, etc.) as well? They might or they might not want you to do this, but you won't know if you don't ask. If you ask three or four patients these questions, you are likely to get one letter by the next week. If you ask the patients who initially said yes but then forgot to bring in or send a letter, you are likely to get at least one more, and that's all you need. You should try to get one or two new letters each year, minimum.

➤ Articles and research

There are many sources for articles on Oriental medicine, alternative medicine, and acupuncture specifically. If you can search on the internet, the possibilities are endless. If you have to use paper only sources, then clip the article (if it is not from a magazine or newspaper owned by the library!) and make neat, clearly visible copies that are not crooked, smudged, or difficult to read and that fit on normal-sized pieces of paper.

Other things that we have listed for inclusion in your PF do not really require any explanation. So, let's discuss how to put this all together and what to do with it when completed.

➤ Putting your presentation folder together

If you go to any good paper supply store, you will find a wide variety of papers and presentation folders. Choose a tasteful color combination and buy some matching large envelopes. Start with purchasing only 10-15 of these.

If possible, design your pieces so that they are easy to see in the folder. Perhaps some can be taller and others shorter so that they are staggered in height, with the taller ones behind the shorter ones. If you do this, cut them carefully or get that done at a professional copy shop so they are not crooked across the bottom. We have seen some very classy looking folders that used some variation of this technique. Use the same paper and choose a consistent typeface or faces throughout as much as possible. Obviously some pieces will not "match" and that is OK as long as many (at least all the ones that you create yourself) of them do. If you have a color printer, be a little conservative on your use of colors unless you are marketing yourself as wild and outrageous on purpose.

Once you are sure that there are no spelling errors, print out one set of all your pieces and put it together. Get some feedback from a friend before you make all the remaining copies. Then organize your cover letters depending upon where you are sending them. Obviously, a media person cover letter would emphasize your knowledge about a hot topic they have recently covered or that is being covered a lot in the news. A letter to an assisted reproductive technologies clinic would be different from a letter to an orthopedist.

➤ Final steps

Don't handwrite your envelope labels. Get some labels that can go through your inkjet or laser printer. Get relatively large-sized labels. Both MS Word and WordPerfect have label specs for almost all sizes of labels. Type in the addresses for where you want to send these or pull them from your mailing list (see Chapter 4 above).

Take one completed presentation folder to the post office, get it weighed for postage, and buy some beautiful stamps, the largest sized ones that work. Don't have your folders metered! People love beautiful stamps and are more likely to take notice of your folder. If you are hand-delivering any of these (and that is quite okay), dress your best for this sojourn. When you are well dressed, you look and feel more confident. What's true is that when you feel more confident, others notice it and respond accordingly.

➤ Who gets your presentation folders?

If you are on a budget, choose carefully to whom you will send these. They will have cost you a lot of time and a couple of bucks (at least) apiece. However, one good medical referral relationship, one supportive HR director, one interested hospital director, or one great media contact can make a $250–300 expenditure completely worth your while. And, once sent out, you never know under whose eyes your folder will pass. Send them to:

- MDs and DCs whom you have researched in your community as likely to be friendly to alternative medicine or who have been referred to you by family or patients. How about your own family practitioner?

- All the media people we discussed in the "Community Marketing" chapter above.

- Call the local hospital(s) in-service or community coordinator and see if there is an opportunity to connect. If there is an interest or you can actually talk to someone who has an open mind, send that person a folder.

- If you are interested in working in a very specific medical niche, definitely send folders to all the medical practitioners who specialize in that niche. Remember, in this case, give them evidence of malpractice insurance.

- If you happen to live in a town with one or more large corporations or unions, find out the names of the medical insurance provider PPO or HMO, Worker's Comp insurance provider, or Human Resources directors and send a folder. For these type of people, do your homework first. Call and see if you can get a specific decision maker's name. Make your cover letter specific to the kinds of injuries or health complaints you believe to be most common in their world.

- During political campaigns to expand your scope of practice, you may want to send your PF to some governmental body or to specific politicians.

- Remember, again, that much of the content of this piece can also become content on your website.

Also, keep a few of these in reserve for spur-of-the-moment public relations opportunities. Add to or change items in your folder as your professional situation evolves. Presentation folders are a great way to help grow the use of acupuncture and

Oriental medicine in the U.S. by educating the people who are most likely to either influence or control where people go for medical care.

POINTS TO PONDER FROM CHAPTER 5

- Presentation folders (PF) are a useful component in your outside marketing toolbox. They have many components, some optional, some mandatory.

- When designing a PF, use consistent design elements such as papers, fonts, colors, and logo as much as you can.

- Write several different cover letters for different audiences—the media, specific health care professionals, hospital directors, corporate Human Resource directors, Worker's Comp administrators, or politicians. Keep your cover letter to one page with a specific request for a follow-up step.

- Make sure you have at least 5–6 different pieces in your PF.

- Plan to spend a minimum of $2 and a maximum of $10 per unit on a good PF.

Using Press Releases | 6

Press releases are how the media get a lot of their news. Either the media run the release with their own editing or they follow up on the release to develop their own story. Press releases are a way of garnering free advertising. They are typically the first step in getting your name in an article in the paper or a piece done about you on radio or TV. Because press releases are relatively easy to write and send, they should be a regular part of your overall marketing plan. Below are 10 keys to writing a good press release—one that will translate into free media coverage for you and your clinic.

1. **Use an active headline to grab the reporter's attention.**
   Your headline should be short, active, and descriptive. For instance, instead of "Honora Wolfe Receives Award," use "Honora Wolfe Named Boulder's Best Acupuncturist."

2. **Put the most important information at the beginning.**
   The reporter needs to know who, what, when, where, why, and/or how in the first two paragraphs. In a busy newsroom, that's often all that gets read.

3. **Avoid hype and unsubstantiated claims.**
   If you make a claim, be sure you have some evidence to back it up. In most, if not all, states, it is illegal for a licensed health professional to promise a cure. Whatever you say, be sure it's true.

4. **Be active and to the point.**
   Try not to use passive voice. Use active verbs as much as you can. Also get to the point quickly. Don't meander. All you really need to do is answer the questions: Who, What, Where, When, Why, and/or How.

5. **Keep your release to a maximum of two pages.
   One is better.**

   If you're not stating your point in two pages or less, you're not getting to the point. Reporters tend to be busy people. They're not going to hunt through a poorly written, meandering four page release. The only file such an unfocused, poorly written release is going to go in is the circular kind.

6. **Include a contact.**

   If your release strikes an interest, the reporter is going to want to know how to get more information, how to followup. Therefore, every release should have the name and numbers of a contact person on the bottom. But be sure that A) the contact person is knowledgeable about the topic of the release and B) knows releases have been sent with their name on the bottom.

7. **Keep jargon to a minimum.**

   Try to keep any technical terms to a minimum. You know what qi, yin, and yang are, but the general public does not. Also try to use more simple Anglo-Saxon words and less words that come from Latin. Remember, journalists write for the average 6th grade reader. So keep it simple. Communication is more important than showing off your education.

8. **Stress benefits.**

   Everyone wants to know what's in it for me. Don't tell people that Chinese medicine is 2,000 years old, is ancient, great, wonderful, or the best. People want to know what benefits they are likely to experience. A better approach is to tell them about freedom from side effects, low cost, proven healing effects, or anything else which expresses a benefit to the prospective patient. Maybe that's something as prosaic as convenient parking and weekend office hours. Telling them how good Chinese medicine is or how good you are is not a direct benefit to the reader.

9. Be specific and detailed.

Don't assume that the reporter already knows anything about Chinese medicine and/or acupuncture. Don't be afraid to say that acupuncture refers to the insertion of very thin, sterile, stainless steel needles into certain specific points on the body for the purpose of re-establishing metabolic harmony and balance. In the foregoing sentence, I was very specific and detailed about my description of the needles most of us use. The reader should be able to visualize what you are talking about. Saying that acupuncture is an ancient system of health care from the Orient which re-establishes balance and harmony in the body just doesn't have the same effect. People have nothing concrete yet to visualize.

10. Proofread.

Be absolutely sure you *and someone else* proofreads your press release before sending it off. Proofread your release for spelling and also for grammar. Then proof it again to check to see if you've followed the previous nine pieces of advice. Nothing can sink a press release faster than a sloppy, unprofessional presentation. As a corollary of this, don't use fancy typefaces or dingbats (cute little graphic symbols). They're hard to read and look amateurish.

On the following page is a sample press release.

➤ Formatting

Standard format for a press release is double-spacing on one side only of white 8 1/2 x 11" paper. Put your name and address on the top of the page. If only sending to one publication, tell them it's "first run" in addition to "for immediate release." Be sure to use a typewriter or computer to compose the release. No handwriting.

In terms of topics for press releases, there is no end to the things you can announce. If you go to a seminar, tell people what you

Stillwater Health Clinic
3001 Baseline Ave.
Boulder, CO 80301
303-447-8367

Press Release

For immediate release.

Honora Wolfe Named Boulder's Best Acupuncturist

July 19, Boulder, CO: Local acupuncturist, Honora Lee Wolfe, received the Best of Boulder Award as acupuncturist of the year for 2002. This award was given by the Daily Camera yesterday at a ceremony held at the Broker Inn. Each year, the Daily Camera holds a contest for determining the Best of Boulder in 35 different categories. Ms. Wolfe, who is also a Fellow of the National Academy of Acupuncture and Oriental Medicine, has won this award two times before, once in 1997 and the other time in 1995. Ms. Wolfe has practiced acupuncture and Chinese medicine in Boulder since 1988. She is a student of Dr. Eric Tao of Denver and Bob Flaws of Boulder and has attended trainings at the Shanghai College of Chinese Medicine in the People's Republic of China in 1984, 85, and 87. Besides obviously having the support of her many satisfied patients, Ms. Wolfe has taught at the Southwest Acupuncture College in Gunbarrel and is the author or translator of several books on Chinese medicine, including Better Breast Health Naturally with Chinese Medicine and Managing Menopause Naturally with Chinese Medicine. Ms. Wolfe currently conducts a private practice at Stillwater Health which is a multipractitioner alternative health care clinic located at Baseline and 30th in Boulder. For the last several years, Ms. Wolfe has specialized in the treatment of chronic pain and sports injuries.

END-END-END-END

For further information, Ms. Wolfe can be contacted at: 303-447-8367 or by e-mail at: honora@stillwater.com.

learned and how it could potentially help them. If you go to a convention or symposium, tell them about the new techniques, information, or instruments you've brought back. If you receive an award or certificate for anything, for sure tell people about that. Let's say you were recently elected as Secretary of your state acupuncture association. You and I know that's mostly a lot of work and an honor of dubious distinction, but it sounds good to those who don't know any better. You might think these things are no big deal, and they aren't if that's the way you couch them. But put another spin on them and they're news with benefits for you to market. Instead of telling people that you address and lick the stamps of your state association's newsletter, you tell them you've been elected to the Board of Directors. Now you're one of the head honchos of acupuncture in your state.

POWER POINT

Resources for writing press releases:

1. *Six Steps to Free Publicity* by Marcia Yudkin, Plume, 2008. As the title describes, this book provides practical advice for a small business' publicity campaign.

2. *The Associated Press Stylebook and Libel Manual,* Addison-Wesley, 2008. A guide for spelling, punctuation, as well as information on avoiding libel and respecting copyright.

3. *The Elements of Style* by William Strunk & E.B. White, Macmillan, Revised 1979. This little book is the time-honored guide to clear writing.

4. Public Relations Society of America, 33 Irving Place, New York, NY 10003; 212-995-2230. A national organization for PR professionals that also sponsors educational seminars.

POINTS TO PONDER FROM CHAPTER 6

- You can help out the local media, become a local expert, get free publicity, and build your business, using press releases.

- Create a good media mailing list.

- Whenever you do anything that is interesting, remarkable, even a seminar with an interesting topic, write a press release and send it to all the local media.

- Follow the rules: one page, double-spaced, with Who, What, When, Where, Why and/or How statements.

- Is it Breast Cancer Awareness Month or National Diabetes Week, or The Great American Smoke Out? Find a timely hook, create a marketing activity in your community, and let the media know you are a mover and shaker in your town.

Marketing Your Practice on the Internet | 7

ere are some revealing statistics about computer and internet usage. More than 77% of US households were connected to the internet by the end of 2010. At the time of this writing, over 85% of businesses are connected, there are over 1.6 billion internet users worldwide, Facebook is the third largest "country" in the world, and over 200 million laptop computers were sold worldwide in 2010. Sales of products and services on the internet were up by more than 11% in 2009 over 2008 and 62% of all off-line purchases are influenced on online research. Throughout 2011, there will be over *200 million Google searches per day*. You, too, can use this amazing tool to grow your practice. This chapter is an attempt to give you the basics of what you need to know (at this swiftly-changing moment in time) to maintain some type of internet presence, create a simple website, and/or do basic internet marketing.

➤ What does it cost to create a simple website?

There are three basic ways to get a website built. 1. Use online web creation tools that walk you through the process. (See Web Resources listed below for leads.) 2. Do it with free share-ware if you are very comfortable with your computer and your first question is not, "What is shareware?" 3. For the technologically faint of heart or those who know that tinkering with html code is not for them, I suggest you hire a good web designer and create a long-term relationship with them. Tech-nerds need acupuncture, too, so at least a partial trade may be possible! Lets look at these three in more depth.

Online Web Creation Tools are

+Very cheap (possibly free)
- Require a learning curve for most of us
- Lack flexibility of design

+Often come with cheap site-hosting

\- There is little or no tech support

+May be great if you are computer savvy. VistaPrint, Weebly, Yahoo, Network Solutions are some of these. Others are www.designer360.com, www.register.com, you can find tons more by doing a web-search.

Do It Yourself with Shareware or Web services

+These are more flexible; you can create pretty much anything you want.

\-They take more time and have a steeper learning curve

1. Find free HTML (web computer language) editing or web publishing shareware at www.tucows.com
2. Pay for "assisted" software www.zyweb.com, www.2createwebsite.com
3. Buy Adobe Dreamweaver (complete around $200 for the student version at the time of this writing)
4. Take a Community College or online class in website creation. There are lots of these out there. Check out Weebly if you like to take online courses.

Hire a web designer

+ With good communication, you can get exactly what you want *plus good Search Engine Optimization* (vital)

+ With a good contract, you should have good tech support

\- Costs $ (but less than you might think). Try www.Elance.com and ask for bids from the freelance web designers just to see what you get.

Check references and look at the company or person's work!! You should be able to get a simple 5-page website for $360+or- You can get a simple, low-cost website at Acufinder.com AcupunctureClinicWebsite.com, TCMDirectory.com, and ChineseMedicineTools.com, but these may or may not meet all your criteria. More of these pop up all the time, so search and compare prices, services, tech-support, and longterm contracts.

➤ What about my domain name?

- A domain name is not expensive anymore. Unless you are choosing something really generic, *e.g.,* www.SeattleAcupuncture.com, you should be able to get a good domain for a few dollars per year ($10-25).
- Start with a visit to fatcow.com, godaddy.com, or justhost.com and see if the domain name you want is available.
- Try to choose a domain name that includes key words, e.g., www.Dallasathleticacupuncture.com says what you do and where you are.
- Names like www.crazyhorseclinic.com are fun but will not help your search engine rankings
- .com and .net are better than other designations; .org is only for non-profits; .edu is only for schools
- It's cheaper and easier to buy a multi-year contract if you are fairly sure to be staying where you are for a while.

➤ What about hosting?

Online site creators like those shown above offer hosting packages along with web creation tools, but little or no customer service. Prices start as low as $6-10 per month for minimal services (static pages + an email account) and go up from there. Get more of what you need for $20-30 per month, *i.e.,* a decent bulk email feature to send newsletters and capture names. Again, visit sites like justhost or fatcow for a decent package.

There are lots of smaller local and regional companies that do hosting. Start with price shopping, but mostly ask about their tech support, which is a good reason to stay local. You can always visit with the people in person and keep your money and networking in your city or town.

The main feature you need is to be able to capture visitor information, especially email addresses and to send bulk emails.

You may also want to sell a few products on line and there is more about that further in this chapter. Also ask about marketing support costs, such as key words on the homepage, metatags, and search engine optimization and submission.

➤ What should my site include?

A good website is meaningful, unique, succinct, and laced with key words. If you are not a good writer, hire a copywriter to help you create content and proofreading services to help you keep typos to a minimum. I [HW] can tell you that your web designers will be unhappy if you cannot or do not create the content you have agreed upon and that they require for building your website, and on the schedule that you create together. Remember that "content is king" is practically a mantra for web marketing gurus. I suggest going to a few practitioner's websites and see what they have included. It will help you save money when you visit a designer or, even if you build a site yourself, if you have an outline and some files written, photos taken, color scheme ideas, etc., completed before your start.

You can draw up paper "dummy" pages showing your designer some basic layout ideas, an outline for what opens up when you click on various items. If you can dump your completed article files and pictures from a thumb drive to their computer (already proofread, of course), you'll find this can go pretty quickly and easily and not be too expensive. The more you write/sketch/design in advance, the better the price will be.

The first sentence or two at the top should have all the **key words** you can think of that people would use to find your site. Example, "Back to Life Acupuncture Clinic in Boulder, CO specializes in treating people with all types of back pain." This has the words "acupuncture," "Boulder," and "back pain" which

SECTION FOUR: MARKETING YOUR PRACTICE

will help search engines and, thus, your prospective customers find you easily. Write a list of key words you want on your home page and as many other pages on your site as possible; *i.e.,* the words you think people will use to search for services like yours.

Your site should look and read like your biz card, company brochure, letterhead, etc. In other words, it should have an integrated look and feel in terms of colors, fonts, photos, and design elements, along with everything else that you print to promote your practice.

A photo or two of you working, or of the inside and outside of your clinic, or of your pharmacy, are good additions and give visitors a sense of who you are and what your practice feels like.

If you really cannot afford to have a website but you want one, maybe you can sell ad space to related businesses to help pay for your site if you are strapped for cash. For example, if you sell books or simple herbal products, you might be able to get the manufacturer of those products to place an ongoing ad at your website which would pay for the hosting fees.

Building link popularity

The best way to get higher search engine rankings is for your site name to show up on lots of other people's sites. How do you do that? One way is to provide content for other people's sites in exchange for a mention of your URL (web address) at the end of each piece. If you like to write, offer your content for free to as many other sites as possible. For example…

- *Boulder Parents Magazine* has a website. Most magazines do. Offer to write a health-wellness piece for their website every other month in exchange for mentioning your name and URL address in their print magazine and on their website.
- Do the same thing with as many other publications and

P O W E R P O I N T

Examples of Good Site Content

People want and expect some value added content. For example, on my Back to Life Clinic website, I want a short article (I really mean short) such as the following: "Research on Back Pain and Chinese Medicine"

- 3-5 bullet points on things to do at home and what to avoid
- Maybe some photos or a YouTube style video of you demonstrating a couple of exercises.
- At the end of the article describe how acupuncture has proven in research to help many types of back pain.
- At the very end is your phone number, email address, and an "Ask the Acupuncturist" form for questions or to book an appointment.

I might also include the following:

- Several articles on different, related subjects, especially conditions you prefer to treat.
- A "Links" page allows you to request to trade links with other people's sites. Link trading is a good way to increase "link popularity," which helps you get higher in search engine lists. More on that below.
- An "opt-in" email sign-up form that gets them something free (a quarterly video newsletter on health, discount coupons for classes you teach, specials on seasonal herbal products, etc.) Opt-in means they choose to sign up or not. This is vital because it gives you an inexpensive way to stay in touch with your potential patients!! By the way, each communication you send out must have instructions at the bottom on how to "opt-out" if they so choose.
- Information on any products you might be selling on your site is optional but possible.

websites as you have time to contact. If you really want to use the Web as your main marketing medium, this is how you do it without spending lots of cash.

- Get your name/URL on as many listing services as possible.
- Offer to trade links with other practitioners websites in other cities. The more of these links you can create, the better your "organic" search engine placement (good search placement that you have not paid for) will be.
- If you can create short articles about acupuncture, Chinese medicine, alternative health, the benefits of exercises, etc., all day long, offer these articles to other people for their websites in trade for your URL link appearing with the article.

➤ What are listing services?

There are lots and lots of these out there! Your website can be listed at your state association website, the AAAOM website, AcuFinder.com, AcupunctureToday.com, www.gancao.net, www.byregion.net, http://alternative-doctor.com/links, www.citysearch.com, and www.Chinesemedicinetimes.com. Look for local, regional, and national places to list your website. Some are free and some not. It's worth it to spend some cash here if you are serious about web marketing, but do a Google search for "Alternative Health Listing Services" and only pay for ones that come up on the first page of your search or you are wasting your money.

➤ Search-based web ads

The best of this type of advertising are probably small ads on Google Maps or CitySearch. The way this works is that when someone searches for an address in your city, your little ad appears along the side of the page when the local map pops open if someone searches for anything within a certain radius of your address. Or, when someone searches for anything to do with healthcare in your city on CitySearch, your ad appears. This is not cheap, but if used over time, it could be very effective. This type of add can be done on Facebook and other social networking sites as well, with costs per click-through.

Google Places

One absolutely vital place for you to be listed on the internet, irrespective of having a website, is claiming your business on Google Places. To see what that is, go to Google and do a search for acupuncturists in your town. See the map that comes up with the little red markers for various clinic locations? Well, you need to be there, too. This is easy and need not cost you money, although you can enhance placement of your listing through the use of AdWords on Google if you want more exposure.

Google gives you all sorts of straightforward tutorials for creating and enhancing your listing. Just do what they say, create the listing as per their instructions and then search on Google by using the key words you'd expect potential patients to use. Remember that over 60% of non-internet purchases are made after people did internet research! In other words, they may call you and come in person, but the research that made the decision about who and where to call was done online! So check this out and do it as soon as you have a physical address!

Using bulk email blasts

You can purchase opt-in email lists of people interested in alternative health. More importantly, you should be collecting email addresses of all your patients and anyone who attends a class or lecture that you do; these addresses should be in your web database. The two most important website hosting services totally worth paying for are visitor data collection and group emailing for you to easily and accurately keep track of and stay in touch with interested visitors. As stated above, all outbound communication from you must have an opt-out statement of what people do if they are no longer interested.

Here's another option for those without a website. If you have an email "address book," hire an online bulk-email-sending company to send e-communications for you. These are easy to find online (MailChimp*, ConstantContact, iContact) or your email service provider may already include this service. Always include contact and opt-out info every time you send anything.

Keep email communications short. People don't scroll down very far unless they are really interested in something. A basic formula is an intro headline to capture interest, then some bullet points, and then a call to action (call you, attend a class, watch your new video, attend a webinar, etc.) No more than a one or two of these emails per month or people will start to tune you out or opt out altogether.

> **Blogging**

A blog and a social network profile at places such as Facebook are your virtual representatives. These are where people can maintain anonymity yet make that first contact in a potential relationship with you. It's important to remember

> **POWER POINT**
>
> For more help with blogging and how to do it really well, you might check out articles to get you started at sites like Thoughts.com, Blogspot.com, and ProBlogger.com. There's tons of help out there for almost any online activity such as blogging.

that, especially for many non-Asians, coming the first time for acupuncture or Chinese medicine requires a great deal of trust. Few people will come to you without some belief that they can trust you. A blog is a great way to help you establish credibility and enough trust for people to make that first call or send you that first email. The best news is that there are ways to create an internet presence in the blogosphere for free (at the time of this writing), notably at *Blogger*, which is so easy to use that some people adapt it as a basic "website" as well. I suggest you poke around and check out various blogs there for samples of how to use this software to the best advantage. Another good thing about *Blogger* is that it allows you the opportunity to use the right margin of the screen as a "brochure" about you and your services. This includes your contact information, what services you offer, general information about acupuncture and Chinese medicine, etc.

Besides using *Blogger* as a brochure, you should actually post blogs there and at other blogs as well! There are tons of health-related blogs out there. For example, if you do a search for "hay fever blogs," "fibromyalgia blogs," "infertility blogs," or "stomach disease blogs" (you get the idea) you will come up with tons of blog sites where your knowledge would be appreciated and well received; just don't make them "ads" about you. With your (hopefully regular) posts, potential clients get a

---

Resources for going further with your website marketing
Books to help you with Web-based marketing

The Zen of Social Media Marketing: An Easier Way to Build Credibility, Generate Buzz, and Increase Revenue by Shama Kabani and Chris Brogan

Successful Website Marketing by Peggy Ridgway

Self-Promotion Online by Ilise Benun

Internet Marketing for Less than $500 A Year by Marcia Yudkin

Get Clients Now: A 28 Day Marketing Program for Professionals by C.J. Hayden

Online Promotion Services

While you can find hundreds of these by doing an online search, I would start with local companies. That way you can interview both the owners and get local referrals to see how they have measured up to expectations and how well they fulfull their contracts.

---

chance to "meet you" and know a great deal about your personality as well as your skills, history, knowledge. Your blog posts can establish you as an expert and create a virtual person for people to relate to directly. If people feel like they know you through your posts, you'll greatly increase your success in attracting clients. You might say to me, "People from anywhere on the planet could read my blog. How do I know if any of them will become my patient?" And I would respond that the world is getting smaller every day and you never know where the next patient or referral will come from.

Another positive thing to remember is that blog posts do not have to be long or scholarly. They can be short, personal, simple informational tidbits or even questions, about which people are encouraged to comment and dialog with you. Do try to spell correctly and use complete sentences, however, since your purpose is to sound both personable and intelligent!

Sites like *Blogger, Blogspot, CafeMoms, Wordpress,* and other large blog centers are also great because search engines love blogs. Having a blog that you post at regularly helps your rankings in the search results when someone searches online for what you do or what you blog about. So, if you want to create a web presence in less than an hour and for no cost, try *Blogger.* And remember, if you already have a website, a blog increases your opportunities for communication with potential clients, gives them a way to get to know you, and increases site traffic in the search engines.

Squidoo is another free and easy website-alternative or internet-promotion tool, which was started by the marketing genius Seth Godin. Because of Mr. Godin's insight and communication skill, *Squidoo* includes almost everything you need to get started marketing yourself on the internet, website or not.

On *Squidoo* you build what is called a "lens" on any subject, as broad or narrow a subject as you want, and including as much or as little as you want. For example, there could be a lens on "My Acupuncture Practice in Miami," or one on "Everything You Wanted to Know About Acupuncture," or whatever subject you think might interest the clients you want to attract. The lens is actually a collection of absolutely anything digital that you want to share on this subject. In addition to answering questions about your practice, your education, your knowledge, etc., you can link to any web-based resource that seems useful, informative, fun, or relevant. This should include YouTube videos, books at Amazon, blog posts and articles by you and others, photos, and your and others' websites. Your *Squidoo* lens can even serve as a website alternative until you decide to create one of those as well.

The marketing value of *Squidoo* is that search engines love it the way they love blogs. From a potential client's perspective, your presence here can establish you as an expert and someone they may want on their healthcare team. For example, if you are a tai chi teacher, you would insert links to your favorite tai chi books, your personal tai chi teachers, tai chi videos on YouTube, other tai chi websites or blogs, articles about tai chi that you find in the online press, and anything you yourself write about tai chi. While this may seem like potentially giving business away, usually the contrary is true. For example, videos absolutely don't compare to working with an actual tai chi teacher and most people visiting your *Squidoo* lens are likely to be seeking something beyond video instruction. By referring to related, useful resources beyond yourself, you make it clear that you know the industry, your motivation is client-centered and all about providing great content to people whether they buy from you or not. That makes you the open-hearted and generous sort of person people want to study with. *Squidoo* is also free, user-friendly, and fast.

➤ Social network marketing

There are marketing experts who say that all the patients you could ever need are friends, colleagues and acquaintances of all the people that you already know. With the rise in popularity of internet social net-working sites like *Facebook, Brightkite, Naymz, LinkedIn,* and other similar sites, you have potential access to several degrees of separation through all your friends and acquaintances. There are several ways you can use social network sites to help you market your practice.

On *Facebook* you can do things as simple as write Chinese-medicine-specific messages or quotes on your "wall" and your friends' "walls," let all your networked friends know about upcoming classes, speeches, events, special offers you are giving, or great books on CM that you have recently read. You can start a fan-club for yourself; you can ask your *Facebook* friends for referrals; you can create Facebook events. You can, for a small amount of money that you control, avail yourself of marketing tools at the *Facebook* Marketplace, although you must follow their rules quite specifically or your ads will not be placed. Similar opportunities exist at *LinkedIn, Brightkite,* and others.

> **POWER POINT**
>
> To see a comprehensive list of social networking opportunities, check out "social networking sites" at Wikipedia.com. There are literally hundreds of them, many quite subculture-specific. An interest in treating children or families, for example, might lead you to join networks such as CafeMom.com. Check this out for sure! 200,000 Moms talking to each other about everything; .join the conversation!

This discussion could be endless, so if you have a real interest in it, or if you already have a healthy social network presence on the web, I suggest you check out articles on social network marketing at sites such as www.ehow.com, www.geeknews-central.com, and other similar websites by typing in something

416

like "marketing your services on social networking websites." This discussion is huge and all over the internet, so poke around, read some stuff, and decide how to connect. One suggestion from me [HW] is to keep your personal Facebook presence separate from your business presence, *i.e.*, have two Facebook pages.

Other Online opportunities

People love to talk about things and services they like. Online this has been "formalized" through websites such as *Yelp* and *Angie's List*. You can ask your best patients to "yelp" about you, but do not be tempted to fake another name and do it yourself. You'll get "busted" for this by *Yelp* in a heartbeat. Go to their site, type in "acupuncturist" for any city and see who your competition is.

If you want to know what the press and online world is saying about acupuncture, Chinese medicine, your clinic name, or any other subject, go to *Google Alerts* and sign yourself up be alerted by email any time these subjects appear in the news. This is an excellent way to collect articles for your waiting room scrapbook and see what new research is being reported in our industry. You'll be surprised how often we are in the news!

Got photos or video of your trip to China to study medicine?? or of you working in your clinic? Share them at *Flickr* or *YouTube*. and link them to your site, your *Facebook* page, your *Blogger* page, Say that these are open source and that anybody can use your photos as long as you are given attribution. More people visit *YouTube* and *Flickr* than most of all the other sites put together in the whole universe.

Prefer Live Contact?

Prefer face to face marketing? Go to *Meetup.com* and see what's happening in your area in the coming days (or hours!) that you might attend for fun or volunteering and networking. Or, create an event yourself and post it there. This can be really easy... something like "Interested in the Politics of Food (or March Madness....or whatever subject you like)? Meet me at the XYZ Bar at 5 PM for a rousing conversation."

▶ The wonderful world of E-commerce

If you want to sell anything on your site, the easiest way to do it is to create a "merchant account" at *PayPal*. That way, people can pay you either with credit cards or their *PayPal* account. All the tools you need in order to add the *PayPal* information and capability onto your site are available at *PayPal* and they have online help if you get stuck. You can sell books, herbal products, facial or personal care products, aromatherapy candles, soap, CDs or DVDs, or offer sign-up for live or online classes.

If, by any chance, you are a shy person, selling yourself on the internet may be a great place to start. While you still must try to find some comfort level with people when they call, write, or come in to see you, there is a huge potential audience out there on the Worldwide Web, just waiting to find out about you and your services, without the requirement of standing up in front of groups and giving lectures.

▶ Conclusion

This chapter could, of course, go on for many, many more pages. It may also be the case that, within a year (or even a few days!) of the publication of this book, something in this chapter will no longer be accurate or there will be new services that we should have discussed. We will try to add new things that seem relevant on the website. The main thing to know is that the internet is a huge and constantly growing resource for almost all types of businesses. Don't be overwhelmed; pick a couple of these suggestions to start and add on as seems relevent. While no easier to use as a marketing tool than any other type of marketing, if you are comfortable on a computer and on the internet, this is one way that many practitioners are using successfully to get new patients. You can, too.

POINTS TO PONDER FROM CHAPTER 7

- Since the use of the internet is growing exponentially, this can be a great way to market your services.

- There are many ways to get a website built. The easiest is to hire someone to do it for you ($500-$1500 for the least expensive and simplest sites), or you can do all or part of it yourself with purchased software or free shareware for the most techno-savvy.

- Domain names (your URL) need not cost more than $10 per year.

- Hosting services may cost as little as $10 per month, but make sure you have three things:
  1. Opt-in information gathering ability
  2. Group email blasting ability
  3. Ability to add PayPal® or other E-commerce options

- Blogging is an effective way to market yourself online for free. Get started at Blogger and "disease-specific" blogs. Use Squidoo to create digital credibility.

- Social network sites can also be a source of patients through your friends and your friends' friends.

Marketing Odds and Ends | 8

As we said at the beginning of this section, it is more difficult to decide what to exclude than what to include when talking about marketing. Marketing is, from one point of view, the sum total of everything you do. As Seth Godin, one of our favorite marketing gurus, says, it can be the way you answer the phone, launch a new service, paint your rooms, or organize your schedule that will make the positive difference. Getting in the habit of excellence and of exploring the limitless possibilities for a great clinic should be a daily goal. Being the most expensive instead of the least, the fastest or the slowest, the hottest, the easiest, the most efficient, the oldest or the newest, or just the most, you should test the limits of what works to grow your practice every chance you get. If you can think of a way to overwhelm those you serve with your remarkability, you're there.

Meanwhile, here are a few more tips.

- Silent auctions are an opportunity to use your services to market your services and support your community at the same time. Donate a series of treatments. Think how many people will walk by the bidding tables deciding what to bid on.

- When you do a speaking engagement, after the lecture, follow up with a thank you card to the person who was in charge. Let them know they can contact you any time for lectures on other related subjects.

- Donate the proceeds of one treatment per month to a specific local cause. Send a press release to the local media announcing that you are doing this and what the cause of the month is.

- Never go anywhere without a stack of business cards in your pocket. Take every opportunity to talk to anyone who will listen about what you do.

- Develop an "elevator speech," *i.e.,* one minute or less about what you do so that, when you are in line at the grocery store, you've got something compelling and interesting to say to anyone who asks, "What do you do for a living?" Practice until you've got it memorized.

- Give free treatments during "The Great American Smoke Out" to people trying to quit. Send a letter to social services offices in the city health department as well as doctors in town citing the success of acupuncture for dealing with addictive behaviors and offer to help their patients quit.

- If you are giving a lecture somewhere that you've never seen before, go and check out the room in advance. You'll be more comfortable when you arrive for the talk and do a better job.

- Start and maintain a support group of businesspeople and related professionals. Meet once per month for an early breakfast. At each meeting, two people get to discuss an issue or problem they have and ask for everyone's opinion. This is very powerful and can energize your business in ways you can't imagine. Napolean Hill calls this your "mastermind" group.

- When there are no patients, don't always sit and read clinical books. Go out and meet others in your building or on your block. Introduce yourself and pass out your cards. If you practice in a high-rise office building, does every receptionist in that building know you on a first name basis?

- Speaking of high-rise offices, what about the building janitor and the guy who runs the coffee shop in the lobby? These guys talk to a large percentage of the people who work in your building. They both should also have some of your cards in their pocket or by the cash register!

- Cruise over to www.morenewpatients.com for ideas you have not yet thought of. Originally for chiropractors, this website is a goldmine of new ideas when you need to be energized.

- When you are in a waiting room anywhere, read the magazine only for the advertising. Which ones do you like and why? Which ones would get you to spend your money? Are there any ideas that you can translate into marketing ideas for your own written marketing pieces, ads, or brochures?

Finally, as much as you can for as long as you can, keep your intellectual curiosity alive. This will help you stay interested in and passionate about what you are doing professionally. Go to seminars, read books, research what is out there. Really learn and understand this medicine to the limit of your ability. Don't be lazy. This type of passion and true skill are magnetic and seductive. The universe supports it and will support you because of it. At the end of the day or the end of a career or the end of a life, you have only yourself and your own integrity to answer to. If you truly love and understand this medicine and you can communicate that love to your patients through everything that you and your clinic embody, you will be successful. That, exactly that, is the essence of good marketing.

POWER POINT

If you want more marketing ideas, you may occasionally want to cruise over to read my [HW] blog at www.bluepoppy.com/blog/blogs. Mostly I write about practice management and success issues and there is an archive (right side of the blog pages, toward the bottom) of my blogs and our other writers blogs as well. Maybe I can give you a bit of inspiration from time to time!

We all wish you a successful and happy professional life. Think more, do good work, and stay in touch!

OK, let's say you have your practice off the ground enough to pay the rent, heat, insurance, and phone bill. Most of your practice days are busy and your referrals are good. Now you have to decide how large and busy a practice you want to create. The point of a private practice is to help your patients and support yourself financially and emotionally, not to create practitioner burnout. If this is you or if it will be you in another several months, your situation is pretty good and you should feel proud of yourself. You are in the minority in our profession. However, we hope this book will help more practitioners be effective and successful businesspeople. With that in mind, we feel it is important to talk about handling a large, busy, and successful practice so that the growth is managed in a way that supports you and doesn't make you crazy.

So how do you keep a balance and how to keep growing without making yourself sick? Here are several ideas to consider:

➤ Raise your prices

This is one way to make sure that the patients who are coming to see you really want to be getting their therapy from you. Send out a notice to all your active patients or put a flyer in their herb prescription bags announcing that, on the first of the following month, your prices will go up $10, $15, or $20 per treatment, exam, and/or intake, and that you will charge $25 for a 15 minute phone consultation. State gently that, if these prices are too high for anyone, you are happy to refer to one of a number of other practitioners in the area. You may lose a few people, but probably not many. At least this may slow your growth for a while.

SECTION FOUR: MARKETING YOUR PRACTICE

➤ Hire an assistant

In the chapter about getting a job (see Section 1, Chapter 7), we discussed all the reasons it might be great to hire a new graduate to work with you. Another reason is that you may be able to have one or more assistant practitioners to whom you refer within your clinic for specific types of ailments without your clinic losing all the income or the herbal therapy income. This help may be supervised or not, but, even if and when it is unsupervised, as the boss, you can set very clear guidelines about patient care in your clinic. That way, if you are charging $90 for your treatments and $60 for your assistant's treatments, but paying the assistant $40, you are still making money. You will, of course, have to figure out what the other costs may be involved in having an employee to make certain that there is profit for you in the deal. Such an arrangement may also require that you have some type of corporate structure because fee-splitting is illegal in many states. If you are growing at this rate, it is probably time to consider incorporation if you have not already done so. That means your helper(s) have to be employees unless they are merely renting space from you on a per hour basis, which is a completely different sort of arrangement.

P O W E R   P O I N T

Tips for Hiring an Associate

- Make sure you hire someone who is as like-minded as possible when it comes to patient care.

- Pay them enough that they will want to stay with you for at least one year. Two years is better.

- Run the numbers carefully to make sure that you are making some money from the assistant's work. One key to capitalism is hiring other people's labor to make you money. Giving jobs to people is also a wonderful thing to be able to do.

➤ Hire a professional specialist

Another way to hire help and lighten your load is to find a specialist who offers services completely different from your own. If you wish to move your personal practice largely in the direction of gynecology, for example, and have fewer other types of patients, you might hire a new practitioner who does not wish to specialize in anything specific but get a wide range of experience, at least for a while. If you pay them a fair wage and provide a pleasant working environment, this can be a good solution for limiting the growth of your practice. Such an arrangement also gives you someone to cover your patients when you want to take time off or need to go out of town. You may need a lawyer-written contract that discusses the minimal length of time the practitioner must work for you, how the relationship will be severed or how a future partnership may be created, what benefits in addition to salary you will pay, or who gets the profits from herb and product sales.

In this case, you would contact your existing clientele to announce that you will only be taking gynecology cases in the future and that you are proud and happy to have so-and-so as the new practitioner joining your practice to take care of all other types of complaints and what new skills or services you will now be able to offer. They need to feel assured that they will still be well taken care of and that you will be there to consult with the new practitioner about their personal history and specific needs. While you may lose a few patients through this type of transition, you will keep most of them if you market it well. You could also manage this slowly, only channeling new patients to the new practitioner while keeping your current patients and allowing natural attrition to take care of slowing the growth of your practice.

Another possibility is to hire a young MD who is still a resident and looking for a moonlighting job. This may cost less than you think and will add prestige to your clinic and allow you to offer some basic medical screening services that could be very valuable to your patients. See Section 1, Chapter 7 for more information about a practitioner who has had success with this option.

We also realize that such a plan may require a larger space and more treatment rooms, but, if your practice is growing, you may consider moving into a larger clinic space in any case.

➤ Interns or treatment aides

Another possibility is to hire a graduate or even someone who has not yet graduated from school to assist you directly in treating your patients. This intern's jobs include doing moxa, tuina, removing cups, taking out needles, cleaning up the treatment rooms after each patient, checking on patients while you are off doing an intake on the next patient, taking blood pressure or doing other basic intake and exam procedures, pulling out files, making follow-up phone calls, or whatever else you feel you can delegate. This person is not the same as your receptionist or front desk staff. They help you directly in the treatment room, streamlining each patient's therapy and, thereby, allowing you to see more patients without losing quality of care. At the same time, this new practitioner is receiving excellent on-the-job training. Pay scale can be $10–15 per hour for such work.

PRACTITIONER POINTER

"Follow through with what you say you will do. Arrive on time. Look people in the eye. Make it easy for people to come to see you. Don't forget to get treatments and take herbs yourself. You can be much more effective in marketing Chinese medicine when you are doing the things you'd like your patients to do."

—Elizabeth Liddell
Philadelphia, PA

➤ Close your practice for a specific period of time

This is an extreme measure, but we have heard of it. Alternatively, you may have your front desk tell people that you are not taking new patients until such-and-such a date and then create a call-back system for anyone who wants to be put on a waiting list.

Want to sell your practice? Get a free quote and selling ideas from Professional Practice Specialists, Inc., www.practicesales.com, 800-645-7590.

➤ Conclusion

Of course it is our hope that all practitioners will become so successful that they need to consider options for limiting or channeling the growth of their practice or hiring a younger practitioner to work for them in order to maintain their personal health while still growing their income. We hope that any practitioner out there who has managed this phase of their professional life in some creative way that we have not discussed here will get in touch with us. We will post your story on our website and include it in the next edition of this book.

It is our personal goal that thousands more acupuncturists become financially and personally successful beyond their wildest dreams.

POINTS TO PONDER FROM CHAPTER 8

- Once you are running a full, successful practice, you need to think about how to keep your patients happy and your income growing without leading to personal burnout, which does neither you nor your patients any good.

- You can raise your fees significantly and see who drops out of your practice. This will only work for a short while if you are good, so do this first.

- You can hire an associate, a specialist, or an MD to serve some of your patient overload.

- You can hire a treatment assistant to take out needles, do tui na, cupping, and/or moxibustion.

- You can limit your hours and take a waiting list for new patients.

- You can close your practice altogether for a month or two, taking no new patients until you feel there is space in your schedule.

- Take care of your health while you are taking care of others.

Conclusion | 10

At the beginning of this book we suggested that you try to think and work "from your dreams," visualizing the life, working environment, and income that you desire with as much clarity and intensity as you can. Everything we have included in this book is created to help you do just that. If you are clever, hardworking, and persistent enough to become wealthy (and we hope you are), we'd like to suggest that you also take some time to consider how you'd use that resource.

We believe that being a wealthy person carries with it great responsibility. There are only so many ways to spend money on yourself, and, ultimately, that is not what makes for a truly successful life. So, what would you do with your money if all your own needs and wants were met? How would you go about leaving the world a better place than you found it? What we are suggesting is to also formulate some meta-goals for after you have become materially comfortable and secure—in other words, reasons for becoming wealthy beyond shear materialism.

We leave you with those thoughts and we thank you for purchasing and, hopefully, reading and using this product to help you fulfill your goals and dreams. Please let us know how we can continue to help you with our courses, newsletters, websites and any other future products. We appreciate your feedback. Best wishes to you for great and happy success. Do good work and stay in touch.

Honora Lee Wolfe
Eric Strand
Marilyn Allen

Resources for Going Further (books, classes, websites)

• Also go to http://pointsforprofit.bluepoppy.com •

➤ **Resources for Entrepreneurship**

Websites

http://www.youngentrepreneur.com/forum Young Entrepreneurs Organization has a really good biz plan template

http://www.weainc.ws/ Women Entrepreneurs of America has a blog, local chapters for business, referral, and moral support

www.entrepreneurship.org articles, resources, hot links, bookstore, glossary, media resource center

www.tannedfeet.com resources, legal forms, marketing, PR, human resources, humor

www.entrepreneurs.com resources, articles, web guide, marketing services

www.startupjournal.com Wall Street Journal Center for Entrepreneurs, business plan tools, trademark search, bookstore, articles, how-to, financing, running a business

Books

Steps to Small Business Start-up by Linda Pinson & Jerry Jinnett

The Real World Entrepreneur's Field Guide by David H. Bangs & Linda Pinson

The Entrepreneur's Guide to Finance & Business: Wealth Creation Techniques for Growing a Business by Steve Rogers *et al.*

Entrepreneurs: Talent, Temperament, Technique by John Thompson & Bill Bolton

What No One Ever Tells You About Starting Your Own Business by Jan Norman

Start Your Own Business: The Only Start-up Book You'll Ever Need by Rieva Lesonsky *et al.*

Thinking Like an Entrepreneur by Peter I. Hupalo

Working for Yourself: Law and Taxes for Independent Contractors, Freelancers and Consultants by Stephen Fishman

How to Start and Run Your Own Corporation by Peter I. Hupalo

The Young Entrepreneur's Guide to Starting and Running a Business by Steve Mariotti *et al.*

Defying the Odds by Marcia Israel-Curley

Free Money and Help for Women Entrepreneurs by Matthew Lesko *et al.*

Entrepreneur's Ultimate Start-up Directory by James Stephenson

Think & Grow Rich by Napolean Hill

➤ **Resources for Writing a Business Plan**

Web resources

www.bplans.com sample plans, software, legal advice, market research, "ask the experts," web directory

www.sba.gov/starting/indexbusplans.htm business plan basics
www.businessplans.org software, resources, consulting, examples, tools
http://home3.americanexpress.com/smallbusiness/tool/biz_plan/index.asp creating
    an effective business plan step-by-step
www.business-plan-maker.com 250 plus pages of templates and guides
www.planigent.com customizable, downloadable, do-it-yourself
www.ibpConsultants.com professional business plan writers
www.morebusiness.com/templates_worksheets/bplans/ templates, tools, books
www.planware.org software to try and buy, white papers to read, things to do

Books
Anatomy of a Business Plan by Linda Pinson
Successful Business Planning in 30 Days by Peter J. Patsula
Business Plan Kit for Dummies (with CD-Rom)
    by Steven J. Peterson & Peter E. Jaret
The Ernst & Young Business Plan Guide by Ernst & Young LLP
The One Page Business Plan by Peter J. Patsula
The Successful Business Plan: Secrets & Strategies by Rhonda Adams
Business Plans for Dummies by Paul Tiffany & Steven J. Peterson
How to Write a Business Plan by Mike McKeever
The Complete Book of Business Plans by Joseph A. Covello
Writing a Convincing Business Plan by Art Dethomas *et al.*
The McGraw-Hill Guide to Writing a High-impact Business Plan
    by James B. Arkebauer
Writing Business Plans that Get Results by Michael O'Donnell

➤ Resources for Lowering Taxes & Legitimate Business Deductions

websites
www.Kiplinger.com
http://taxes.about.com/od/taxplanning/Lower_Your_Taxes.htm
www.Taxsaveronline.com
www.articlesbase.com/business-articles/tax-advantage-strategies-of-a-home-based-
    marketing-business-878620.html

Books
422 Tax Deductions for Businesses and Self-employed Individuals
    by Bernard Kamoroff
The Complete Idiot's Guide to Tax Breaks & Deductions by Lita Epstein
Lower Your Taxes—Big Time! By Sanford C. Botkin
Your Federal Income Tax (Publication 17), *Tax Guide for Small Business*
    (Publication 334) and *Guide to Free Tax Services* (Publication 910) are all free
    from your local IRS office at 800-829-1040

Year Round Savings by Julian Block is $16 from J. Block, 3 Washington Square, #1-G, Larchmont, NY 10538
Taxes for the Self-Employed audiotape
   by Noelle Allen $49.95 at 408-252-1367

▶ Resources for Finding a Job

Job search websites

www.acupuncturetoday.com www.careerbuilder.com
www.alternativehealthjobs.com www.job.com
www.monster.com www.overseasjobs.com
www.hotjobs.com www.summerjobs.com
www.postdocjobs.com www.nationjob.com
www.tcmstudent.com www.jobsonline.com

▶ Resources About "Buzz," Word-of-Mouth Marketing

Books

Buzz: Harness the Power of Influence and Create Demand
   by Marian Salzman *et al.*
The Buzz on Buzz by Renee Dye
The Anatomy of Buzz by Emmanuel Rosen
Unleashing the Idea Virus by Seth Godin & Malcolm Gladwell
What Clients Love: A Field Guide to Growing Your Business
   by Harry Beckwith
Permission Marketing: Turning Strangers into Friends and Friends into Customers
   by Seth Godin
The Tipping Point: How Little Things Can Make a Big Difference
   by Malcolm Gladwell
Leap! A Revolution in Creative Business Strategy by Bob Schmetterer
How Customers Think by Gerald Zaltman
Why We Buy: The Science of Shopping by Paco Underhill
Creating Customer Evangelists by Ben McConnell & Jackie Huba
Love is the Killer App: How to Win Business and Influence Friends
   by Tim Sanders
The Secret of Word-of-Mouth Marketing by George Silverman

▶ Resources for Learning the Art of Negotiation

Books

Getting to Yes: Negotiating Agreement Without Giving In by Roger Fiske *et al.*
The Only Negotiating Guide You'll Ever Need: 101 Ways to Win Every Time in Any Situation by Peter B. Stark & Jane S. Flaherty
Getting Past No: Negotiating Your Way from Confrontation to Cooperation by William Ury
Secrets of Power Negotiating by Roger Dawson

Negotiating Rationally by Max H. Bazerman
A Woman's Guide to Successful Negotiating by Lee E. Miller & Jessica Miller
Negotiate This! By Caring, But Not T-H-A-T Much by Herb Cohen

➤ Resources to Improve and Inspire Your Marketing

Websites
www.marketingtips.com
www.successmagazine.com
www.success-solution.com
www.powerfulpromoter.com
www.marketingsurvivalkit.com
www.clickz.com

Books
Shameless Marketing for Brazen Hussies: 307 Awesome Money-making Strategies for Savvy Entrepreneurs by Marilyn Ross
How to Give a Damn Good Speech by Philip R. Theibert
Chase's Calendar of Events published by Contemporary Books at 719-395-4790
Purple Cow: Transform Your Business by Being Remarkable by Seth Godin
The Art of Possibility: Transforming Professional and Personal Life by Rosamund Stone Zander
Creating Customer Evangelists by Ben McConnell & Jackie Huba
Raving Fans: A Revolutionary Approach to Customer Service by Ken Blanchard and Sheldon Bowles
Marketing Outrageously by Jon Spoelstra
Don't Worry, Make Money by Richard Carlson

➤ Resources for Hiring and Managing Employees

Websites
www.entrepreneur.com
www.assessmentspecialists.com
www.businesstown.com/hiring
www.irs.gov/businesses/small/article/0
www.entrepreneur.com/humanresources/index.html
www.howtomanagepeople.com/

Books
Finding & Keeping Great Employees by Jim Harris and Joan Brannick
Perfect Phrases for Performance Reviews by Douglas Max and Robert Bacal
Happy Employees Work Better by rp4rp, a worker
1001 Ways to Reward Employees by Bob Nelson and Kenneth Blanchard
Why Employees Don't Do What They're Supposed to and What to Do About It by F. F. Fournies

First Break All the Rules! What the World's Greatest Managers Do Differently by Marcus Buckingham and Curt Coffman

Resources for Working with Your Money Neuroses

Websites
www.prosperityplace.com
www.lifemanual.net
www.flyingsolo.com.au/
www.growingwealthy.com
www.artofabundance.com

Books
The Millionaire Course: A Visionary Plan for Creating the Life of Your Dreams by Marc Allen
The Start-Up Garden: How Growing a Business Grows You by Ehrenfeld and Collins
I'd Rather Laugh: How to be Happy Even When Life Has Other Plans for You by R. L. O'Donnell-Richman
Making Peace with Money by Jerrold Mundis
The Advisor's Guide to Money Psychology by Olivia Mellan
Money and the Meaning of Life by Jacob Needleman
Your Money or Your Life by Joe Dominguez

Resources for Billing Insurance

Books
Playing the Game: The Acupuncturists' Guide to Billing Insurance and Getting Paid by Dr. Greg Sperber and Tiffany Andersen
The Acupuncture Code Book by H.J. Ross & Co.

For lots more resources and live links, go to:
http://pointsforprofit.bluepoppy.com

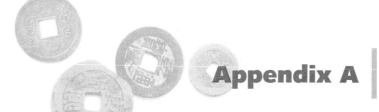

Appendix A

Getting a National Provider Identifier (NPI) Number

All health care providers, whether an individual or a group practice, that provide medical or other health services or supplies, must now be assigned an NPI ten position numeric identifier. This NPI is a unique identification number that will be used by all health plans. It will be required on all CMS 1500 forms, on superbills, and may be required on some HIPAA related forms as well.

There are three ways to apply for an NPI:
- Online at https://nppes.cms.hhs.gov
- Mail to request an application from NPPES, PO Box 6059 Fargo, ND 58108-6059
- Phone NPPES to request that an application be sent to you at 800-465-3203 or 800-692-2326

Health care providers must notify NPPES within 30 days of an office relocation. Since your NPI will be used for billing purposes and other transactions, it should be kept private and secure.

10 Things to Consider When Creating a Work Agreement with a Hospital

These questions need to be at least discussed, and better yet written in to your contract or work agreement with any hospital or other public health facility.

1. How much should you charge? If you had no overhead at all, how much would you need to make per patient or per hour to be comfortable? That's where you might start. If most of your patients will be billing insurance, discuss how much you will be reimbursed for various codes.
2. Who will order supplies and who will pay for them? How will needles and other biohazard materials be handled? If you are required to pay for these items, could you be reimbursed?
3. How many treatment spaces do you want or need to work efficiently? If you need more than one treatment space at a time to be efficient or make an adequate living, will that always be available?
4. Be collegial and neither arrogant nor intimidated. If you value what you do but start from a position of building a positive relationship with the other practitioners and administrators in the hospital team, trust is likely to be easier to build. Also remember that, to get along most effectively, you need to dress in professional medical style and speak medical-speak comfortably.
5. How will your services be marketed and who will be

Appendix B continues on the next page

responsible for that marketing? Will you have access to other departments to put out brochures, put up signage, give in-service lectures, attend meetings, and meet others who are potential referral sources? Will you be allowed to use the hospital name on your card to help you market outside the hospital?

6. How long will you work there before your contract is up for renewal? Under what conditions can you terminate the contract legally? Is it transferrable to another practitioner?

7. Are there any other duties for which you will be responsible in addition to just doing acupuncture? Do any of these require training?

8. Will you be permitted to prescribe herbal medicine in appropriate situations? If so, how will it be paid for?

9. Will you be salaried, an independent contractor, paid by the hour or by the patient? Will you have any benefits such as health insurance or paid vacation? If not right away, when might such benefits begin and how do you apply for them?

10. If most or all patients are billing insurance for your services as well as other services in the hospital, how will that billing be handled and how does it relate to what you are paid.

For more in depth information on working in hospitals, see the business-related or miscellaneous articles at the Blue Poppy Website/Free Articles section and look for articles by Marilyn Allen and David Kailin. Also, look for any articles by Kristen Porter and Beth Sommers at *AcupunctureToday.com.*

Index

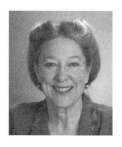

Honora Lee Wolfe

Honora Lee Wolfe has been involved in professional health care education since 1976. Director at the Boulder College of Massage Therapy for five years, Ms. Wolfe went on to study tuina massage at the Shanghai College of TCM and completed her acupuncture training in 1988. She teaches regularly at national and regional acupuncture colleges and conferences in North America and Europe and is the author or co-author of several books, including Prince Wen Hui's Cook: Chinese Dietary Therapy, How to Have a Healthy Pregnancy Healthy Birth with Chinese Medicine, Managing Menopause Naturally with Chinese Medicine, Better Breast Health Naturally with Chinese Medicine, Points for Profit: The Essential Guide to Practice Success for Acupuncturists, The Successful Chinese Herbalist: How to Prescribe Correctly, Gain Patient Comliance, and Operate a Profitable Dispensary, and most recently Western Physical Exam Skills for Asian Medicine Practitioners.

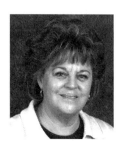

Marilyn Allen

Eric Strand has a diverse background in marketing and management, bolstered by his experience as a leader of Marines. He owns and operates a successful alternative medicine clinic featuring acupuncture, chiropractic and massage in Gresham, Oregon. His most recent project has been the co-creation of affordable practice management software for all healthcare specialties. Eric lives and loves with his wife of 22 years in the beautiful Pacific Northwest.

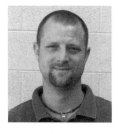

Eric Strand

Eric Strand has a diverse background in marketing and management, bolstered by his experience as a leader of Marines. He owns and operates a successful alternative medicine clinic featuring acupuncture, chiropractic and massage in Gresham, Oregon. His most recent project has been the co-creation of affordable practice management software for all healthcare specialties. Eric lives and loves with his wife of 22 years in the beautiful Pacific Northwest.

IMPERIAL SECRETS OF HEALTH & LONGEVITY
by Bob Flaws
ISBN 0-936185-51-1
ISBN 978-0-936185-51-4

INSIGHTS OF A SENIOR ACUPUNCTURIST
by Miriam Lee
ISBN 0-936185-33-3
ISBN 978-0-936185-33-0

INTEGRATED PHARMACOLOGY: Combining Modern
Pharmacology with Chinese Medicine
by Dr. Greg Sperber with Bob Flaws
ISBN 1-891845-41-1
ISBN 978-0-936185-41-3

INTRODUCTION TO THE USE OF
PROCESSED CHINESE MEDICINALS
by Philippe Sionneau
ISBN 0-936185-62-7
ISBN 978-0-936185-62-0

KEEPING YOUR CHILD HEALTHY WITH
CHINESE MEDICINE
by Bob Flaws
ISBN 0-936185-71-6
ISBN 978-0-936185-71-2

THE LAKESIDE MASTER'S STUDY OF THE PULSE
by Li Shi-zhen, trans. by Bob Flaws
ISBN 1-891845-01-2
ISBN 978-1-891845-01-7

MANAGING MENOPAUSE NATURALLY WITH
CHINESE MEDICINE
by Honora Lee Wolfe
ISBN 0-936185-98-8
ISBN 978-0-936185-98-9

MASTER HUA'S CLASSIC OF THE CENTRAL
VISCERA
by Hua Tuo, trans. by Yang Shou-zhong
ISBN 0-936185-43-0
ISBN 978-0-936185-43-9

THE MEDICAL I CHING: Oracle of the Healer Within
by Miki Shima
ISBN 0-936185-38-4
ISBN 978-0-936185-38-5

MENOPAIUSE & CHINESE MEDICINE
by Bob Flaws
ISBN 1-891845-40-3
ISBN 978-1-891845-40-6

MOXIBUSTION: A MODERN CLINICAL HANDBOOK
by Lorraine Wilcox
ISBN 1-891845-49-7
ISBN 978-1-891845-49-9

MOXIBUSTION: THE POWER OF MUGWORT FIRE
by Lorraine Wilcox
ISBN 1-891845-46-2
ISBN 978-1-891845-46-8

A NEW AMERICAN ACUPUNTURE By Mark Seem
ISBN 0-936185-44-9
ISBN 978-0-936185-44-6

POCKET ATLAS OF CHINESE MEDICINE
Edited by Marne and Kevin Ergil
ISBN 3-131416-11-7
ISBN 978-3-131416-11-7

POINTS FOR PROFIT: The Essential Guide to Practice
Success for Acupuncturists 4rd Edition
by Honora Wolfe, Eric Strand & Marilyn Allen
ISBN 1-891845-25-X
ISBN 978-1-891845-25-3

PRINCIPLES OF CHINESE MEDICAL ANDROLOGY:
An Integrated Approach to Male Reproductive and
Urological Health by Bob Damone
ISBN 1-891845-45-4
ISBN 978-1-891845-45-1

PRINCE WEN HUI's COOK: Chinese Dietary Therapy
By Bob Flaws & Honora Wolfe
ISBN 0-912111-05-4
ISBN 978-0-912111-05-6

THE PULSE CLASSIC:
A Translation of the Mai Jing
by Wang Shu-he, trans. by Yang Shou-zhong
ISBN 0-936185-75-9
ISBN 978-0-936185-75-0

THE SECRET OF CHINESE PULSE DIAGNOSIS
by Bob Flaws
ISBN 0-936185-67-8
ISBN 978-0-936185-67-5

SECRET SHAOLIN FORMULAS FOR THE
TREATMENT OF EXTERNAL INJURY
by De Chan, trans. by Zhang Ting-liang & Bob Flaws
ISBN 0-936185-08-2
ISBN 978-0-936185-08-8

STATEMENTS OF FACT IN TRADITIONAL
CHINESE MEDICINE   Revised & Expanded
by Bob Flaws
ISBN 0-936185-52-X
ISBN 978-0-936185-52-1

STICKING TO THE POINT: A Step-by-Step Approach
to TCM Acupuncture Therapy
by Bob Flaws & Honora Wolfe   2 Condensed Books
ISBN 1-891845-47-0
ISBN 978-1-891845-47-5

A STUDY OF DAOIST ACUPUNCTURE
by Liu Zheng-cai
ISBN 1-891845-08-X
ISBN 978-1-891845-08-6

THE SUCCESSFUL CHINESE HERBALIST
by Bob Flaws and Honora Lee Wolfe
ISBN 1-891845-29-2
ISBN 978-1-891845-29-1

THE SYSTEMATIC CLASSIC OF ACUPUNCTURE &
MOXIBUSTION
A translation of the Jia Yi Jing
by Huang-fu Mi, trans. by Yang Shou-zhong & Charles Chace
ISBN 0-936185-29-5
ISBN 978-0-936185-29-3

THE TAO OF HEALTHY EATING: DIETARY
WISDOM ACCORDING TO CHINESE MEDICINE
by Bob Flaws   Second Edition
ISBN 0-936185-92-9
ISBN 978-0-936185-92-7

TEACH YOURSELF TO READ MODERN
MEDICAL CHINESE
by Bob Flaws
ISBN 0-936185-99-6
ISBN 978-0-936185-99-6

TEST PREP WORKBOOK FOR BASIC TCM THEORY
by Zhong Bai-song
ISBN 1-891845-43-8
ISBN 978-1-891845-43-7

TEST PREP WORKBOOK FOR THE NCCAOM BIO-
MEDICINE MODULE: Exam Preparation & Study Guide
by Zhong Bai-song
ISBN 1-891845-34-9
ISBN 978-1-891845-34-5

TREATING PEDIATRIC BED-WETTING WITH
ACUPUNCTURE & CHINESE MEDICINE
by Robert Helmer
ISBN 1-891845-33-0
ISBN 978-1-891845-33-8

TREATISE on the SPLEEN & STOMACH: A
Translation and annotation of Li Dong-yuan's
Pi Wei Lun
by Bob Flaws
ISBN 0-936185-41-4
ISBN 978-0-936185-41-5

THE TREATMENT OF CARDIOVASCULAR DIS-
EASES WITH CHINESE MEDICINE
by Simon Becker, Bob Flaws &
Robert Casañas, MD
ISBN 1-891845-27-6
ISBN 978-1-891845-27-7

THE TREATMENT OF DIABETES MELLITUS WITH
CHINESE MEDICINE
by Bob Flaws, Lynn Kuchinski &
Robert Casañas, M.D.
ISBN 1-891845-21-7
ISBN 978-1-891845-21-5

THE TREATMENT OF DISEASE IN TCM, Vol. 1:
Diseases of the Head & Face, Including Mental &
Emotional Disorders   New Edition
by Philippe Sionneau & Lü Gang
ISBN 0-936185-69-4
ISBN 978-0-936185-69-9

THE TREATMENT OF DISEASE IN TCM, Vol. II:
Diseases of the Eyes, Ears, Nose, & Throat
by Sionneau & Lü
ISBN 0-936185-73-2
ISBN 978-0-936185-73-6

THE TREATMENT OF DISEASE IN TCM, Vol. III:
Diseases of the Mouth, Lips, Tongue, Teeth & Gums
by Sionneau & Lü
ISBN 0-936185-79-1
ISBN 978-0-936185-79-8

THE TREATMENT OF DISEASE IN TCM, Vol IV:
Diseases of the Neck, Shoulders, Back, & Limbs
by Philippe Sionneau & Lü Gang
ISBN 0-936185-89-9
ISBN 978-0-936185-89-7

THE TREATMENT OF DISEASE IN TCM, Vol V:
Diseases of the Chest & Abdomen
by Philippe Sionneau & Lü Gang
ISBN 1-891845-02-0
ISBN 978-1-891845-02-4

THE TREATMENT OF DISEASE IN TCM, Vol VI:
Diseases of the Urogential System & Proctology
by Philippe Sionneau & Lü Gang
ISBN 1-891845-05-5
ISBN 978-1-891845-05-5

THE TREATMENT OF DISEASE IN TCM, Vol VII:
General Symptoms
by Philippe Sionneau & Lü Gang
ISBN 1-891845-14-4
ISBN 978-1-891845-14-7

THE TREATMENT OF EXTERNAL DISEASES WITH
ACUPUNCTURE & MOXIBUSTION
by Yan Cui-lan and Zhu Yun-long, trans. by Yang Shou-zhong
ISBN 0-936185-80-5
ISBN 978-0-936185-80-4

THE TREATMENT OF MODERN WESTERN
MEDICAL DISEASES WITH CHINESE MEDICINE
by Bob Flaws & Philippe Sionneau
ISBN 1-891845-20-9
ISBN 978-1-891845-20-8

UNDERSTANDING THE DIFFICULT PATIENT: A
Guide for Practitioners of Oriental Medicine
by Nancy Bilello, RN, L.ac.
ISBN 1-891845-32-2
ISBN 978-1-891845-32-1

WESTERN PHYSICAL EXAM SKILLS FOR
PRACTITIONERS OF ASIAN MEDICINE
by Bruce H. Robinson & Honora Lee Wolfe
ISBN 1-891845-48-9
ISBN 978-1-891845-48-2

YI LIN GAI CUO (Correcting the Errors in the Forest of
Medicine)
by Wang Qing-ren
ISBN 1-891845-39-X
ISBN 978-1-891845-39-0

70 ESSENTIAL CHINESE HERBAL FORMULAS
by Bob Flaws
ISBN 0-936185-59-7
ISBN 978-0-936185-59-0

160 ESSENTIAL CHINESE READY-MADE
MEDICINES
by Bob Flaws
ISBN 1-891945-12-8
ISBN 978-1-891945-12-3

630 QUESTIONS & ANSWERS ABOUT CHINESE
HERBAL MEDICINE:
A Workbook & Study Guide
by Bob Flaws
ISBN 1-891845-04-7
ISBN 978-1-891845-04-8

260 ESSENTIAL CHINESE MEDICINALS
by Bob Flaws
ISBN 1-891845-03-9
ISBN 978-1-891845-03-1

750 QUESTIONS & ANSWERS ABOUT
ACUPUNCTURE
Exam Preparation & Study Guide
by Fred Jennes
ISBN 1-891845-22-5
ISBN 978-1-891845-22-2